Occupational Health Nursing

Mary Louise Brown, R.N., M. Litt., Certified Occupational Health Nurse, is the former Regional Consultant for Occupational Safety and Health in the U.S. Department of Health and Human Services Regional Office II. A graduate of the Western Pennsylvania Hospital School of Nursing, Pittsburgh, Miss Brown has a B.S. in nursing education and an M.A. in mental health from the University of Pittsburgh. After working as a chief industrial nurse and teaching at Yale, Miss Brown joined the U.S. Public Health Service as Chief of the Occupational Health Nursing Section of the Bureau of Occupational Health. As Chief of the Health Maintenance Branch of the Division of Training of the National Institute for Occupational Safety and Health, she was involved in developing and conducting courses for occupational health nurses and in helping develop educational opportunity for occupational health personnel in support of the Occupational Safety and Health Act of 1970. An internationally known authority in her field, Miss Brown is the Chairman of the Nursing Committee of the Permanent Commission, International Association on Occupational Health. She has written two books, *Occupational Health Nursing* (Springer, 1956) and *Occupational Health Nurses: An Initial Survey*, and has authored numerous articles.

Occupational Health Nursing

Principles and Practices

Mary Louise Brown, R.N., M. Litt.

Springer Publishing Company
New York

Copyright © 1981 by Springer Publishing Company, Inc.

All rights reserved

No part of this publication may reproduced, stored in a retrieval system, or transmitted in any form or by any means, electronic, mechanical, photocopying, recording, or otherwise, without the prior permission of Springer Publishing Company, Inc.

Springer Publishing Company, Inc.
200 Park Avenue South
New York, New York 10003

81 82 83 84 / 10 9 8 7 6 5 4 3 2 1

Library of Congress Cataloging in Publication Data

Brown, Mary Louise
   Occupational health nursing.

   Includes bibliographies and index.
   1. Industrial nursing. I. Title. [DNLM:
1. Occupational health nursing. WY141 B879oa]
RC966.B73   610.73'46   80-21024
ISBN 0-8261-2250-7
ISBN 0-8261-2251-5 (pbk.)

Printed in the United States of America

This book is dedicated to the occupational health nurse-leaders who on May 26, 1972, signed the papers for incorporation that established the American Board for Occupational Health Nurses, Inc., and whose courage, dedication, and standard of excellence will increasingly influence the practice of occupational health nursing and the education of those who will work in the field:

Marguerite S. Ahern	Edna May Klutas
Dorothy Benning	Jane A. Lee
Marie M. Carrell	Iva Edwards Pleasants
Anita M. Harris	Anne J. Murphy
Jeanne T. Healey	Marjorie D. Schmidt
Rosemary Huffman	Sara P. Wagner

Contents

Preface ix

Acknowledgments xi

PART I: NURSING PRACTICE IN THE WORK ENVIRONMENT 1

Chapter 1: The Nature of Occupational Health Nursing 3

Chapter 2: Occupational Health as a Field of Practice 12

PART II: ENVIRONMENTAL MONITORING 31

Chapter 3: Occupational Hygiene 33

Chapter 4: Occupational Safety 46

Chapter 5: Occupational Ecology 56

PART III: HEALTH SURVEILLANCE 69

Chapter 6: Health Assessment 71

Chapter 7: Medical Surveillance 89

Chapter 8: Occupational Health Maintenance, Conservation, and Promotion 98

PART IV: PRIMARY CARE 111

Chapter 9: Occupational Primary Care 113

Chapter 10: First-Aiders in an Occupational Setting   121

Chapter 11: Occupational Illnesses and Injuries   125

Chapter 12: Workmen's Compensation Laws   144

Chapter 13: Nonoccupational Health Problems of Workers   154

Chapter 14: Occupational Mental Health   163

Chapter 15: Alcoholism and the Worker   178

Chapter 16: Health Insurance   191

PART V: HEALTH AND SAFETY EDUCATION   197

Chapter 17: Education for Health and Safety   199

PART VI: MANAGEMENT OF THE OCCUPATIONAL HEALTH UNIT AND PROGRAM   219

Chapter 18: Administration of Occupational Health Services and Units   221

Chapter 19: Administrative Reports   245

Chapter 20: Records   251

PART VII: THE OCCUPATIONAL HEALTH NURSE   267

Chapter 21: The Nurse as Person and Professional   269

APPENDIXES:

Appendix A: Acronyms and Abbreviations   281

Appendix B: Glossary   284

Appendix C: Occupational Safety and Health Resources   298

Appendix D: Sample OSHA Standard   321

Appendix E: Excerpts from Public Law 91-596   332

Index   335

Preface

The concepts expressed in this book have evolved from two major influences: the practice of nursing and the team relationship so essential to the practice of occupational safety and health. The focal point of their interaction is and always will be worker health and safety.

Because of proximity to the worker, occupational health nurses are the first to see the injured or ill worker and make a decision on care required. Information nurses collect and use to make nursing diagnoses determines what they and also in large part what others on the occupational safety and health team must do. Establishing the cause-and-effect relationship between workers' health and a safe work environment is the essence of the team relationship in occupational safety and health. Prevention of illness and injury requires the application of engineering and public health principles and practices. Needed are the skills and understanding of the safety professional, the industrial hygienist, the health physicist, the toxicologist, and the physician.

The challenge for occupational health nurses is to be capable of functioning independently and with a high degree of proficiency at all three levels of prevention, yet also to be able to function cooperatively as a team member in planning, implementing, and evaluating a comprehensive occupational health and safety program that meets the special needs of the employing establishment and its workers. Since workers are free to accept or reject the health program provided by management, they must have sufficient information to make decisions about taking responsibility for their own health maintenance and participating in medical surveillance programs.

The importance placed on health and prevention of illness today requires that occupational health professionals be involved. In this book I have attempted to explicate when and how occupational health nurses can be involved most effectively. The book provides the framework for nurses' participation in the major parameters of an occupational health program.

The workers' right to know presents a very real challenge to all members of the team. Because of their frequent contacts with workers and their understanding both of how people learn and how toxic substances and physical hazards can and do cause harm, nurses are the professionals of choice to teach workers. In my earlier book *Occupational Health Nursing*, I delineated, with the assistance of Dr. J. Wister Meigs, my colleague at Yale, the doctor-nurse relationship. That relationship—based on the physicians' responsibility for medical practices—was and is the keystone in the role of occupational health nurses caring for injured and sick workers. It is equally important to fulfillment of the medical surveillance requirements of the Occupational Safety and Health Administration Standards. The management of the establishment that employs safety and health professionals is ultimately accountable for the provision of a safe and healthful work environment. Their delegation of this responsibility to the occupational safety and health team must be done in such a way as to create a legally and ethically sound physician-nurse relationship that permits the utilization of the professional competence of both. When there is a collaborative relationship, nurses can and do provide much of the care workers require.

Increasingly in the future a similar relationship must exist between the industrial hygiene and safety professionals on the occupational health team and the nurse. When nurse, safety professional, and industrial hygienist work as colleagues, a team relationship is possible. Neither of these relationships should be such that the physician or any of the other specialists supervises the nurse. They must expect the nurse to be able to function independently yet work cooperatively with them in those activities that require their expertise.

The Occupational Safety and Health Act of 1970 has become a shaping force in the practice of occupational health nursing. The creation of the American Board of Occupational Health Nurses in 1972 and the process of certification have set a standard of excellence that will require occupational health nurses to have the academic preparation and professional competence to function as expert practitioners.

The impact of the work environment on worker health is the major influence that determines not only what nurses must know but what they must be able to do with and for workers. In the future, nurses entering this field may have the opportunity to learn this, not by trial and error, as has happened so often in the past, but through preservice education in both undergraduate and graduate programs.

This book has two aims: to enable nurse members of occupational safety and health teams to function at a high level of competency and to help students of nursing or of occupational health nursing understand the extent of the occupational safety and health field and the many facets to the role of occupational health nurse.

Mary Louise Brown

Acknowledgments

This book was written by Mary Louise Brown in her private capacity. No official support or endorsement by the U.S. Department of Health and Human Services, Center for Disease Control, National Institute for Occupational Safety and Health is intended or should be inferred.

I want to acknowledge the help I received from Dr. J. Wister Meigs, my collaborator on *Occupational Health Nursing*, published by Springer Publishing Company in 1956. I also want to thank once more those occupational health nurses I have worked with over the years because it is they who have helped me to delineate the dimensions of the occupational health nurse practitioner's role. They have adapted nursing practices to the special needs of the industrial establishments where they work, and their professional behavior gives evidence of their belief in prevention and of their ability to help others to know how to protect and to improve their own and their families' health.

The Occupational Safety and Health Act of 1970 has focused attention on environmental hazards and on federal standards of what constitutes a safe and healthful work environment. This emphasis requires a working relationship among industrial hygienists, safety professionals, and nurses. At present, in only a few industrial settings do the occupational safety and health personnel truly function as a team. To them I say thank you for demonstrating that a team relationship results in a more comprehensive and effective health care program for workers than is possible when representatives from each discipline work independently. Their experience has helped me to identify the nurse's role on an occupational health team and the nurse's work ecology functions. I acknowledge that I have used these teams as my role models when writing Part II of this book, "Environmental Monitoring." I say a special thank you to my colleague Jacqueline Messite, M.D. for sharing her knowledge of occupational toxicology and her experiences as a member of an occupational health team that investigated the impact of the industrial environment on workers' health. She has helped me to delineate what nurses need to know about the nature of occupational diseases and what they can do about them.

Just as I have learned about occupational health and occupational health nursing from working in the field and from others working in it, I acknowledge that I have learned about writing a book while working on this one. Without editorial assistance from Helen Duncan Behnke this book would not have the cohesiveness that it does, and without Helen's ability to keep me at the task of writing it, there would not be a book. If the book is useful it is because Mrs. Behnke helped me make it so.

PART I

Nursing Practice in the Work Environment

The synthesis of nursing practice and the application of the basic principles and practices of occupational safety and health to the end that worker health is conserved, maintained, and, it may be hoped, improved, is the focus of this book. How this influences the role of the occupational health nurse is presented in Part I.

CHAPTER 1

The Nature of Occupational Health Nursing

The Nurse on the Occupational Health Team

The team relationship that is so essential to the practice of occupational safety and health requires that the nurse:

1. Participate in the formulation of the occupational health unit's protocols that determine the extent of the primary care that is given and the medical surveillance programs that are undertaken.
2. Provide primary care for workers who have been injured or become ill at work.
3. Counsel and/or provide crisis intervention for workers who are experiencing interpersonal, family and/or work related problems that interfere with or have the potential for interfering with a person's ability to carry on regular work.
4. Consult on health and safety matters with management, workers, and the representatives of the health community.
5. Participate in the health surveillance program that includes the assessment and recording of the health status of persons at time of job placement and at specific intervals thereafter.
6. Participate in the environmental control program that aims to identify, eliminate, and/or control health and safety hazards.
7. Teach workers how they can protect their own health, use health resources, and utilize safe work practices.
8. Participate in planning, conducting, and evaluating the many activities that contribute to the maintenance of the health of the worker.
9. Fulfill an ombudsman's role for those workers who require help in understanding their rights and how they may benefit from the legal, social, and health resources that are available to them, and assist workers to enter and utilize the health care system.

The following activities which support those in the foregoing list and assure the efficient management of the health service require that the nurse:

1. Participate in planning and evaluating the occupational health program which aims to meet the needs of the workers and the industry.
2. Participate in the evaluation of and, when required, the use of a disaster plan, and in teaching and coordinating the activities of the first-aid personnel.
3. Develop and maintain a health record for each individual worker.
4. Prepare reports that reflect the range of activities of the occupational health service; permit drawing conclusions as to cause, frequency, and severity of illnesses and injuries; identify needs; and propose program plans that permit an evaluation of the effectiveness of the occupational health service.
5. Establish and maintain liaison with community health and social agencies.
6. Maintain and improve her or his own professional competence.

Profile of Occupational Health Nursing

Over the years definitions of nursing have reflected the changing role of the nurse and changes in the health care system. These definitions have increasingly identified the independent nature of nursing practice, the accountability of nurses for their actions, and the relationship between nurses and their clients. In occupational health, the nurse's client is not a patient in the usual sense but a worker whose work environment can be and frequently is hazardous to health. These two factors, the work environment and the health of the person who is a worker, determine the role of the occupational health nurse.

The primary goal of occupational health nursing practice is to assist the worker to attain and maintain optimal physical and psychological functioning. Occupational health nurses are called upon to provide this assistance to many persons who may be old, middle aged, or young adults, many of whom do not believe that they "need a nurse." The health problems they must be able to help workers solve extend along the entire health-illness continuum. Occupational health nurses are called upon to perform a very wide range of tasks from the very simple, such as redressing simple second-degree burns, to complex procedures such as attempting to defibrillate the heart of a worker who has had a heart attack. They need to understand and take part in the medical surveillance programs implemented for specific exposures in the work area. Their handling of each situation has as its purpose the enhancement of workers' health. They teach by word and example. They give emphasis to the importance of care for minor health problems and to the development of health and safety habits that prevent illness and injury or the aggravation of already existing health problems.

The Nature of Occupational Health Nursing

The men and women who are clients of occupational health nurses frequently bring their home and family problems to work with them. Thus the nurses have many opportunities to help people involved in crisis situations. These problems may be acute but are usually temporary in nature; they are the response to situational difficulties that people cannot understand or handle by themselves. The nurses provide an opportunity for workers to air their feelings and their problems. They listen to what the workers say and also try to understand their nonverbal communications. They make a conscious effort to understand what a problem or situation means to a worker, meanwhile being aware of and understanding their own behavior, attitudes, and feelings. They work hard at being "listening" rather than "telling" persons.

Nurses may intervene in crisis situations on the basis of their understanding that a helping person can influence the resolution of a crisis. They encourage workers to examine problems and think about how they can handle them. They give envouragement and support and, at times, anticipatory guidance. They use the anxiety of the moment to help people accept their need for care or for changing their behavior. They help clients identify alternative ways of handling a problem and to select solutions they consider most satisfactory. These nurses know the importance of work to a client's mental health and how essential it is to the person, the family, the industry, and the community that the client continue to be a productive, employed person. Occupational health nurses work hard at creating an environment in which the workers feel safe, one in which they can and do ask questions and get answers. These nurses also recognize that they must earn the workers' trust.

Occupational health nurses must not take on duties for which they are not prepared. The converse is also true in that nurses must be involved and must accept every opportunity to learn more about the work environment and the work practices. They must look for relationships between ill health or injury and the job or work environment of the employee. They must risk the indignity of being told that some work situation they may be investigating is "none of their business" when they believe that it is, and especially when they believe that by being involved they will be able to help workers to understand or cope better.

In 1895 Florence Nightingale said, "Nursing is not only a service to the sick, it is a service also to the well. We have to teach people how to live."[1] When nurses working in occupational health perceive their role in the light of these words, the workers to whom they give care and the other members of the occupational health team with whom they work will see the nature of occupational health nursing to be participation in significant, positive health programs and therapeutic care for injured or ill workers. They will also be aware that there is a meaningful interpersonal relationship between the worker and the nurse as they identify problems and work out solutions that are compatible with the work environment, management policy, and the health system on the one hand and with the special health, social, and environmental needs of the workers on the other.

Occupational Health Nursing and Community Health Nursing

Occupational health programs have an increasing relevancy for community health programs and an ongoing, direct relationship to other community health resources. Health programs that are supported by industrial management closely resemble school health programs for children, and they operate for the mutual benefit of industry and the community. Modern occupational health could not be practiced without community health resources. Likewise most community health resources would be used less by adults were workers not referred to them through occupational health programs.

Community health resources must be utilized for workers in small businesses and industrial establishments that find it financially impossible to maintain occupational health programs. This has led to a developing interest of community health professionals in the health status of employed adults and is resulting in some experimentation. For example some hospitals and health maintenance organizations have developed occupational health clinics which sell services to the small industries in the area. These services include performing physical examinations and coordinating the medical care of injured workers. Progressive health departments are providing certain services already available to some workers at their places of employment. For example, immunization, health education programs, and health counseling may be provided by public health nurses who visit industrial establishments on an appointment basis. A few community agencies have developed part-time nursing-in-industry programs which they sell to various employers. The nurses in these programs provide some of the services of an occupational health program for the employees.

Part-time Occupational Health Nursing Services

The Occupational Safety and Health Act of 1970 established that industrial management is responsible for providing a safe and healthful work environment. The Department of Labor's Occupational Safety and Health Administration (OSHA)* promulgates standards some of which require that the worker be provided with a medical surveillance program. It may be antici-

---

*Appendix A is a list of acronyms and abbreviations used in this book.

pated that such surveillance programs will be mandated in increasing numbers in the near future. OSHA has established the workers' right to know the safety and health hazards of their work environment, the precautions to be taken, and the procedures to be followed in case of accidental high exposure to a toxic substance. The responsibility for carrying out these requirements belongs to industrial management personnel, who frequently need the help of those health professionals who can teach health and safety practices. This creates a serious problem for the management in smaller businesses and industries that do not maintain an occupational health service. More than half of the labor force in the United States is employed in establishments that employ less than 100 workers and do not employ a full-time occupational health nurse. Many such establishments, however, could use the part-time services of a nurse to good advantage. An occupational health nurse who wishes to work only part-time may be employed by a single establishment, but occasionally a nurse will contract to serve two or more industries on a part-time basis. Unless the agreement between the nurse and these different companies is carefully worked out in advance, problems may arise as to who will pay the nurse for travel time, sick leave, and vacations, to name only a few of the administrative details of this type of agreement.

The administrator of the public health nursing agency is usually in a much better position to work out a satisfactory agreement for a part-time occupational health worker than is an individual nurse. Part-time occupational health nursing programs can be developed by public health nursing agencies based on a contract between the agency and one or more industrial concerns. It is important that the agency set the same high standards for these services as it does for all of its other services. Several factors are of special importance. The staff of the agency must be large enough to carry the agency's increased load. There needs to be a nurse supervisor and also staff nurses both interested in and with preparation and experience in occupational health nursing so they can function with a high degree of proficiency. An in-service education program and the services of an occupational health nursing consultant increase the efficiency of the service and the skills of the staff. Each in-plant health service must have a licensed physician to whom the nurse may turn for consultation when workers require medical care.

The advice and guidance of a committee made up of representatives of the community and the professional sanction of a medical advisory committee are as important to the part-time occupational health nursing program as they have proved to be to the agency's other programs. Cost of the service to the industry should be based on the agency's cost per visit, plus necessary adjustments to cover the extra expense of maintaining an appointment service. Equally important and in order to keep the cost to the industry affordable, those special services and specialized staff not required for the occupational health service should not be included in the formula to determine costs.

Guidelines for Initiating a Part-time Service

I. Establish responsibilities of the agency and the industry.
   A. Provider to supply:
      1. Qualified nurse and relief nurse for the plant.
      2. Adequate nursing supervision.
      3. The same consultant and advisory services as are available to all nurses in the agency.
   B. Industry to supply:
      1. Medical supervision.
      2. Administrative supervision through top management.
      3. Qualified first-aider(s) for hours when the part-time nurse is not on duty.
      4. Adequate facilities (room, equipment, supplies, etc.).
      5. Service and maintenance for facilities.
II. Establish policies, for example:
   A. The nurse's hours on duty shall be not less than 6 hours a week for each 100 employees, in blocks of at least 2 hours whenever possible.
   B. Medical direction and signed standing procedures shall be provided by a physician who reports to the plant at least 1 hour per week at a time when the nurse is on duty.
III. Provide for orientation of nurses to:
   A. The company.
      1. Number of employees. Age, sex distribution, and types of jobs.
      2. Type of industry, its products or services, and associated hazards.
      3. Insurance plan (sickness, compensation).
      4. Sick leave policy.
      5. How workers are to be transported to home, doctor's office, or hospital when ill or injured.
      6. Lines of communication.
      7. How the announcement of new health program is made to workers.
   B. The role of supervisory personnel.
   C. The establishment, by tour and explanation of process.
IV. Determine responsibilities of the part-time nurse.
   A. To plan a program designed to meet both the special needs of

the industry and the worker and the requirements of the OSHA Standards.
B. To provide or to arrange for physical examinations of workers.
 1. Take history.
 2. Prepare workers for the examination.
 3. Keep records.
 4. Carry out follow-up programs.
C. To give primary care to workers who become ill or injured when nurse is on duty.
D. To reevaluate care given by first-aider.
E. To provide or to arrange for medical surveillance for workers at special risk.
F. To provide health counseling and health education sessions.
 1. Individual.
 2. Group.
G. To maintain the health facilities.
 1. Order supplies.
 2. Supervise maintenance of department and equipment.
H. To observe the environment for unsafe conditions, scheduling 1 or more hours per month in the plant to do plant tour and to participate on safety committee.
I. To keep the necessary records.
 1. Workmen's compensation forms.
 2. Individual employee records.
 3. Monthly reports to physician, management, and public health nursing agency.
 4. Periodic review by nurse and physician of health and accident experience in records of the occupational health service.

Interdependency

The relation of existing occupational health programs to community health programs is ideally one of mutual support. Health education for employed adults is an occupational health service but without the support and assistance of community health agencies may be meaningless. The best counseling and health education is of little value to workers unless there are also community health services available to workers and their families. The whole system of periodic examinations, case finding, and screening programs utilized in effective occupational health programs would fall apart without the backup of community services. Increasingly those in community health work will be involved in planning how to extend their activities so that these are more readily available to adults at their places of employment.

The health of the employed adult is a responsibility of both the community and industry. To realize the full potential for worker health and community health, the professionals working in occupational and public health programs must be aware of the responsibilities and services provided by both industry and the community. Occupational health nurses who do not work closely with other community health nurses, especially with those who go into the homes of people who work for their companies, miss opportunities to contribute to comprehensive care. For example, when at work, a first-line supervisor of Company A has a heart attack. An occupational health nurse sees this person first, makes a nursing diagnosis, and transfers the supervisor to the hospital. Time passes and the supervisor is now at home recuperating, being visited by a community health nurse and talking about going back to work. The more the community health nurse and the occupational health nurse can plan together for this person's care and return to work, the more comprehensive and effective the nursing care will be.

Reference

1. Nightingale, F. *Selected Writings of Florence Nightingale*. Comp. by Lucy R. Seymour. New York: Macmillan, 1954, Chap. 2, "Notes on Nursing; What It Is and What It Is Not" (1895), pp. 123-220.

Selected Readings

AAOHN. *Standards for Evaluating an Occupational Health Nursing Service*. New York, 1977, p. 7.

ANA, Special Committee of Nurses Engaged in Occupational Health Nursing. *Functions, Standards, and Qualifications for an Occupational Health Nurse in a One-Nurse Service*. Kansas City, Mo.: 1968, p. 4.

"A.N.A. Board Approves a Definition of Nursing Practice," *American Journal of Nursing*, Vol. 55, No. 12, Dec. 1955, p. 1474.

Brown, M. L. "A Profile of Occupational Health Nursing," *Occupational Health Nursing*, Vol. 18, No. 2, Feb. 1970, pp. 16-18.

Brown, M. L. "The Extended Role of the Nurse in Occupational Mental Health Programs," *Industrial Medicine*, Vol. 40, No. 9, Dec. 1971, pp. 17-23.

Collings, G. H. "Managements' View of the Nurse," *Occupational Health Nursing*, Vol. 27, No. 2. Feb. 1979, pp. 9-12.

Igoe, J. B. "The School Nurse Practitioner," *Nursing Outlook*, Vol. 23, No. 6, June 1975, pp. 381-384.

ILO. *Encyclopedia of Occupational Health and Safety*, A-K, Vol. 1, 1971; L-Z, Vol. 2. Geneva, 1972.

Indiana State Board of Nurses' Registration and Nursing Education Act, Sec. 1(b), 1973.

Joint Practice Committee of North Carolina Medical Society and North Carolina Nurses' Association. *Occupational Health Services,* Rep. of Task Force. Raleigh, N.C., 1976.

Kerr, L. E. "Occupational Health—A Discipline in Search of a Mission," *American Journal of Public Health,* Vol. 63, No. 5, May 1973, pp. 381–385.

Lee, J. A. *The New Nurse in Industry.* Washington, D.C.: GPO, 1978.

New York State Educational Law, Title VIII, Art. 139, Sec. 6902. Albany, 1972.

Peterson, E. *Industrial Health.* Englewood Cliffs, N.J.: Prentice-Hall, 1977.

"The President's Reports of Occupational Safety and Health," Washington, D.C.: GPO, 1972, 1973, 1974.

"The Role of Medicine within a Business Organization," *JAMA,* Vol. 210, Nov. 24, 1969, pp. 1446–1450.

Schilling, R. S. F. (ed.). *Occupational Health Practices.* London: Butterworth, 1973.

Selbeck, H. B. *Occupational Health in America.* Detroit: Wayne State University Press, 1962.

Special Task Force to Secretary of HEW. *Work in America.* Cambridge, Mass.: M.I.T. Press, 1973.

Tabershaw, I. R. "Occupational Medicine: The Search for Identity," *Journal of Occupational Medicine,* Vol. 13, No. 7, July 1971, pp. 325–330.

Zenz, C. (ed.). *Occupational Medicine: Principles and Practical Applications.* Chicago: Year Book Medical Publishers, Inc. 1975.

CHAPTER 2

Occupational Health as a Field of Practice

As a field of practice, occupational health is broad and complex. It requires the skills, understandings, and interaction of many different professionals and disciplines to accomplish a wide variety of activities. Hazards that may harm workers' health need to be identified and controlled. The toxicity of substances used in manufacturing certain products and their potential for harm must be studied. The impact of the work environment on the health of workers needs to be identified and modified if it is found to be hazardous.

Basic Principles of Occupational Health Practice

There are seven basic principles that underlie the effectiveness of an occupational health program:

1. The occupational health program should be in conformity with the provisions of the Occupational Safety and Health Act of 1970 (PL 91-596).
2. Occupational health care is essentially an interdisciplinary team effort.
3. The occupational health unit must be staffed by qualified professional personnel, must have administrative stability, and must have the understanding and support of both management and labor.
4. The quality of the work environment is of vital importance and is central to the prevention of disease and injury.
5. The workers themselves must participate in achieving a common goal: a high level of wellness as a measure of the quality of life.
6. Occupational health professionals must understand the dynamics of the American labor movement and work cooperatively with the union leaders in their establishment.
7. Occupational health is an essential component of community health; they are interrelated and interdependent.

Principle 1: Regulatory Requirements

The occupational health program should be in conformity with the provisions of the Occupational Safety and Health Act of 1970 (PL 91-596). When the U.S. Congress enacted this law they declared that its purpose was "to

Occupational Health as a Field of Practice

assure so far as possible every working man and woman in the nation safe and healthful working conditions and to preserve our human resources."[1] This was to be accomplished by authorizing the Secretary of Labor to set mandatory occupational safety and health standards applicable to businesses affecting interstate commerce and by encouraging employers and employees in their efforts to reduce the number of hazards in their places of employment.[2] The act states that its purpose was to be achieved by 13 separate means (see App. E for the other 11 statements). The act created OSHA within the Department of Labor (DOL) and the National Institute for Occupational Safety and Health (NIOSH) within the Department of Health and Human Services (DHHS). The responsibility for promulgating and enforcing occupational safety and health standards rests with the DOL.

OSHA Responsibilities

- Conducts the inspections of work places and the investigations of working conditions
- Promulgates and modifies mandatory occupational safety and health standards
- Prescribes the regulations that determine what records and reports concerning work-related injury, illness, and death the employer must maintain
- Certifies and monitors state occupational safety and health programs
- Conducts, or has others conduct, educational and training programs to help employers and employees understand the act and how to fulfill their responsibilities under the act
- Maintains a system for collecting and analyzing OSHA statistics.

NIOSH Responsibilities

- Develops criteria for dealing with toxic materials and harmful physical agents, indicating safe exposure levels for workers for various periods of time
- Conducts research on which new standards can be based
- Implements education and training programs to provide for professional manpower to carry out the purposes of the Act
- Makes toxicity determinations on request of employer or employee groups
- Publishes annually a list of all known toxic substances and the concentrations at which toxicity is known to occur
- Implements a grant program for research on occupational safety and health problems and for educational programs to train occupational health and safety personnel.

In addition, a 12-member National Advisory Committee on Occupational Safety and Health (NACOSH) was created by PL 91-596 to advise, consult, and make recommendations to the Secretary of Labor and the Secretary of Health, Education, and Welfare. This committee is composed of representatives of management, labor, occupational safety and health professions, and the public. The act also created the Occupational Safety and Health Review Commission appointed by the President, which deals with disputes arising from enforcement of the act. This Commission appoints hearing examiners, who are called administrative law judges, to hear any contests of OSHA's citations. Both the Secretary of Labor and the contesting party have access to the U.S. courts.

The National Commission on State Workmen's Compensation Laws was established to make a comprehensive study and evaluation of all worker compensation laws and to report its findings to the President and the Congress. This commission was concluded in 1972. Some of its recommendations have been incorporated into state programs. There are great differences among the various states in regard to laws concerned with workers' compensation (see Chap. 12).

The right of OSHA to make an inspection without a warrant as set forth in section 8(a) of the Occupational Safety and Health Act was challenged in the courts. The U.S. Supreme Court ruled that "warrantless inspection was in violation of the Fourth Amendment to the U.S. Constitution." This was finalized in May 1978.[3] This decision has caused the most major change in the administration of the act since its inception in 1970. Since the ruling by the Supreme Court the compliance officers must get a court order if admittance is not permitted when the OSHA compliance officer presents his or her credentials as the first step in making an inspection. The Supreme Court in handing down this decision defined the probable cause for obtaining "a warrant to be a showing that a specific business has been chosen for an OSHA search on the basis of a general administration plan for the enforcement of the Act, derived from neutral sources such as, for example, dispersion of employees in various types of industries across a given area, and the desired frequency of searches in any of the lesser divisions of the area . . . "[4] (see App. E for sec. 8(a) of the act).

Principle 2: Team Effort

Occupational health care is essentially an interdisciplinary team effort. Occupational health services exist because individuals have occupations and work together in groups. The size of the group, the nature of the organization (service, manufacturing, commercial, or governmental), and the willingness of management to provide an occupational health service at the place of employment determine whether there will be such a service. It is a truism that the needs of workers to have a health and safety program at their place of employment are the same whether they work for a company that employs 20,000 or 20 persons, and the need is related more to hazard of the operation than to size of the work force. However for the same industry quantitatively, the need is usually less in the small establishment and also is less likely to be met.

The Occupational Safety and Health Act of 1970 requires that the employer provide a safe and healthful place of employment for the employees and places the responsibility for compliance with current occupational safety and health standards on the employer. The Act does not require the employer to maintain a health service. However federal regulations do require that the employer have a plan for providing medical care for workers who have industrial injuries or illnesses and a program of medical surveillance for employees whose work brings them into contact with specified chemicals. In addition the regulations require that at least one person who has had first-aid training be on duty during working hours.

The American Medical Association's Department of Environmental, Public, and Occupational Health identifies seven activities that support the objectives of an occupational health program: "(1) maintenance of a healthful work environment; (2) preplacement examinations and/or screening; (3) periodic health appraisals; (4) diagnosis and treatment; (5) immunization programs; (6) medical records; and (7) health education and counseling."[5]

Staffing Patterns

The number and variety of personnel who staff occupational health services depend upon the size and type of the industry. Occupational health departments of very large manufacturing and service industries employ a full complement of staff. Full-time medical directors are often members of top management. Nonmedical administrators are sometimes employed as managers of the health departments. The medical staff is made up of full-time and part-time physicians, including a selected list of consultants. The nursing staff includes staff nurses who report to a director of nursing services.

When the service is operational for more than 8 hours, sometimes head nurses are employed for the various units and shifts. In many chemical plants and heavy manufacturing establishments, the occupational health units are staffed for 24 hours a day throughout the year. Licensed practical nurses may be employed, although most of the nurses working in occupational health are registered professional nurses.

The occupational health teams in large industries include X-ray and clinical laboratory technicians, and certified personnel to perform the audiometric and pulmonary function tests when the work load for these procedures is heavy. There is also a clerical staff and, in the very large units, a record librarian or supervisor of the health records. Industrial hygienists, health physicists, and safety professionals are sometimes an integral part of the occupational health department, but more often they are assigned to a separate environmental health department.

The number of persons on the staff of the environmental facet of the occupational health program often exceeds that of the medical personnel. In addition to the occupational safety and health staffs, there frequently is a special staff whose members are concerned with the administration of the workmen's compensation and health insurance programs. Some industries have their own industrial hygiene laboratory staffed by qualified personnel and certified by the American Industrial Hygiene Association (AIHA).

The laboratory work on industrial hygiene samples usually is done, however, by commercial or governmental laboratories on a fee-for-service basis. Only in the very large establishments is a complete staff employed. As the size of the establishment decreases, so does the number and variety of full-time professional health care personnel. Another factor that helps to determine the composition of the occupational health unit staff is the type of establishment and the nature of its hazards. A chemical industry is much more apt to employ an industrial hygienist than is a retail store, even though the latter may employ many more workers.

Data gathered in 1972 for the Survey of Public Health Nursing, which was carried out by the Division of Nursing of the Health Resources Administration of the DHEW, permit an estimate of the number of occupational health nurses and occupational health units in the United States, as shown in Table 1. As can be seen in the table an estimated 21,406 occupational health nurses (19,784 full-time plus 1,622 part-time) were employed in 8,484 occupational health units in the United States, Puerto Rico, Guam, and the Virgin Islands as of January 1, 1972. For this survey an occupational health unit was defined as a "facility which gives nursing services under general medical direction to employees of a factory or other establishment," and industry was categorized as manufacturing, nonmanufacturing, or governmental. Manufacturing industries employed 71% of the 21,406 occupational health nurses and ranked as the largest employer of occupational health nurses. Of these, 94% were registered nurses and the remaining 6% were licensed practical nurses. Employed on a full-time basis were 92% of the registered nurses and 97% of the licensed practical nurses.

The survey collected information concerning the position level of nursing personnel, and from these statistics it can be inferred that 2%, or 841, of the 21,406 nurses employed in occupational health units were classified as administrators. Over 92% of these administrative-level nurses were further classified as supervisors, while the remaining 8% were directors (3.6%), consultants (3.1%), and coordinators (1.3%).

Table 1
Distribution of Full-time and Part-time Occupational Health Nurses and Occupational Health Units by Size of Nursing Staff, January 1972

Size of Staff	Full-time Nurses	Part-time Nurses	Occupational Health Units
Total	19,784	1,622	8,484
1	4,384	117	4,505
2–4	6,375	686	2,852
5–9	4,885	468	874
10–24	2,388	297	215
25–49	802	29	25
50–99	950	25	13
100 or more			

Source. DHEW. *Survey of Public Health Nursing 1968–1972.* Washington, D.C.: GPO. 1973, p. 123. Tab. 93.[6]

The employment of adult health nurse practitioners and physician assistants is a new development in occupational health. Some industries have released nurses from their responsibility for day-to-day provision of care so that they can enroll in a training program and work under the proctorship of the health unit's physician in order to develop their skills in performing physical examinations.

The Nurse on the Team

In many occupational health programs, especially those in the smaller and medium-sized industries, the nurse is the only professional member of the occupational health team who works full time. He or she functions as an expert occupational health nurse, never as a pseudophysician, safety professional, or industrial hygienist. The skills and understanding of an occupational health team must be available whether personnel providing these skills and understanding are drawn from an official agency, insurance company, university, or private consulting firm. The success of these programs depends on the nurse's conception of his or her role and on his or her ability to involve other health professionals in the total occupational health program.

Occupational health nurses function ethically and legally as nurses when they work with a physician responsible for the medical aspect of the health service. It is estimated that approximately two-thirds of all occupational health nurses work in establishments that cannot support the employment of a full-time physician. In such instances the physician is part-time, on call, a member of a panel, or perhaps only a voice on the other end of a telephone. Many of these physicians do not come into the plant on a regular schedule. Under such circumstances the nurse becomes the only full-time member of the occupational health department staff. The employer who employs a nurse to staff the health service should also employ a physician to provide medical direction. Employers who do not do so ask nurses to carry responsibilities for which they have neither the legal right nor the professional training.

The work environment and the people with whom nurses work influence, in part, their role. A nurse as the only full-time staff person in the occupational health unit works with someone who is assigned the responsibility for safety. This person may or may not be trained as a safety professional and usually works out of a department other than the occupational health unit. Effective practice requires that the nurse be able to participate in the accident prevention program. It is essential that both the nurse and the safety professional recognize each other's special contribution to worker health and safety. If and when an industrial hygienist is employed, the position is often that of corporate industrial hygienist. Other nurses work with a consultant from a private consulting firm, insurance company, or official agency. When there is such separation of team members, implementation of a comprehensive health program and the establishment of a team relationship are difficult. Occupational health nursing is best practiced when nurses work with or have access to the skills and abilities of the others on an occupational health team. If they are the only full-time people employed, it is their responsibility to make recommendations to management when a situation arises that requires the expertise of one or more of the other members of an occupational health team.

It is essential that nurses understand the principles of industrial hygiene and accident prevention and know how to apply them. Equally important, the nurses need to be able to communicate with first-line supervisors and top-level management people who have the responsibility for production of the product or the service. Participation in activities designed to protect workers who are at an increased risk is one factor that gives the occupational health nurse's role its speciality classification. To work effectively nurses must know the health hazards of the industry and how these can be and are controlled. They recognize that prevention of injury and disease from work-connected causes requires knowledge of safe handling of materials and of body mechanics, engineering principles, public health practices, and motivational techniques. Furthermore, if the health service is to be complete, someone at the policy-making management level of the business or industry must understand the need and provide the administrative framework for such a service. Because it controls the budget, management determines the extent of the health service that can be provided. Within the frame created by medical direction, safety and industrial hygiene measures, and administrative controls, the occupational health nurse can and does have a significant part to play in the achievement of the objectives of an occupational health service.

It is essential that both nurses and employers recognize the nurse's responsibility as a member of the occupational health team. As professional people, nurses are responsible for what they do or do not do. They must restrict their functions to the extent and degree for which they have had preparation. When they identify the health needs of workers and then take action to meet these needs, and when they teach workers who then take action based upon their understanding of safety and health, nurses are carrying in large part their share of the occupational health team's responsibility. They perform these duties with the competence of nurse specialists.

It had been said that "occupational health nursing is the easiest job in the nursing profession to do badly, and one of the hardest and most satisfying to do well."[7] This is true because occupational health nurses give care to workers, not patients. They deal with the many factors that influence the physical and mental health of people at work. They must work cooperatively with health personnel from community agencies, physicians and others on the occupational health staff, management, the workers and their union representative, and at times with families of workers.

Principle 3: Qualified Professionals and Administrative Stability

The health unit must be staffed by qualified professional personnel and must have administrative stability. Administrative stability makes possible the credibility of the staff, since it is founded on policies that have the support of management and are understood by the workers. The professional staff participates with management and the workers in developing policies that determine in large part the staff's conduct. A policy provides the basic framework and, like a law, a well developed policy determines what is to be done, for whom, and at what frequency, thus eliminating differences in the services offered, which can happen if each professional makes individual decisions.

Administrative policies that are well conceived and faithfully followed help to create trust in the occupational health service and the personnel who provide health care. Trust is vitally needed if the workers are to use the service and to consider the professional staff competent. The occupational health program and the staff must not be viewed as tools of management but should be seen as providers of a service to the workers. Trust by the workers is not easily won; however, it is essential, and it can be achieved.

An individual at the policy-making level of management must provide administrative direction to the health care staff. This person should participate in the health service planning sessions, voice management's view on policy, and approve the health unit's budget. Such a person must assure the autonomy of the professional staff in all health-related decisions. This includes appointing a physician to provide medical direction and to determine the necessary extent of the health services. It also includes allowing the nursing staff to set standards for nursing practice and to perform nursing activities under the supervision of a nurse designated by management as the nurse supervisor. The only nurse must be expected to be self-directive in nursing matters and have the opportunity to call into the health unit a nurse consultant when such services are necessary.

Principle 4: Quality of Work Environment

The quality of the work environment is of vital importance and is critical to the prevention of disease and injury. The professional members of the occupational health team must remember that it is the employer who is required to be in compliance with the Occupational Safety and Health Act of 1970. Management has the utlimate responsibility to assure its employees that hazards in the work place are identified and controlled so that the lives of the employees are not lost or shortened. Because it is management's responsibility to see to it that safe work practices are followed, first-line supervisors are much involved in occupational safety and health care activities.

The industrial hygienist and the safety professional, as members of the occupational safety and health team, apply their expertise to the identification and control of health and safety hazards and to the development of safe work practices. The roles of these members of the team are explained in Chapters 3 and 4.

The nurse with a high index of suspicion can be the most valuable co-worker that the occupational health physician, the industrial hygienist, and the safety professional can have. The nurse's desire to know the ecology of the work environment and ability to spot possible relationships between the physical and mental ill health of workers and the stresses of their jobs are essential characteristics of the occupational health nurse. The nurse must be able to recognize and identify the environmental factors associated with the industrial establishment in which she works and to understand their effects on health.

Principle 5: Worker Participation and Quality of Life

The workers themselves must participate in achieving the common goal of a high level of wellness as a measure of the quality of life. Providing care for people who consider themselves as workers, not patients, is the most demanding of all the activities of the occupational health professionals.

Many workers are of the opinion that they do not need help from the nurse unless they have been injured or become ill at work. Since much of what the nurse and others on the team must do with and for workers relates to prevention, it is essential that they understand that the occupational safety and health professionals cannot promise good health for the employees. The professionals must be able to help workers understand this and, most importantly, they must be able to help workers to want to protect, maintain, and improve their own health status. Chapter 17 considers the how and why of this principle.

Principle 6: The Unions and Health Care

The unions are an acknowledged force in American society. A labor organization, a union, is a free, voluntary association of workers organized for the common purpose of attaining the workers' and the union's objectives through collective bargaining with employers in both the public and private sectors. Today's union leaders are more administrators than agitators. They are the heads of business organizations that have many branches scattered all over the country.

The strike is the method used to force the issue. The economic gains of the American worker have been impressive. Those in today's labor movement have benefited from the generations of workers in the early trade unions who, at a considerable cost of lives and property, in a hostile atmosphere, gained job security and higher wages. The interest and concern of some of the labor leaders with the hazards of the work environment and their ability to influence legislation contributed to the enactment of the Occupational Safety and Health Act of 1970, sometimes referred to as the "Workers Bill of Rights."

History of the Union Movement in America

The union movement in the United States has a long and interesting history. As early as 1791, craftsmen joined together in small local unions. The Noble Knights of Labor, the first big union organization, was started in 1869 as a small local union of garment workers. It grew as other craft unions joined and was the forerunner of modern day unions. It had approximately 10,000 members in the early years, and by 1886 it claimed 700,000 members in the United States.[8]

The American Federation of Labor (AFL) was founded in 1881. This organization had as its goal to improve wages of the worker members and to improve working conditions. Samuel Gompers was the first president. Six craft unions—printers, workers in iron and steel, molders, cigar makers, carpenters, and glass workers—joined together to form the new organization.[9]

As the labor movement began to emerge as an influential economic factor, there was great opposition. There then followed a long period of great unrest. The Homestead strike in 1892 came during this period.[10] The Amalgamated Association of Iron and Steel Workers tried unsuccessfully to get the Carnegie Steel Company to recognize their demands. Armed detectives hired by the company fought a pitched battle with the strikers, and 10 people were killed before the National Guard of Pennsylvania restored order. The strike of the American Railway Union against the Pullman Palace Car Company of Illinois in 1894 resulted in many deaths and injuries. Antiunionism continued, and some was still evident during World War I. The labor shortage of this period brought about a rapid growth of the unions. The National War Labor Board was created by the government to promote union-management cooperation in order that disputes would not interfere with production of war materials.

The Congress of Industrial Organizations (CIO) was formed in 1935. Six AFL-affiliated unions, and officers of two other unions, formed the Committee for Industrial Organization. The issue between this group and the AFL was industrial versus craft unionism. The many new mass-production industries in the United States were not organized, and the CIO was formed so that all workers from an industry could be organized into one union. This was thought necessary because many of the workers in these industries were not eligible for membership in the existing craft unions.

The National Industrial Recovery Act (NIRA) was passed in 1933. Unions regained their importance and influence because this Act guaranteed the rights of workers to organize into unions of their own choice and to bargain collectively with their employers. The National Labor Relations Act, better known as the Wagner Act, was passed in 1935. This again guaranteed the workers the right to organize. It also prohibited the employer-dominated or employer-financed company union. The Fair Labor Standards Act was passed in 1938. This set minimum wage, overtime, and child labor standards for employees engaged in interstate commerce or in the manufacture of goods for interstate commerce. When this was enacted in 1938 the minimum hourly wage was $ .40. This was raised in 1950 to $.75, in 1956 to $1.00, to $2.00 in 1964, and to $2.90 in 1979.

In 1947 a new labor law, the Labor Management Relations Act, more often referred to as the Taft-Hartley Act, was passed. The unions expressed strong opposition to this new law. The Taft-Hartley Act upheld collective bargaining, as did the Wagner Act. It also listed unfair labor practices forbidden to employers, and for the first time it listed unfair labor practices that applied to unions. This Act provided rules governing strikes that imperiled the nation's health and safety, and it set up the 80-day cooling-off period. This law is an example of social action to influence labor-management relations at a time when union strength had surpassed that of many industries.[11]

There are over 200 autonomous national and international unions. Most are affiliated with the AFL or the CIO. In 1955 these two separate organizations joined together and are now the AFL-CIO. Unions that do not belong to the AFL-CIO are known as independent unions.

The local union is the foundation of the union movement structure. The local may be large or small. It may be a craft union whose members all work at a single trade or related trades, such as the Carpenters Union, or it may be an industrial union, all of whose members are employed by one industry. Steelworkers and coal miners belong to an industrial union.

The Industrial Union Department of the AFL-CIO publishes a quarterly, *Spotlight on Health and Safety*. The following quotation from it and from a speech made by the Secretary-Treasurer of the AFL-CIO at the Oil, Chemical and Atomic Workers (OCAW) Convention in 1977 gives an indication of the concern about and the importance given to occupational safety and health by the AFL-CIO:

every responsible union leader and union member has a job to do in seeing that OSHA is observed and enforced and that the workers of America get the protection of life and limb and health that they need and deserve and that they are guaranteed by federal law. And the greatest responsibility lies on the local officers and committeemen and stewards on the actual job site where the hazards exist and the violations take place and the corrections have to be made.[12]

Health Insurance

Labor unions have long been interested in the health of their workers and in health programs for union members. The first of the union sick-benefit programs was established in 1866 by the Granite Cutters Union.[13] After 1949, collective bargaining agreements provided for medical coverage insurance, pensions, and other fringe benefits. It was in 1949 that the courts ruled pensions and group insurance programs to be a condition of employment and a form of compensation on which employers are required to bargain with the union. Today approximately 11 million workers have fringe benefits.[14] Their employers contribute over $1.25 billion per year to these programs.

The New York locals of the International Ladies Garment Workers Union started the first union-sponsored service type of medical care plan in 1913. The Health Center was incorporated in 1917. The Krug-Lewis agreement, which was signed in 1946, set up the health and pension fund for workers in the bituminous coal industry. A DOL study shows that by mid-1950 practically every major union in the country, excluding unions representing railroads and governmental employees, for whom special federal, state, and municipal legislation exists, had negotiated pensions or health and welfare programs providing one or more of the following: (a) life insurance or death benefits; (b) accidental death and dismemberment payments; (c) accident and sickness benefits (but not sick leave or workmen's compensation); (d) cash or services covering hospital, surgical, maternity, and medical care, and in some contracts, dental care.

There is no standard pattern of medical care provided through union plans. Most agreements provide for some form of insurance, or for Blue Cross and Blue Shield programs to provide protection for their members. A limited but growing number of unions handle their own programs. These unions have established health centers to provide preventive, diagnostic, and treatment services for their members. The services provided at the union health centers are usually supplemented by insurance programs to cover hospitalization costs and the fees of the physician who gives care to the person in the hospital. All union health programs provide for some form of employer financing. Under the collective bargaining agreement, the employer contributes to the fund. The amount is based in some cases on a given percentage of the payroll, while in others the contribution is based on the number of workers employed or the units produced or mined. Certain contracts specify that benefits are to be provided without reference to their cost or method of financing except that the employer will pay. Under the Taft-Hartley Act the funds appropriated for health programs must be administered by boards with equal representation from labor and management.

The Union Representative and the Nurse

The shop steward is the grassroots elected union leader. This person maintains a close working relationship with the members of the union. This union representative is frequently in contact with the foreman in the industrial establishment. Sometimes the business agent of the union is also the shop steward.

All unions have a grievance committee. Its responsibility is to process all grievances and to assure the proper administration of contractual items. Increasingly unions have negotiated for the establishment of a safety and health committee to deal with grievances related to safety and health matters.

Affiliated with the Consumer Commission on the Accreditation of Health Services, Inc., in New York, the Labor Safety and Health Institute was formed in the late 1970s. It provides guidance for union members on occupational safety and health problems. An occupational safety and health workbook was developed by the institute's director and published in 1977. It has had wide distribution. In Berkeley, Chicago, and Philadelphia, to name only three of the better-known and active committees or labor occupational health programs have been established. Unions like the Interna-

Occupational Health as a Field of Practice

tional Association of Machinists have employed a medical consultant, and the United Rubber, Cork, Linoleum, and Plastic Workers of America and several others have an industrial hygienist on their headquarters staff, as does the United Auto Workers Union. Oil, Chemical and Atomic Workers have established research units in two universities. The United Auto Workers, the International Union of Electrical Workers, and others have developed publications dealing with occupational safety and health.

Nurses, like the foremen, need to work closely with the shop steward. Often the nurses have to learn to do so, and frequently they have to prove to the steward their concern about the workers' health and safety. All too often these nurses and shop stewards have difficulty communicating effectively. Nurses need to know the health provisions of the contract. They should have a copy of the information provided the workers concerning the extent of the health insurance package. They should understand this to be able to help workers and their families with questions about their health insurance benefits. Nurses' attitudes about organized labor must not be permitted to interfere with their ability to provide care for the workers. The shop steward and the nurse need to respect each other and the roles they each play in worker health and safety.

Principle 7: The Relationship between Occupational and Community Health Services

In a sense there is no such thing as "worker" health as distinct from "community" health. Workers are not just workers; they are productive members of the community. The worker population of an industry varies just as the adult population of a community varies. Included are male and female, skilled and unskilled, the well-educated and those with little education, and the healthy and those with health problems.

People who work in industry spend about one-third of their time at work. They spend the rest of their time at home and in the community, shopping, playing, eating, participating in or viewing sports, traveling from place to place, and so on. The men and women of the labor force are the community's greatest resource. They are the voters; they pay a large proportion of the taxes; they give voluntarily to good causes. They are the parents of the school children, and they are the people who, when ill, use the community health care facilities. Individuals in this age group are at the most risk of developing chronic illness, partly because such diseases as diabetes, glaucoma, hypertension, and cancer characteristically develop most often in adults. We have recently become more aware that elements in the work environment can and do contribute significantly to the death rolls for cancer. We should also note that similar exposures in the community or at home are additive in producing their noxious effects. Thus it can be seen that industry and workers in industry are an integral part of the community, and it is essential that there be a collaborative relationship between occupational health and community health personnel.

Scope and Objectives

As industrialization has spread, the workers' health has become increasingly important. Social legislation, in the form of worker's compensation laws, established employers' responsibility for providing treatment for workers who suffer work-related injuries or illnesses. Industry's concern with the care of workers who were injured on the job provided the foundation on which broader programs of worker health maintenance have been built. Although some programs continue to be held fast in the bedrock of first-aid or emergency care, the full potential of occupational health care is realized only when such care takes a place of relative importance in the complex of a total occupational health program.

Unfortunately, not all workers have access to a comprehensive occupational health service. About half of the work force is employed in small establishments which do not have occupational health units. In these establishments, injured workers are sent to local hospital emergency rooms or to a doctor's office for treatment and workers receive little or no health education or instruction in disease and accident prevention. Less than 10,000 industrial organizations maintain occupational health services in which approximately 21,000 nurses are employed.[15] How to provide occupational health services to workers who presently do not have access to such services is a perplexing problem. That no realistic solution has yet been found does not detract from the value of the services for those who have them, nor does the difficulty in organizing such services negate the need for them for workers to whom they are not now available.

The benefits of modern occupational health programs are felt far beyond the walls of industry. For instance the preemployment physical examination that was formerly done to screen out all but the fit has given way in many industries to a preplacement examination which aims to match the worker and his or her abilities to the job. Periodic physical examinations of workers as part of an occupational health program permit the reevaluation of the workers' health and often detect disorders before symptoms are present.

Health education programs for workers and counseling services that result in referrals to appropriate community health and social resources are occupational health activities that help to maintain good health. The value of these services has been demonstrated repeatedly, but it is impossible to calculate the full benefits of such services to workers, their families, and the community. The woman worker who is also mother and housewife carries home information about nutrition and meal planning and about child care given to her by the occupational health nurse. She integrates into her household duties knowledge about eye protection which she has acquired in an industrial safety session. The problem drinker who is a problem to her or his employer and family will become a problem to society if not helped; counseling and early referral to a community alcoholism clinic may save the person from losing a job and will probably improve the family life.

When a worker is seriously injured in an industrial accident, the immediate and perhaps lifesaving care is given by the occupational health personnel. Following this the injured worker is sent not to a company hospital but to a community hospital or clinic, or to a doctor's office. The costs are paid by the workmen's compensation insurance company, and the worker's family receives workmen's compensation payments in lieu of the person's salary. While these community services are being utilized, the patient's care should be coordinated by the occupational health personnel at the person's place of employment. For example the worker with a cardiac disorder who is discharged from the hospital and approved for return to work by the workers's own physician may be referred by the occupational health physician to the cardiac evaluation clinic of the local heart association to assure that he is now physically capable of meeting the demands of the job.

Occupational health practice is concerned with all the many factors that influence the health and safety of workers. There are as many points of view about it as there are disciplines involved. This field is practiced by those who work in a safety and health program provided by the employer to deal constructively with the health of employees in relation to their work. It is also practiced by those who work for federal, state, and other governmental agencies to fulfill the aims and objectives of the Occupational Safety and Health Act of 1970.

Occupational health practice is the science and art of promoting the physical and mental health and the well-being of workers. It includes activities to prevent work-connected disease and injury, and to treat and rehabilitate workers who have been injured or become ill from work-connected causes. It requires a multidisciplinary team of specialized professional personnel—physicians, nurses, industrial hygienists, health physicists, and safety professionals—to work with management and employee representatives in planning and conducting activities that ensure the provision of medical care; the sanitation, healthfulness, and safety of the work environment; and the education of the employees in the principles of personal hygiene, health protection, safe work practices, and accident prevention.

The basic objectives of an occupational health program as stated by the American Medical Association (AMA) are:

1. To protect employees against health and safety hazards in their work situation.
2. Insofar as practical and feasible, to protect the general environment of the community.

3. To facilitate the placement of workers according to their physical, mental, and emotional capacities in work which they can perform with an acceptable degree of efficiency and without endangering their own health and safety or that of others.
4. To assure adequate medical care and rehabilitation of the occupationally ill and injured.
5. To encourage and assist in measures for personal health maintenance, including the acquisition of a personal physician whenever possible.[16]

Four sets of correlative activities comprise a comprehensive occupational safety and health program:

ENVIRONMENTAL MONITORING

Evaluation of the work environment to identify and measure safety and health hazards	Corrective action to eliminate or control hazards; preventive maintenance and good housekeeping procedures to maintain a safe and healthful work environment

HEALTH SURVEILLANCE

Physical assessment of the worker to determine the worker's state of health and to identify as early as possible any potential health problems	Health promotion initiatives to maintain and to improve the worker's health

PRIMARY CARE

Identification of occupational or general health problems by medical and/or nursing diagnosis to determine care required	Management and continued care of the individual as an ambulatory consumer or referral for specialized care and rehabilitation

WORKER EDUCATION

Continuing awareness of employee needs and environmental conditions to determine what are safe work practices and good health procedures	Instruction to increase the worker's understanding of the nature of the exposure and its effects and of preventive health measures and to develop the worker's ability to follow safe work practices and good health procedures; supervision of work practices and follow-up of health-related behavior to ensure each worker's continued well-being

The effectiveness of each set depends upon the carrying out of the required activities for both parts of each set. Moreover, since these sets are interrelated, failure to carry out any one set will result in an ineffective program. The activities listed in each set suggest the roles of the professional members of the occupational health team and their contributions to a comprehensive occupational health program. Parts II, III, IV, and V of this book deal with these four sets of correlative activities that are the parameters of an occupational health program. The nurses' role is developed in terms of their team relationships with the others members and in terms of their professional competencies and independent functioning.

References

1. 29 CFR. 651 et seq. Occupational Safety and Health Act of 1970, PL 91-596. Washington, D.C.: GPO, 1970, p. 1.
2. Ibid., pp. 1–2.
3. U.S. Supreme Court Decision No. 76-1143: *Ray Marshall, Secretary of Labor, et al., Appellants v. Barlow's, Inc*, May 23, 1978, majority opinion delivered by Mr. Justice White, pp. 1–2.
4. Ibid., p. 13.
5. AMA, Department of Environmental, Public, and Occupational Health. *Scope Objectives and Functions of Occupational Health Programs*. Chicago, 1971, p. 1.
6. DHEW. *Survey of Public Health Nursing 1968–1972*. Washington, D.C.: GPO, 1973, p. 125.
7. Copplestone, J. F. *Preventive Aspects of Occupational Health Nursing*. London: Edward Arnold, 1967, p. 16.
8. DOL. *Brief History of the American Labor Movement*, Bulletin No. 1000. Washington, D.C.: GPO, 1957, p. 67.
9. Ibid., p. 68.
10. Wolff, L. *Lockout*. New York: Harper & Row, 1965, p. 126.
11. DOL, op. cit., p. 35.
12. "Washington Focus," *I.U.D. Spotlight on Health and Safety* (Indianapolis), Vol. 4, No. 2, 1977, p. 4.
13. Banta, H. D., and Bosch, S. J. "Organized Labor and the Pre-paid Group Practice Movement," *Archives of Environmental Health*, Vol. 29, No. 7, July 1974, pp. 43–49.
14. DOL, Bureau of Labor Statistics. *Major Collective Bargaining Agreements: Safety and Health Provisions*. Washington, D.C.: GPO, 1976, p. 16.
15. DHEW, op. cit., p. 124.
16. AMA, op. cit., pp. 3–6.

Selected Readings

AAIN. *The Nurse in Industry: A History of the American Association of Industrial Nurses, Inc*. New York: AAOHN, 1976.

Brodeur, P. *Expendable Americans*. New York: Viking, 1974.
Brodeur, P. *The Zapping of America: Microwaves, Their Deadly Risk and the Cover-Up*. New York: Norton, 1977.
Capell, P. T., and Case, D. B. *Ambulatory Care Manual for Nurse Practitioners*. Philadelphia: Lippincott, 1976.
Charley, I. H. *The Birth of Industrial Nursing*. London: Baillière, Tindall, 1978.
Craig, J. "A Practical Approach to Cost Analysis of an Occupational Health Program," *Journal of Occupational Medicine*, Vol. 16, No. 7, July 1974, pp. 445–448.
DOL, *The Anvil and the Plow*. Washington, D.C.: GPO, 1963.
Flanagan, L. *One Strong Voice*. Kansas City, Mo.: ANA, 1976.
Horsley, B. "A Registered Nurse as an OSHA Compliance Officer," *Occupational Health Nursing*, Vol. 20, No. 9, Sept. 1972, pp. 7–9.
Hunter, D. *The Diseases of Occupations*, 6th Ed. Sevenoaks, Kent, England: Hodder & Stoughton, 1978.
Joint Practice Committee of North Carolina Medical Society and North Carolina Nurses' Association. *Occupational Health Services*, Rep. of Task Force. Raleigh, N.C., 1976.
Lee, J. A. *The New Nurse in Industry*. Washington, D.C.: GPO, 1978.
Mancuso, T. F. *Help for the Working Wounded*. Washington, D.C.: The Machinist, 1976.
Morris, R. B. (Ed.). *Bicentennial History of the American Worker*. Washington, D.C.: GPO, 1976.
Murchison, I., Nichols, T. S., and Hanson, R. *Legal Accountability in the Nursing Process*. St. Louis: Mosby, 1978.
Murphy, J. F. "Role Expansion or Role Extension: Some Conceptual Differences," *Nursing Forum*, Vol. 9, No. 4, 1970, pp. 380–389.
Nelson, N. "Critical Problems in Environmental and Occupational Health," *Journal of Occupational Medicine*, Vol. 16, No. 9, Sept. 1974, pp. 581–583.
O'Toole, J. (Ed.). *Work in America*. Cambridge, Mass.: M.I.T. Press, 1973.
O'Toole, J. (Ed.). *Work and the Quality of Life*. Cambridge, Mass.: M.I.T. Press, 1974.
Page, J. A., and O'Brien, M. W. *Bitter Wages*. New York: Grossman, 1973.
Ramazzini, B. *Diseases of Workers (De Martus Artificum)*, New York Academy of Medicine History of Medicine Series No. 23. Trans. by W. C. Wright. New York: Hafner, 1964.
Randall, W. S., and Solomon, S. D. *Building Six*. Boston: Little, Brown, 1977.
Sax, N. I. *Dangerous Properties of Industrial Materials*, 5th Ed. New York: Van Nostrand Reinhold, 1979.
Scott, R. *Muscle and Blood*. New York: Dutton, 1974.
Stellman, J., and Daum, S. *Work Is Dangerous to Your Health*. New York: Random House, Vintage, 1973.
Tabershaw, I. R. "Occupational Medicine: The Search for Identity," *Journal of Occupational Medicine*, Vol. 13, No. 7, July 1971, pp. 325–330.
Wallick, F. *The American Worker: An Endangered Species*. New York: Ballantine, 1972.

PART II

Environmental Monitoring

The healthfulness and safety of the work environment depends in large part on the recognition by the employer that the work environment may be hazardous to the health of the workers; that the work environment must be evaluated to determine what, if any, hazards exist; and that controls must be put into place if health and safety problems are to be identified. These facts determine the establishment's need for occupational safety and health professionals. Part II of this book deals with what nurses must know, whom they must be able to work with, and what contribution they can and do make to the fulfillment of the first of the four parameters that determine the scope and objectives of an occupational safety and health program for employees:

ENVIRONMENTAL MONITORING

| Evaluation of the work environment to identify and measure safety and health hazards | Corrective action to eliminate or control hazards; preventive maintenance and good housekeeping procedures to maintain a safe and healthful work environment |

The nurse as a member of the occupational safety and health team:

- Participates in an environmental control program that aims to identify, eliminate, and/or control health and safety hazards
- Consults on health and safety matters with management, workers, and representatives of the health community.

CHAPTER 3

Occupational Hygiene

The evaluation and control of the occupational environment form the keystone of occupational health and safety and are basic to primary prevention. In line with this philosophy, the Occupational Health and Safety Act of 1970 (PL 91-596) was enacted and is being administered as a work environment law. Industrial hygiene involves: (a) the recognition of environmental factors associated with work and work operations; (b) the evaluation, with the aid of quantitative measurements, of the magnitude of these factors in terms of their ability to affect workers' health and impair their well-being; and (c) the prescription of methods to control or eliminate such factors or to alleviate their effects. The basic principles that underlie industrial hygiene practices are those that are incorporated in the correlative activities associated with environmental monitoring.

The Environmental Control Team

The safety engineer and/or the safety professional and the industrial hygienist are the professionals who carry the major responsibility for accident prevention and control and for industrial hygiene. In addition there are other professionals whose numbers are less but whose contributions are essential. The chemist who works in the industrial hygiene laboratory identifies and determines the amount of potentially harmful substances that may be present in the samples collected by the industrial hygienist. The health physicist applies special expertise to the control of environmental problems associated with atomic energy, ionizing radiation, and nonionizing radiation (microwaves, laser, etc.). The physicist has much in common with the industrial hygienist in that they both use similar techniques for testing and control and both are involved in the control of health hazards associated with nonionizing radiation.

The epidemiologist studies worker populations for cause-and-effect relationships between occupational diseases and injuries and the work environment. Another area of expertise that is involved is ergonomics and biomechanics. The ergonomist is concerned with designing industrial operations and equipment to facilitate the safe implementation of work operations and the minimization of their harmful effects.

The Industrial Hygienist

The industrial hygienist is the health professional who is most often identified with environmental control of toxic chemicals and physical agents that are associated with work operations. Within his sphere of responsibility, the industrial hygienist:

1. Directs the industrial hygiene program.
2. Inspects the work environment and environs.
3. Makes appropriate measurements of toxic substances to determine the magnitude of exposure of workers and the public.
4. Conducts tests or has tests performed on materials associated with the operations to determine their content and toxicity.
5. Interprets the environmental monitoring data in terms of the amount of a toxic substance present and its ability to impair health.
6. Recommends and conducts appropriate environmental surveillance programs.
7. Establishes and maintains a system for recording the industrial hygiene data generated by environmental monitoring activities.
8. Assures the compatibility of the environmental data system with the systems for recording medical surveillance data.
9. Recommends control measures to assure that the hazards in the work environment are controlled.
10. Selects appropriate personal protective equipment and instructs workers in the use and care of such equipment, especially respirators.
11. Conducts in-service training for members of the occupational safety and health team.
12. Conducts training sessions for first-line supervisors and for workers, especially those who work with hazardous substances.
13. Prepares reports that reflect his participation in the occupational safety and health program and makes recommendations as to what modifications are necessary to keep the establishment in compliance with proposed OSHA Standards.
14. Actively participates in the activities of local and national industrial hygiene organizations—the American Industrial Hygiene Association (AIHA) and, when appropriate, the American Conference of Governmental Industrial Hygienists (ACGIH).
15. Prepares and presents scientific papers for oral presentation and/or publication.

Evaluating the Occupational Environment

Inspections and surveys of the work environment are conducted to identify safety and health hazards. The correlative to finding a health and/or safety hazard is action to correct or eliminate the hazard. There are few if any industrial operations that do not involve materials or processes that can cause harm to workers' health unless used properly and controlled by proper engineering methods. The three most common types of surveys performed by industrial hygienists and/or health physicists or chemists on the occupational safety and health team are the preventive survey, the trouble-shooting survey, and the survey for checking compliance with OSHA regulations.

Methodology

As the first step in an industrial hygiene survey, the industrial hygienist observes the environment and evaluates the work practices. He wants to know what the workers' complaints are, what the union's concerns are in regard to the work environment, and what environmental problems are seen by the safety professionals, the supervisor, and the physician or nurse(s).

Essential to an industrial hygiene survey is the procedure sometimes called a "walk-around" or a "walk-through." This is a preliminary survey that includes taking a good look, with educated eyes, at all the processes, the work environment, and the work practices. The industrial hygienist usually starts where the process starts—with the raw materials—then follows along to see what happens to make the product. He makes a list of all chemicals used, the products produced, and any by-products. This involves a great deal of detective work. The industrial hygienist seeks information from the purchasing agent, reads the signs and labels on drums and containers, and asks suppliers about their products. The industrial hygienist identifies substances in the work environment that are toxic and to what degree, and checks the current threshold limit values (TLVs) and time-weighted averages (TWAs) for each. See Appendix B for additional information about these.

The industrial hygienist identifies by visual observation the areas in the establishment where there are dusty operations and where processes are used that give off fumes or generate mists and also uses his nose because many vapors and gases can be detected through the sense of smell. The industrial hygienist knows that when a substance can be smelled the threshold for safety may be passed. The industrial hygienist also checks for sources of radiant heat, abnormal temperatures and humidity, and for noise and areas that are inadequately illuminated. It is essential that he find any sources of ionizing or nonionizing radiation.

Sampling

Following the walk-through, the industrial hygienist first uses direct reading instruments to determine what and how much of substances used in production are in the environment, especially in the breathing zone of the workers, and in what form, then, when indicated, uses appropriate methods to collect samples, both at the workers' breathing zone and in the general work area, so as to be able to obtain the data needed to determine whether there are areas that do not meet the criteria for a safe and healthful environment. The industrial hygienist often discusses the number, type, and method of collection of samples with the chemist who will do the analysis because the substance may be present in very small amounts and its chemical properties may not be known.

Samples may be taken for any of several reasons in addition to determining the level and type of exposure of workers: (a) to investigate complaints or the cause of illness; (b) to determine the effectiveness of control measures; or (c) to determine the degree of compliance with OSHA Standards.

The samples taken by the industrial hygienist or health physicist are sent for analysis to a specialized laboratory accredited by the AIHA. In 1967 a federal law, the Clinical Laboratories Improvement Act, was passed. Responsibility for the administration of this act is centered in the Center for Disease Control (CDC) in Atlanta.

When persons not certified as industrial hygienists are involved in collecting environmental samples and can not have assistance from an industrial hygienist, the results will be more reliable if that person will contact the laboratory to which the samples are to be sent for analysis and request guidance as to how to collect the sample, as well as what media it is to be collected on, for what time period, and at what sampling flow rate, and how the sample should be transported to the laboratory. Similar advice occasionally is requested by industrial hygienists. Because of the nature of the samples, these can be easily contaminated by substances from nearby work sites; the sampling media can be overwhelmed if the level of contamination is high; or an insufficient amount can be collected if the level in the air is very low. The correct filter and sampling rate are essential to an accurate measurement. The industrial hygiene chemist and the industrial hygiene laboratory represent essential environmental control specialists and specialized services, respectively.

All the information generated by observations and by sampling must be taken into consideration, and the industrial hygienist uses his own knowledge and understanding of work ecology to determine the extent of the hazard, if any, to the workers.

The Preventive Survey

The preventive survey is performed when a new material or operation is introduced or a change in a process or material is made. The survey is done to evaluate the nature and the degree of the potentially hazardous exposure that may be created by the change. A preventive survey is also done periodically to assure the continued safety of the environment and to comply with the monitoring requirements of OSHA. The preventive survey gives the industrial hygienist a firsthand knowledge of what the employees are working with, what the hazards are, how much and what hazardous substances are in the work area, and what modifications are needed and where. Some industries schedule a total preventive industrial hygiene survey at least once a year because they are prevention minded and believe that if the health professionals don't look for hazards they will not find them and get them under control.

The Trouble-shooting survey

The trouble-shooting survey is carried on when a problem arises and the cause and effect need to be determined. For example several workers may have become ill, or there may have been reports of increased deaths among exposed workers, or workers may have reported changes in body functions or evidence of excessive absorption of toxic substances. A trouble-shooting survey may also be ordered when a significant change in environmental exposure is discovered by a preventive survey.[1]

The Compliance Survey

The third type of industrial hygiene survey is that carried on by the plant industrial hygienist and/or the industrial hygienist who works for OSHA and/or a state agency approved by OSHA. This survey is done as outlined in *The OSHA Industrial Hygiene Field Operations Manual* to determine whether the establishment is or is not in compliance with the OSHA Standards. Copies of this manual are available for sale from the U.S. Government Printing Office (GPO) in Washington, D.C.

Corrective Actions

There are few if any industrial operations that do not involve materials or processes that can cause harm unless they are used properly or are controlled by proper engineering methods. The industrial hygiene survey is conducted to identify such hazards. Four methods recommended for use singly or collectively by industrial hygienists to protect workers from occupational hazards are:

1. Substitution of a less toxic substance
2. Isolation or enclosure of the process
3. Installation of a ventilation system
4. Protection of the individual worker through the use of personal protective equipment.

Substitution

Substitution of a less toxic substance is the most effective corrective action. The literature abounds with interesting and exciting accounts of the work of leaders in occupational medicine and industrial hygiene who have identified hazardous materials and who have worked out safe, equally effective substitutes. The match industry, in which white or yellow phosphorus is an occupational hazard, is an example. Early on, many of the workers exposed to this material while making matches died of an occupational disease known as "phossy jaw." The substitution of red phosphorus effectively controlled the hazard. In many processes, toluene or xylene can be used instead of benzene. Steel shot or ground walnut husks can be used in many cleaning operations to eliminate the workers' exposure to silica.

Isolation

Isolation or enclosure is another means of modifying an occupational hazard. This may consist of such a simple procedure as putting a lid on a container or it may be as complicated as the isolation procedures designed to control exposure to atomic radiation or the closed system designed to control exposure during the manufacture of some drugs or vinyl chloride. Isolation of a process limits the exposure to an area and/or to as small a number of personnel as is feasible.

Ventilation

Ventilation systems are engineer designed to carry hazardous materials associated with the manufacturing process away from the breathing zone of the worker. For example the ventilation in a spray-painting booth is designed to eliminate the worker's exposure to solvents, or an exhaust hood may be placed around a grinding wheel. The principles of ventilation and isolation may be combined, as when the sandblasting of small castings or granite memorial monuments is done in a shatterproof box or tent enclosure with armholes through which the worker handles the objects and the nozzle of the sandblasting device.

Ventilation provides a large percentage of the worker's protection from toxic and hazardous materials. This may be achieved by a general ventilation system or one that provides ventilation for a single operation. A local exhaust system will remove an airborne contaminant such as a dust, fume, vapor, or gas near the source of its generation by using hoods and ductwork to trap the material at its source. In such a system adequate make-up air must be brought in to replace that which is exhausted or the system will not work to capacity. A general exhaust system removes air from the room after the contaminant has spread from the source where it was generated.

The terms *general ventilation* and *dilution ventilation* are often used interchangeably, but "the Committee on Industrial Ventilation of the American Conference of Governmental Industrial Hygienists (ACGIH) uses general ventilation to refer to the removal (or supply) of air from a general area, room, or building for the purpose of comfort control. Dilution ventilation refers to dilution of contaminated air with uncontaminated air in a general area, room, or building for the purpose of health hazard or nuisance control."[2] The latter term refers to a system that utilizes natural convective currents through open doors, windows, or exhaust fans located on the roof. Dilution ventilation works only when the air contamination is not excessive and when the contaminant is released at a distance from the worker's breathing zone.

The American National Standards Institute's (ANSI) Standard Z9.2-1971 provides the guidelines for ventilation, as does the ACGIH *Industrial Ventilation*, a *Manual of Recommended Practice* (see App. C for address).

Use of Personal Protective Equipment

Personal protective equipment can be a useful means of protecting worker health. However, industrial hygienists recommend its use only as a last resort when engineering controls cannot be used or as an interim measure until such controls can be put into place. Personal protective equipment is also useful in mobile or transient operations. When the exposure involves a substance that can be absorbed through the skin, protective clothing is used. The selection of the equipment depends on how it works to provide protection for the worker. The National Institute for Occupational Safety and Health (NIOSH) publishes a list of approved personal protective equipment.

Selection of respiratory protective devices depends upon whether the person is to be protected from dusts or from fumes. There are schedules of approved respirators for protection against (a) pneumoconiosis-producing dusts, (b) toxic dusts, (c) metal fumes, and (d) various combinations of dusts and fumes. ANSI's Z88.2-1969 *Practices for Respiratory Protection* is a useful publication. The requirements for respiratory protection are specific in the OSHA Standards, as are the requirements for teaching the worker about how to use and maintain the respirator.

The General Industry Standards of OSHA contain five sections in the 1910 series that relate to personal protective equipment:

- 132 General Requirements
- 133 Eye and Face Protection
- 134 Respiratory Protection
- 135 Occupational Head Protection
- 136 Occupational Foot Protection.

Most of these requirements are based on ANSI codes and indicate the many kinds of personal protective equipment that may have to be used by workers for health protection. The use of safety shoes, eye protectors, and ear defenders is usually ordered by the safety professional. When an industrial hygienist is employed, this professional deals with the selection and use of respiratory protection equipment and also develops the work practices and instructs the worker in the use and care of the protective equipment. Cleanliness and proper maintenance of respiratory protection equipment is esential for its proper functioning. When exposures cannot be controlled by primary prevention activities, when it is not possible to carry out these activies immediately, or when spills or other emergencies arise, the use of personal protective equipment is mandated.

Personal protective equipment must be properly maintained and someone must be responsible for overseeing this maintenance. It is useful to have a schedule for checking such equipment and to keep a record of the date and condition of the equipment. In the case of respirators used for protection against certain substances, OSHA requires that such a record be kept.

Although the use of personal protective equipment as a means of protecting workers is never the method of choice, when such equipment is necessary it can be most effective The nurse can and should be involved in helping the workers to understand the health hazard, why the equipment must be used, and how to use and care for it.

Control through Occupational Toxicology

"Toxicology is the study of the nature and action of poisons."[3] It is the capacity of something to produce injury or harm. All substances have the potential for being toxic, but the term *toxicology* is generally used by occupational health personnel in reference to a substance that would or could be encountered in an industrial environment. Toxicity may be regarded as the net effect of two opposing actions: (a) how the toxic substances act on the body and (b) how the body acts on the substances.

The industrial hygienist recognizes, and so must the nurse, the meaning of the dose-response curve. "In simple terms, the dose-response relationship indicates how a biological organism's response to a toxic substance changes as its exposure to the substance increases."[4] For example a small dose of carbon monoxide will induce drowsiness; a larger dose can induce death. With the exception of exposure to the carcinogens (for which any amount no matter how small may be too much), for a substance to be hazardous to health it must be in sufficient quantity and in a physical state that permits entry into the human body, and exposure of the worker must be for a sufficient period of time. "A cardinal principle to remember is that the intensity of toxic action is a function of the concentration of the toxic agent which reaches the site of action."[5]

Health Physics in Environmental Control

The Health Physics Society describes the health physicist as a nuclear scientist with the responsibility to protect humans and their environment from the hazards of radiation. Protection of worker health is based on a deep appreciation of how radiation can and does cause harm. Knowledge of the route of entry is essential, since external radiation creates one type of health problem and internal radiation another. Breathing air contaminated with particles of gaseous radionuclides is the most common route of entry, but ingestion and skin absorption are also routes of entry. A skin puncture can result in implantation of a radioactive source in the wound. Once inside the body radionuclides are absorbed, metabolized, and distributed throughout the tissues and organs according to the chemical properties of the elements and compounds in which they exist.

Ionizing radiation is energy in the form of particles (alpha particles, beta particles, protons, and neutrons) or waves (X-rays or gamma rays) emitted from radioactive materials, X-ray machines, and high-energy accelerators. Radioactive chemicals are chemicals that possess one or more atoms that can spontaneously emit alpha or beta particles, or gamma rays, by disintegration. Radiation is detected and measured by the ionization it produces. This can be measured by conversion to light, which can be measured on a photoelectric cell. The film badge is one means of detecting radiation. Instruments for measuring exposures must be calibrated for the type of radiation to be measured. An understanding of time, distance, and shielding is the basis for the engineering controls. The nurse who works where radioactivity is a potential hazard for the workers has a special need to be knowledgeable about ionizing radiation.

The principles used in the protection of the health of workers whose jobs involve working with physical energies, that is, ionizing radiations, are similar to those for the chemical hazards. At times there may be unique problems which add to the circumstances, and these must be dealt with by the members of the occupational safety and health team. One such problem is fear on the part of workers concerning exposures to ionizing radiation—fear which may be so all consuming as to cause them to want to prohibit any use of atomic energy. Control of radiation hazards requires effective design of equipment, careful planning of procedures, and continued application of safe operating practices. The objective of the activities the health physicist carries on is prevention.

Human Factors Engineering: Ergonomics

In the 1700 edition of his book, *De morbis artificum diatriba*, Bernardino Ramazzini, the father of occupational medicine, stated:

Manifold is the harvest of disease reaped by certain workers from the crafts and trades that they pursue; all the profit they get is injury to their health. That stems mostly I think, from two causes. The first and most potent is the harmful character of the materials they handle, noxious vapors and very fine particles, inimical to human beings, inducing specific diseases. As to the second cause, I assign certain violent and irregular motions and unnatural postures of the body by reason of which the natural structure of the living machine is so impaired that serious disease gradually develops therefrom. . . .[6]

Erwin R. Tichauer, a highly respected professor of biomechanics, cites the foregoing quotation and makes the point that "for nearly two centuries industrial hygiene and related disciplines limited their scope of interest to the first set of occupational disease vectors as discussed by Ramazzini."[7] He also points out that the dire work force needs in the countries of Europe following World Wars I and II forced the women of these countries and men with physical handicaps into the factories. Ergonomics was first applied to overcome the serious and general problems involved in fitting jobs to the physical and behavioral operating characteristics of individual workers. In the United States, interest in the field of ergonomics is increasing because of the number of women in the labor force, and the recognition of the value that results from a better matching of the work environment to the needs of the human body.

Ergonomics is concerned with the design of work. Specialists in this field aim to achieve optimal adjustment between the worker and the work environment in such a manner as to enhance the worker's health, efficiency, and well-being. The fitting of a job or job components to the person's anatomic and/or physiological characteristics is referred to as the biology of work. This involves study of a task in relation to the anatomic and physiological aspects of the person. As seen by the ergonomist there is no clear distinction among the variables in the human-machine-environment system; all are interrelated and interdependent. In the United States the terms *human factors engineering* and *human engineering* are frequently used when referring to ergonomics. These terms are defined as "the application of information about human characteristics, capacities, and limitations to the design of machines, machine systems, and environments so that people can live and work safely, comfortably, and effectively."[8]

By whatever name it may be called, ergonomics is involved with many disciplines, including anthropology, biometrics, biomechanics, and occupational physiology and cybernetics, as witness the definition proposed by the *International Labor Review* in 1961: "Ergonomics is the application of human biological sciences in conjunction with the engineering sciences to achieve the optimum mutual adjustment of man and his work, the benefits being measured in terms of human efficiency and well-being."[9] This mutual adaptation reduces stress, lightens the work load, and increases safety; equipment and plants are used more efficiently and their reliability is improved. An ergonomics program involves:

1. Making an analysis of the job, the tools, the methods, and the materials used in an industrial process. This involves a time and motion study which, when done in detail, will include the identification of the physiological parameters, the dangerous occurrences, the flow lines, and the amount of training the worker requires.
2. Identifying the factors in the work environment that need to be modified and then experimenting to determine which of the feasible alternatives is most acceptable.
3. Making changes in the design of tools and in procedures employed.
4. Checking to assure that the changes are effective.

Nurses' Involvement in Environmental Control

Participation in the many and varied activities basic to environmental monitoring gives to occupational health nursing its specialty classification. Expert occupational health nurses understand and utilize the concept of occupational ecology. They assist the environmental control team in the following ways:

1. Make themselves aware of the potential hazards that exist in the work environment.
2. Consciously look for the relationship between what workers do and the health problems for which they come to the health unit for care.
3. When serving as the only full-time occupational health professional at a plant, identify the special contributions of the industrial hygienists, the health physicists, and the safety professional, and consciously include them when appropriate; when these specialists are full-time members of the occupational health and safety team, work cooperatively with them.

4. Consult with management concerning environmental hazards.
5. When a plant does not employ an industrial hygienist, do the staff work necessary to estimate if there is a possible hazard associated with the establishment and the product or services.
6. Keep informed regarding the requirements of the current and proposed OSHA standards.
7. Identify what needs to be done and what staff and equipment deficits may exist, and suggest to a decision-making member of management what needs to be done and where the special expertise can be found to perform the activities required.

References

1. Kleinfeld, M. "The Trouble-shooting Industrial Hygiene Survey," *AMA Archives of Industrial Hygiene*, Vol. 18, No. 2. Aug. 1958, p. 125.
2. ACGIH, Committee on Industrial Ventilation. *A Manual of Recommended Practice*, 15th Ed. Lansing, Mich., 1978, Chap. 2, p. 1.
3. Amdur, M. O. "Industrial Toxicology," Chap. 7 in NIOSH, *The Industrial Environment—Its Evaluation and Control*. Washington, D.C.: GPO, 1973, p. 472.
4. Ibid., p. 63.
5. Ibid.
6. Tichauer, E. R. "Ergonomic Aspects of Biomechanics," Chap. 32 in NIOSH, *The Industrial Environment—Its Evaluation and Control*. Washington, D.C.: GPO, 1973, p. 431.
7. Ibid.
8. Carpentier, J. "Ergonomics," in *Encyclopedia of Occupational Health and Safety*. Geneva: ILO, 1971, p. 472.
9. Chapanis, A. "Human Engineering," in *Encyclopedia of Occupational Health and Safety*. Geneva: ILO, 1971, p. 677.

Selected Readings

ACGIH. *Guide for Control of Laser Hazards*. Cincinnati, 1976.
ACGIH. *Air Sampling Instruments Manual*, 5th ed. Cincinnati, 1978.
ACGIH, Committee on Industrial Ventilation. *Industrial Ventilation*, 16th ed. Lansing, Mich., 1980.
AIHA. *Analytical Guides, Hygienic Guides, Ergonomics Guides*, and *Non-Ionizing Radiation Guides*, current ed. Akron, Ohio.
AIHA. *Heating and Cooling for Man in Industry*, 2nd ed. Akron, Ohio, 1978.
AIHA. Industrial Noise Manual, current ed. Akron, Ohio.
Ashford, N. A. *Crisis in the Workplace*. Cambridge, Mass.: M.I.T. Press, 1976.
Brief, R. S. *Basic Industrial Hygiene Manual*. Akron, Ohio: AIHA, 1977.
Held, B. J. *History of Respiratory Protective Devices*. Cincinnati, Ohio: ACGIH, 1976.

Hosey, A. D. *History of Development of Industrial Hygiene Sampling: Instruments and Techniques.* Cincinnati, Ohio: ACGIH, 1975.

Linch, A. L. *Biological Monitoring for Industrial Chemical Exposure Control.* Cleveland: CRC, 1974.

NIOSH. *The Industrial Environment—Its Evaluation and Control.* Washington, D.C.: GPO, 1973.

NIOSH/OSHA. *Pocket Guide to Chemical Hazards.* Washington, D.C.: GPO, 1978.

Olishifski, J. B., and McElroy, F. E. (eds.). *Fundamentals of Industrial Hygiene.* Chicago: NSC, 1971.

Patty, F. A. (ed.). *Industrial Hygiene and Toxicology*, 3 Vols. Vol. 1, *General Principles*, Clayton, G. D., and Clayton, F. E. (eds.), 1978. Vol. 2 in preparation. Vol. 3, *Theory and Rationale of Industrial Hygiene Practice*, Cralley, L. V., and Cralley, L. J. (eds.), 1979, Somerset, N.J.: Wiley.

Sax, N. I. *Dangerous Properties of Industrial Materials*, 5th ed. New York: Van Nostrand Reinhold, 1979.

Thomas, H. F. "Some Observations on Occupational Hygiene Standards," *Annals of Occupational Hygiene.* London: Pergamon Press Ltd., 1979, pp. 389–397.

Yaffe, C. D. *The First Forty Years 1938–1978 of ACGIH.* Cincinnati: ACGIH, 1978.

CHAPTER 4

Occupational Safety

The industrial safety movement started in Europe. Governmental regulations for the inspection of factories were passed in England in 1823. Another act, passed in Germany in 1869, required the employer to furnish necessary appliances to safeguard the health and life of employees. This movement, stressing prevention of work injuries and improvement of the work environment, spread to the United States, and in 1867 Massachusets instituted factory inspections.[1] Some American employers became interested in industrial accident prevention before the concept of employee liability was generally accepted. In 1892 the Joliet Division of the Illinois Steel Company formed a safety department; this has been called the birthplace of the American industrial accident prevention movement.[2]

The U.S. Bureau of Mines was created in 1910 to "investigate the cause of mine accidents, study health hazards in mining, and to seek means of correction."[3] The work of this agency in the field of industrial safety has been outstanding. It developed effective mine rescue methods and first-aid training programs that have influenced the care given workers in all industries. The first nongovernmental nationwide effort toward accident prevention was the establishment in 1912 of the National Council for Industrial Safety. This grew out of the efforts of the safety committee of the U.S. Steel Corporation and that of the Association of Iron and Steel Electrical Engineers. In 1915 the name was changed to the National Safety Council (NSC).[4] The activities of this council and its membership have grown steadily over the years. The council seeks to promote safety and to reduce the number and seriousness of accidents in all phases of human endeavor. It maintains a staff of experts who collect, develop, and disseminate safety materials and information and who carry on an information and consulting service for its individual and company members.

The U.S. Bureau of Labor Statistics was organized in 1913 as a division of the DOL.[5] The bureau collects and disseminates information that is useful in labor administration. It annually collects and publishes the general accident experience for American industry. In 1971 OSHA assigned to this bureau the responsibility for collecting and reporting the injury and illness rates of establishments covered by PL 95-596. Workmen's compen-

Occupational Safety

sation legislation gave great impetus to the industrial safety movement. The fact that work injuries are expensive was and still is a motivating factor in accident prevention.

Safety Program Organization

The NSC defines a *safety program organization* as "a method employed by management to assign responsibility for accident prevention and to ensure performance under that responsibility."[6] Responses from 124 personnel executives who were members of the 1976–1977 Personnel Policies Forum of the Bureau of National Affairs, Inc., indicated that more than four-fifths were associated with companies that had a formal safety program. These responses also indicated that separate safety departments are much more common in larger companies (49%) than in small ones (24%) and that the size of the departments ranged from 1 to 34 employees.[7] Seven basic elements of a safety program organization have been identified by the DOL:

1. Assumption of leadership by management
2. Assignment of responsibility
3. Identification and control of hazards
4. Training of employees and supervisors
5. Safety and health record keeping
6. First-aid and medical assistance
7. Employee awareness, acceptance, and participation.[8]

Purposes

The purposes of modern industrial safety programs are (a) to stimulate management employees to take an active interest in promoting safety, (b) to stimulate workers to accept and to follow safe work practices, (c) to identify the cause of accidents, and (d) to take remedial action based on the facts. As used by occupational safety and health personnel the term *safety* means freedom from human-equipment-materials-environmental interactions that result in accidents and injuries. The function of a safety department is to assist management in developing and operating a program which will protect the workers by preventing accidents, whatever their cause.

It is interesting to note that, when personnel in the major disciplines that make up an occupational health team list the basic elements of a safety program, an industrial hygiene program, and an occupational health nursing or medical program, there is a great deal of overlap. This is especially true of lists of elements for industrial hygiene and safety programs. In practice the major difference between these two areas of occupational health is that the activities of the safety professional deal primarily with accident prevention so as to control the number and severity of occupational injuries, while the activities of the industrial hygienist deal primarily with the identification and control of toxic substances that have the potential to cause an occupational illness. Professionals in both areas are involved in record keeping primarily as this relates to environmental controls and the identification of hazards. Both deal with the health unit personnel—doctors and/or nurses—who provide care for workers who have suffered industrial injuries or have symptoms that are suggestive of an occupational disease. The safety professionals and the industrial hygienists are concerned primarily with finding and correcting the cause when injuries happen or people become ill from work hazards. There is a very real need for good team relationships and every effort must be made to foster cooperation, not competition.

Leadership

A successful safety program for industrial workers depends upon there being someone at the management level who states the establishment's safety policies that are to be followed by all employees. In larger organizations the responsibility for conducting the safety program is delegated to the safety director and his staff. Sometimes this delegation is to a single safety professional. The term *safety professional* is generally used to identify the person who is concerned with the prevention and control of trauma arising from accidents, and with hazard control systems based on environmental and human factor analyses. This person and the nurse are the two professionals who have the most direct responsibility for planning, conducting, and evaluating occupational safety and health program activities. They share program planning and health and safety education responsibilities. However they also have separate areas of responsibility based on their own special expertise: the nurse for health care and health assessment, the safety professional for accident prevention and control. Each reports directly to the same management personnel for administrative directions. All too often, however, the nurse is required to report to the safety professional, and this fact frequently causes conflict between these two professionals. Such conflict results from the lack of clearly defined program objectives, of job descriptions for both jobs, and clearly defined lines of communication between the nurse and management, the safety department and management, and the health and safety units. Some nurses report directly to the safety director for administrative directions. This is not recommended as it means that the nurse, and hence the health unit, does not have a direct channel of communication to a decision-making person at the management level. The ideal relationship be-

Occupational Safety 49

tween the safety professional and the nurse is that of co-worker. Both must be expert practitioners who are able to work independently and cooperatively to achieve mutually agreed upon goals.

One of the key people in a safety organization is the first-line supervisor, that is, the foreman. The person in this position provides the most direct interaction of anyone who represents management to the employees. The success of an accident-prevention program depends in large part on the first-line supervisor's understanding of the company's policy and what "the boss" expects to be done about it. Equally important is the supervisor's ability to teach the worker to practice safe work habits and to establish that each employee knows that he or she is responsible for following the prescribed safety and health procedures.

The Safety Committee

OSHA's suggestion that a safety committee can be helpful in detecting unsafe plant conditions and health hazards has resulted in the development of such committees in many industrial establishments. The safety committee can make a valuable contribution to the program of accident prevention. Such a committee is made up of employees who are usually appointed by management to help plan a safety program and to take part in making the program work effectively. Members may be drawn from top management, middle management, and the labor force. Frequently union contracts have clauses that designate joint responsibility for accident prevention, and in those industries the union leader also appoints members to the safety committee. Since all members of the occupational health staff have a part to play in accident prevention, the occupational health nurse is often a member of the committee. The chairman of the safety committee needs to be a person with leadership ability, one who is committed to the safety first concept. The safety committee's activities include:

1. Conducting regularly scheduled meetings at which they deal with:
    a. Suggestions (both negative and positive) made by workers
    b. Accident or injury information so as to identify need for modification of work procedures so as to control recurrences
    c. Safe work practices and rules for working in a safe manner
    d. Personnel protective equipment and recommendations to management concerning those items considered to be most effective
    e. Formulation of policies that outline what personnel protective equipment is required, by whom, and when and where it is to be worn
2. Systematically inspecting the work areas for hazards
3. Conducting studies of employee's working habits and causes of acci-

dents to determine potentially injurious patterns of work in the industry
4. Reviewing audiovisual materials for inclusion in the health and safety training program for the employees
5. Promoting safety training
6. Working cooperatively and in support of the safety and health professionals.

Accident Causes and Their Investigation

Any combination of humans, material, and machines can be involved in an accident, and an accident may cause damage to the machine or the material as well as injury to the worker or another person. Accidents do not always result in injury; but to prevent injuries, accidents must be prevented. Therefore it is wise for the safety personnel to keep a record of the no-injury accidents so that the causes can be eliminated. The causative factors in an accident are an unsafe act or an unsafe physical or mechanical condition or both. To understand an accident one needs to be aware of six factors that contribute to accidents as outlined by the DOL:

1. The agency: the defective object or substance most closely related to the injury and that could have been properly guarded and/or corrected
2. The agency part: the particular part of the agency most closely associated with the injury and that could have been guarded or corrected
3. The unsafe mechanical or physical condition: the condition that could have been guarded or corrected, for example, roughness, sharpness, slipperiness, unsafe storage methods, or poor illumination
4. The accident type: the manner of contact of the injured person with the object or substance or the exposure or movement of the injured person that resulted in injury
5. The unsafe act: the violation of a commonly accepted safe practice that resulted in the accident
6. The unsafe personal factor: the mental or bodily characteristic which permitted or occasioned the unsafe act, such as:
   a. An improper attitude that caused the worker to disregard instructions
   b. Lack of knowledge or skill
   c. Physical impairments such as uncorrected poor eyesight or poor hearing that caused the worker to miss orders or instructions
   d. Lack of knowledge of English, which is needed to understand safety instructions.[9]

Frank C. Bird, Jr., of the International Safety Academy, says that the meaning of the term *accident* has broadened; it is currently interpreted as "an undesired event resulting in personal physical harm, property damage, or business interruption."[10] In this definition, *physical harm* includes both traumatic injury and disease as well as adverse mental, neurological, or systemic effects resulting from work-place exposures.

Hazards are potential sources of harmful contact; consequently a basic component of safety programs is the need to inspect the environment for hazards. In this context the term *hazard* is interpreted as anything that has the potential for causing or contributing to an occupational accident. Bird suggests the following classification system that can be used by the safety committee to rate the hazards found on an inspection:

- *Class A hazard:* A condition or practice with the realistic potential for causing loss of life or body part, permanent health disability, or extensive loss of structure, equipment, or material. *Example:* Barrier guard missing on large press brake used for metal-shearing operation.
- *Class B hazard:* A condition or practice with potential for causing serious injury or illness resulting in temporary disability or property damage that is disruptive but less severe than in a Class A hazard. *Example:* Oil spilled on the floor of a main passageway and not cleaned up so that workers may slip and fall.
- *Class C hazard:* A condition or practice with probable potential for causing nondisability injury or illness or nondisruptive property damage. *Example:* Carpenter not wearing gloves when handling rough lumber.[11]

The supervisor is responsible for the major part of an accident investigation, which should be done as soon as possible following an accident. The purpose of an investigation is not to fix fault or blame but to find out what happened and why in order to take measures to prevent similar accidents in the future. The investigation is, in effect, a study of the accident process; hence it is important that any human factor involved be identified as well as the causative factors. In any accident investigation all of the questions in the well-known list—how, when, what, who, where, and why—must be answered.

Accident Prevention

The tools of a business or industry are workers, machines, and materials. When accidents or injuries happen to any or all of these, the operation of the entire plant is affected. Therefore accident prevention is not something separate or additional to the regular job but is the combination of safe conditions and equipment and safe work procedures interwoven into every phase of the operation. Nurses and others in the occupational health unit know that, when this is not true, workers are injured.

Those who promote the concept that an accident consists of a contact with an energy source propose that accident prevention activities can be directed at the precontact, contact, or postcontact stages. Classifying hazards into the three categories helps put remedial planning in proper perspective, aids in motivating others to take action to correct the more serious conditions, and focuses hazard control attention on the critical areas where removal of hazards requires the greatest concentration of time, effort, and resources.

The Precontact Stage

The most important activity at this stage is inspection to find potential hazards. In his book *Accident Prevention Fundamentals*, M. V. Eninger lists 15 major categories of conditions and items to be considered when making a safety inspection:

1. Atmospheric conditions: dusts, gases, fumes, vapors, illumination
2. Pressurized equipment: boilers, pots, tanks, piping, hosing
3. Containers: all objects for storage of materials such as scrap bins, disposal receptacles, barrels, carboys, gas cylinders, solvent cans
4. Hazardous supplies and materials: flammables, explosives, gases, acids, caustics, toxic chemicals
5. Buildings and structures: windows, doors, floors, stairs, roofs, walls
6. Electrical conductors and apparatus: cables, wires, switches, controls, transformers, lamps, batteries, fuses
7. Engines and prime movers: sources of mechanical power
8. Elevators, escalators, and lifts: cables, controls, safety devices
9. Fire-fighting equipment: extinguishers, hoses, hydrants, sprinkler systems, alarms
10. Machinery and parts thereof: power equipment that processes, machines, or modifies materials, e.g., grinders, forging machines, power presses, drilling machines, shapers, cutters, lathes
11. Material-handling equipment: conveyors, cranes, hoists, lifts
12. Hand tools: such items as bars, sledges, wrenches, and hammers, as well as power tools
13. Structural openings: shafts, pits, floor openings, trenches
14. Transportation equipment: automobiles, trucks, railroad equipment, lift forks
15. Personal protective equipment and clothing: goggles, gloves, aprons, leggings, shoes, hard hats, respirators.[12]

The Contact Stage

The second point at which accidents can be prevented is the contact stage, that is, the point at which the worker comes into actual contact with an accident-causing agent. The safety professional applies the principles of deflection, dilution, reinforcement, surface modifications, segregation, barricading, absorption, and shielding and uses personal protective equipment as the other counter measure at this stage of accident control.

When it is decided that there is a need for workers to wear personal protective equipment, six important considerations deserve special attention:

1. Establishing a policy regarding who must use the equipment and where and when it must be used
2. Informing the workers of the policy and the plans to assure that it is enforced
3. Selecting the proper type of protective device
4. Ensuring that the workers know why they must wear the equipment and how to use the protective devices correctly
5. Ensuring that the equipment is properly fitted
6. Establishing a system for maintaining and sanitizing the equipment.

The Postcontact Stage

The activities associated with the postcontact stage of accident prevention are closely associated with first aid, primary care, and rehabilitation. It is at this point that nurses are most involved. They provide care for injured workers in such a manner as to assure that no further damage is done. For injured workers who can return to work, dressings are applied so as not to create a hazard for them or fellow workers. Seriously injured workers are transported to health care facilities utilizing the best possible medical care modalities. Information about the cause of the injury is collected so as to provide useful data for the safety professional. Nurses capitalize on injured workers' readiness to learn by first finding out what they do not know about how to do the job safely and then filling them in so that they learn from the experience. The postcontact state involves rehabilitation that may require redesigning a job to fit a person's physical handicap, for example following hand injury the machine may be modified so that it can be controlled by foot action, or tools may be selected to fit a person's physical dimensions.

The Nurse's Role

The role of occupational health nurses in accident prevention is five-fold:

1. To participate in the development of a hazard control program geared to the nature and specifics of the work place

2. To participate in the selection, training, and motivation of workers so that they learn how to follow safe work practices and then do so
3. To provide primary care so that workers recover from injury and return to work compatible with their therapeutic care plans
4. To collect and to use data to identify causes and make plans to correct both the situational and the behavioral problems
5. To work cooperatively with the other members of the occupational safety and health team.

Industrial Safety Research

Much of the safety research has looked at three main aspects of safety: hazard recognition, hazard analysis, and hazard control. The first of these, hazard recognition, involves the study of human, task, and environmental variables relative to accident causation. The issue that has challenged the safety professional as well as the safety researcher is how do accidents happen? Many theories have been formulated, the two most popular of which concern behavioral and situational causes. From the behavioral view came the rather well-known but very controversial concept of accident-proneness. This has been disproved, but epidemiologic data show that at any one time a small percentage of the workers have the majority of the accidents. What seems to happen is that the membership in the small percentage of the population that are having the accidents does not stay constant.

Those who have studied the situational model of accident causation include in their studies the human, the machine, and the environment. These researchers have come up with the domino theory; that is, if one of the three elements in accident causation could be changed, then the interaction that could take place would not occur, and the accident would be prevented. Much still remains to be learned about what causes accidents.

References

1. Heinrick, H. W. *Industrial Accident Prevention*. New York: McGraw-Hill, 1941, pp. 376–377.
2. Ibid., p. 368.
3. DOL. *Safety Subjects*. Washington, D.C.: GPO, 1953, p. 24.
4. Ibid., p. 22.
5. Heinrick, op. cit., p. 372.
6. McElroy, F. E. (ed.). *Accident Prevention Manual for Industrial Operations*. Chicago: NSC, 1973, p. 23.
7. P.P.F. Survey No. 17. "Administration of Safety Programs," *Safety Policies &*

Occupational Safety

      The Impact of OSHA. Washington, D.C.: The Bureau of National Affairs, Inc., 1977, pp. 2–6.
8. DOL. *OSHA Handbook for Small Businesses*. Washington, D.C.: GPO, 1977, p. 2.
9. DOL, *Safety Subjects*, op. cit., pp. 44–46.
10. Bird, F. C. "Safety," Chap. 47 in NIOSH, *The Industrial Environment, Its Evaluation and Control*. Washington, D.C.: GPO, 1972, p. 681.
11. Ibid., p. 684.
12. Eninger, M. V. *Accident Prevention Fundamentals*. Industrial Accident Prevention Association (IAPA), Toronto, Ontario, Canada, 1962, pp. 25–34.

Selected Readings

Best's *Safety Directory*. Oldwick, N.J.: A. M. Best, pub. annually.
DOL. *Guidelines for Setting Up Job Safety and Health Programs*, OSHA 2070. Washington, D.C.: GPO, 1972.
Drury, C. (ed.). *Safety in Materials Handling*, NIOSH Pub. No. 78-185. Washington, D.C.: GPO, 1978.
"The Evaluation of America's Industrial Safety Movement," *Occupational Hazards*, Vol. 37, No. 9, Special Bicentennial Issue, Sept. 1975, pp. 51–144.
General Electric. *Materials Safety Data Sheets*. Schenectady, N.Y., 1979.
Gilmore, C. L. *Accident Prevention and Loss Control*. New York: American Management Association, 1970.
Mahmoud, A. "The Problem of Occupational Safety," *Industrial Engineering*, Vol. 7, No. 4. Apr. 1975, pp. 15–23.
Miller, R. "OSHA Compliance Strategies: Decision on Cost-Benefit Analysis," *Occupational Health & Safety 79*, Vol. 48, No. 3, April 1979, pp. 18–22.
Peterson, D. *Techniques of Safety Management*. New York: McGraw-Hill, 1971.
Roland, H. E. "A Fresh Look at System Safety," *Journal of Occupational Medicine*, Vol. 12, No. 3, Mar. 1979, pp. 70–76.
Safety Inspection Manual. Plainview, N.Y.: Man and Manager, 1979.
Scope and Function of the Professional Safety Position. Park Ridge, Ill.: ASSE, 1972.

CHAPTER 5

Occupational Ecology

Ecology is that branch of biology that deals with the relations between organisms and their environment. Occupational ecology deals with the interaction between workers and their work environment. Because of the need to deal constructively with the interaction of the workers and their work environment, occupational health nurses assume duties related to occupational ecology; and as a result the traditional role of the nurse is broadened. Occupational health nurses have a dual level of responsibility: for worker health and for the health and safety of the work environment. They are involved in environmental monitoring, employee education, and epidemiology. The nurses, their employers, and the others on occupation health teams should expect nurses to be concerned about worker health and expert in dealing with health problems. They must also expect nurses to be knowledgeable about the health and safety hazards and to be effective participants in activities that aim to identify and control the hazards of the work environment.

Environmental Monitoring

The interaction between workers and their environment determines the activities associated with environmental monitoring as an essential occupational safety and health activity. These activities are: (a) identifying all factors that have the potential for harm to workers' health and (b) controlling the hazards that arise both from the workers' environment and from the workers' behavior. Environmental monitoring is, in effect, the process of observing, noting, and evaluating for a specific purpose. At times the process of monitoring requires sophisticated means, but at other times very simple means are effective. Occupational health nurses can and should be involved in environmental monitoring. They must be out in the work areas frequently to check the housekeeping, the work practices, the work environment, and the wearing of protective equipment.

Control of toxic or hazardous materials is a job for the expert—the industrial hygienist, the safety professional. This person may recommend a substitution of materials used in a manufacturing process, the redesign or relocation of the work area, the installation of ventilation systems, and/or the selection of personal protective equipment. Once controls are in place, the systems must be checked regularly by the same expert, to assure that they are functioning properly. When the plant employs a full-time industrial hygienist, he or she is responsible for environmental monitoring; when the hygienist is a part-time employee, someone else—perhaps the safety professional or the nurse—is responsible. The nurse should realize that taking on more and more tasks does not necessarily increase his or her contribution to the workers' protection.

Preventive Practice

Prevention as practiced in occupational health is carried out at primary, secondary, and tertiary levels. The activities associated with primary prevention in occupational health programs are designed to promote health and to protect workers from disease agents and/or hazards in their work environment. Secondary prevention activities center on early detection, prompt treatment, and disability limitations. Tertiary prevention in occupational health relates to those activities that contribute to the rehabilitation of injured or ill workers in terms of return to work.

Primary prevention is possible when a known toxic substance is eliminated from the work environment; for example, if a work area is so well-ventilated or the process is enclosed so that workers do not come in contact with the lead in the environment, there is no possibility for them to develop occupational lead poisoning. Providing for the control of such hazards is the true purpose of environmental monitoring. When a health hazard is found, then every effort must be expended to control it and to see that workers are not imperiled.

Work Area Surveillance

To become familiar with the work environment and to see the workers at work, occupational health nurses must leave the health unit occasionally and go out into the work area. How frequently they do this will vary with the size and type of industry, the sophistication of the supervisors, and the magnitude of the health hazards. They can be helpful to both employees and management if they are out in the work area often enough to spot problems. They report any problem to the management, the industrial hygienist, and/or the safety professional. The final responsibility for providing a safe and healthful work environment rests with management.

Nurses must be aware of and look for possible relationships between the work environment and the workers' health problems. When they have a high index of suspicion, they can be most valuable co-workers of managers and industrial hygienists or safety professionals as well as of the physicians with whom they work. Expert occupational health nurses are knowledgeable about the properties of substances used in production and their potential for harm. They are able to spot the possible relationship between workers' ill health and the stresses of their jobs. They alert first-line supervisors and safety professionals if they have reason to believe that there may be a health hazard in the environment.

Health Hazard Clues

When out in the work area, nurses can use the following signals to determine when an expert is needed to determine the presence of a health hazard:

1. An irritation of the eyes
2. An unusual odor
3. A dust cloud coming from an operation into the work area
4. A ventilating system not functioning
5. A fume or mist being produced by a process.

Other indicators that there is need for an industrial hygiene survey include:

1. The need to raise one's voice to be heard, which should arouse the suspicion that the environment is too noisy
2. Mishandling or careless handling of chemicals, for example spills not cleaned up immediately or chemicals kept in open containers or containers without labels
3. Workers not included in a medical surveillance program when hazardous materials such as lead, asbestos, or one of the carcinogens are used in the establishment
4. The development of signs and symptoms of illness in workers from a department where toxic substances are used
5. Workers asking questions and giving other indications of concern as to the hazards associated with their work.

Any or all of these signals and indicators point to the need for an industrial hygiene survey to determine how great the hazard is and what control measures if any should be taken.

Environmental Sanitation

In 1949 the World Health Organization (WHO) Expert Committee on Environmental Sanitation defined *environmental sanitation* as the control of all those factors in man's physical environment which exercise or may exercise a deleterious effect on physical development, health, and survival.[1] Involved are:

- Adequate and safe methods for the disposal of excreta, sewage, and community wastes
- Water supplies that are pure and wholesome
- Housing that is of a character likely to provide as few opportunities as possible for the direct transmission of disease, especially respiratory infections, and to encourage beneficial social habits in the occupants
- Milk and other food supplies that are safe
- Methods for the control of arthropod, rodent, mollusk, or other intermediate hosts of human diseases.

One of the functions of government is to protect the health of the citizens. The principal governmental health agency at the national level is the Public Health Service (PHS) within the U.S. Department of Health and Human Services (DHHS). Each state in turn has a health department, as do most local governmental units. The health department prepares the sanitary code for the state or city. The regulations written into this code have the effect of law, and the code is enforceable by all official health agencies. Other codes empower various official agencies and departments to carry on activities that affect the sanitation of the environment. Local and state agencies may enact codes and pass laws that are more demanding but not less so than a federal law.

The safe handling of food in an in-plant food service requires adequate refrigeration, food storage facilities, and safe dishwashing methods. Any city ordinance in effect for restaurants must be observed since these apply to both in-plant food service and automatic vending machines. Employees who handle food must meet the local requirements for food handlers and for health certification when this is required by law.

The Nurse's Role

Occupational health nurses are not professional sanitarians any more than they are industrial hygienists or safety professionals. As members of a health team, however, they have many opportunities, and hence responsibilities, to identify and meet needs and to be involved in activities associated with the sanitation of the work environment.

On the occasions when a sanitarian is employed by an industry (this rarely happens except in the food or food service industries), it is the nurses' responsibility to call to the sanitarian's attention, or to the attention of management, problems they see or that others have reported to them.

Nurses carry on those activities within their professional preparation; for example they can supervise the sanitation of the food service, the locker rooms, and the rest rooms. As the professionals of choice to educate the workers in the value of sanitation, nurses participate in on-the-job training of nonprofessional personnel responsible for certain aspects of plant sanitation and for the handling of food and eating utensils.

Occupational health nurses must be alert to the possible cause-and-effect relationship between environmental sanitation and the health problems presented by workers. They make investigations and report any suspected condition so that it can be investigated because only in this way is it possible to break the chain of cause and effect. In this aspect of their work nurses act as catalysts; that is, they help start programs and help keep them functioning at top efficiency.

Nurses communicate their interest in and understanding of what the workers are doing, and they use the prestige of their position to reinforce the safety directives and educational efforts of the supervisor and safety personnel. If nurses are not involved to some degree in the safety programs, the relationship is less than ideal. The working relationship between occupational health nurses and safety department personnel centers on control of lost time and injuries. This should be a collaborative effort with nurses being responsible for the care of injured or ill workers and safety professionals being responsible for accident prevention. Together they plan for and do health and safety education.

The occupational health nurse periodically performs a walk-through, sometimes with members of the safety and health committee and/or with other members of the occupational safety and health team, and at other times alone. Good housekeeping in industry, as in home or hospital, is a continuous operation and is achieved only when someone is concerned and tries to get others to follow good practices. This involves keeping things in working order; walls and windows clean and dust free; work benches, aisles, stairs, and stairways uncluttered. OSHA regulations and local fire laws require that exits be unblocked. The OSHA Standard 1910.141 covers the requirements for lavatories, personal service rooms, potable water, toilet facilities, and washing facilities. Part 3 Housekeeping states: "All places of employment shall be kept clean to the extent that the nature of the work allows. The floor of every workroom shall be maintained, so far as practicable, in a dry condition. Where wet processes are used, drainage shall be maintained and false floors, platforms, mats, or other dry standing places shall be provided where practicable, or appropriate waterproof foot gear shall be provided."

Nurses become aware of the personal hygiene practices among the workers. They check the sanitary facilities since good personal hygiene is possible only when adequate facilities are provided and workers know how to use them. Such facilities should include running water, soap, and towels. The workers' clothing also needs to be checked, especially when the operation involves toxic substances that may be carcinogenic or that are very dirty or oily. Workers on these kinds of jobs need protective clothing, and their work clothes must be changed frequently.

Good personal hygiene depends on individual understanding of the need for it and acceptance of responsibility for practicing it. Explaining the principles of personal hygiene and teaching workers how to carry them out is a nursing activity. Nurses will need to give special attention to workers whose home conditions make it difficult to carry out hygienic practices. The importance of workers' not going home in contaminated work clothes must be considered when company policies are developed to deal with the provision of work clothes, changing rooms, and the laundry of clothes worn at work, especially when the work involves exposure to asbestos or any of the chemicals known to cause cancer. This information should be incorporated into the health education program and work orientation sessions for new employees.

Employee Education

This subject (dealt with more fully in Chap. 17) is included here to point up the relationship between the four sets of correlative activities. Employee education is an activity for which nurses can and do have responsibility and which requires that they work in cooperation with others to assure that workers understand the potential for harm that may exist in their work environment and what they must do to protect their health. When exposures cannot be controlled by primary prevention activities or when it is not possible to correct the situation that causes the exposure immediately, or when spills or other emergencies arise, the use of personal protective equipment is mandated. It is essential that workers be instructed in the care and use of the appropriate equipment. They must know where these are stored and be able to get to them when there is need to wear the protective equipment.

The worker's right to know is fundamental to the success of an occupational safety and health program. One aspect of this is helping workers understand the meaning of health. In an article in the issue of *Daedalus* entitled "Doing Better and Feeling Worse: Health in the United States," M. K. Du Val said,

Not long ago, when the World Health Organization attempted to define health, it could do so only in negative terms—that is, it spoke in terms of the absence of physical or mental disease. In my opinion, it is preferable to consider health in positive terms, that is, to define it as a state that permits one to achieve an acceptable accommodation to one's environment and circumstances and to be able fully to join with others in being productive and useful members of society.

When defined in these terms, health is only marginally affected by medical care; indeed, much of contemporary, scientific medicine is almost irrelevant to good health. . . . In the final analysis however, the individual's behavior, his environment, and his living habits have a far greater impact on his health than anything medicine might do for him.[2]

This definition of health requires that occupational health nurses be involved in helping individuals know what is a safe and healthful environment and what are good health practices, and to accept these so as to be able to join with others in being productive and useful members of society.

The impact of the Occupational Safety and Health Act of 1970 and the importance of worker education can be seen in the testimony of Eula Bingham, Assistant Secretary of Labor, at the Manpower and Housing Subcommittee of the Committee on Government Operations: "OSHA has been urged to issue regulations which insure that employees are informed of their exposure to potentially toxic materials. The last two health standards issued by the agency—covering vinyl chloride and coke oven emissions—contain such provisions, as will all future health standards. . . . Clearly, informing employees of the hazards to which they are exposed is an important element in reducing occupational disease and injury and one of the significant purposes of the Act."[3]

Consultation

A consultant is one who gives professional advice or service regarding matters in the field of his or her special knowledge and training. Nurses who work in establishments that do not employ an industrial hygienist will have to consult with the person who provides administrative direction for the health unit. They may do so as to the value of an industrial hygiene survey. For example they may suggest that management consider asking NIOSH to conduct a health hazard evaluation (see page 306 for information about how to request a health hazard evaluation). They may point out that the workmen's compensation insurance company can be requested to send in their industrial hygienist to do a survey. The information nurses provide may help management to decide to engage an industrial hygienist who is a private consultant to identify a suspected hazard and to make suggestions for its control.

When nurses are asked to consult it is essential that they have the necessary information available for the management person to make an informed decision, that is, who can do an environmental survey, where such services are available, and what procedures must be followed to request or to buy the services. In others words nurses need to do the staff work so that they have the information necessary for the decision-making process.

The difference between employee education and consulting on health and safety matters with management, workers, and representatives of the community is one of degree as to the depth of understanding required to do it well. To consult means to seek information, to talk things over. When nurses are in the role of the consultant they are giving professional and technical advice that some one else will use. For example a nurse may be asked for information that she has or can get that the other person needs and will use in carrying out the job responsibilities. This is a consultative function that occupational health nurses must be able to perform.

Increasingly, when changes in processes are being undertaken, management wants to know what hazards if any are associated with the substances to be used. Management wants to know whether there are any recommended exposure limits and where they can find some one to indicate whether the new process will create a hazard to worker health. Knowing where and how to get such information as a staff person is a skill occupational health nurses need to acquire. The old saying, "It is not always what you know but whom you know," applies. For example a telephone call or a letter to the industrial hygienist at one of the educational resources centers established by NIOSH or to the Regional Industrial Hygienist in the DHHS that serves the state in which the industry is located (see App. C for addresses of these sources of help) will get some useful answers. The State Occupational Safety and Health Consultation Service, usually a department of the State Department of Labor and Industries, is another source, as is the insurance company from whom the workers' compensation insurance is purchased.

In 1977 NIOSH published *Guidelines on Pregnancy and Work*. This pamphlet has had a wide distribution. The guidelines were developed (under contract from NIOSH) by the American College of Obstetricians and Gynecologists (ACOG) as a means of helping obstetricians and their patients who are also workers decide if it is safe for them to continue to work. The report contains a schematic format designed to help practicing obstetricians assemble and interpret the information necessary to make appropriate clinical recommendations to pregnant workers. Such information includes what chemicals women work with and the toxicity of the substances they may be exposed to. It can be anticipated that more and more physicians will call the industry for consultation. Depending on the size and complexity of the health unit staff, nurses could be the people who answer these requests for information.

When questions about the hazards of the work area come to nurses from persons outside the industry, it is wise for the nurses to keep a record of the questions and their answers. They should also bring these to the attention of management and the physician. It would be wise for the nurses not to give quick answers; it is also essential when questions are asked that nurses not assume they know what the person is asking. Nurses in turn must ask questions, for example, "Why do you want to have this information?" "Are you ill?" "What are the symptoms?" It is useful to summarize the conversation, saying, for example, "Am I correct in my understanding that Mrs. R. Smith has asked you for advice and you need to know what substances she works with that may be toxic, and what effects if any these substances may have on her health? I don't have this information on hand, but I will get it for you and call you if you will give me your telephone number and tell me when I can call you tomorrow." Few requests for consultation are emergencies. The person being asked to consult is considered to be an expert and/or one who has a channel to expert information; hence the need to be sure that the information used to answer such requests is as correct and complete as possible.

Epidemiology

Epidemiology is the branch of medicine concerned with the cause and control of epidemics. Techniques found to be useful in contagious disease identification and control are equally useful for identification and control of occupational disesases and industrial injuries. Knowledge of the cause and the dynamics of the disease process is required for determining the importance of various factors, such as the host, agent, and environmental conditions, and for estimating the effectiveness of the control procedures. Historically such background has been assembled from three principal sources:

1. The detailed clinical records of each syndrome as it occurs in individuals presenting with apparent reactions
2. The study of the causative agent, whatever it may be—a living organism or its products, a toxic material, or a physical agent such as noise or heat
3. The utilization of observations and analyses of specific conditions associated with the occurrence of the disease and the presence of the alleged causative agent

Scrupulousness and accuracy are imperative when nurses record their observations, including information they gather about the injury or the illness, the environment in which the person works, the health care provided, and the worker's response to it. Such occupational health reports provide the basis for determining what needs to be done and what has been done, not only by the nurse but by others on the team.

The epidemiologic researcher trying to establish cause and effect looks for those factors that appear to be common. The importance of an epidemiologic approach to the use of occupational health records means that those who record information must understand how the information may be used. The need is to be consistent and if certain information is not available to indicate this, so that in the future, there will not be the question, Was it or was it not available? Such care is essential if the data are to have usefulness for research. Occupational health nurses record both the information they have gathered as the basis for giving nursing care and the information they gather as they give care. They use both to evaluate the care they give. All should be in the worker's individual health record.

Epidemiologists are primarily concerned with groups of persons, not separate individuals. They deal with the so-called web of causation, which includes all of the predisposing factors of any type and their complex relations with each other and with the disease or injury under investigation. Epidemiologists consider the many factors that can cause disease: the agent, the host, and the environment.

In epidemiologic studies of workers, such factors as exposure to what, extent of exposure, and smoking, are considered. In one study smoking histories were obtained from 11,657 of a cohort of 17,800 insulation workers. Of 9,591 workers with a history of cigarette smoking, 248 died of lung cancer as compared with 59.5 expected deaths. Among 609 workers who had smoked pipes and/or cigars, 2 lung cancer deaths were observed and 1.24 were expected. Of 1,457 workers who never smoked regularly, 4 lung cancer deaths were observed, while 1.08 were expected. Expected deaths were based on approximate smoking-specific U.S. death rates.[4]

Further analyses of group data have been performed to examine how cigarette smoking and asbestos might be acting together. On a statistical basis it appears that these two independent causes of lung cancer interact positively. In the general population cigarette smokers have a 10- to 15-fold excess risk of developing lung cancer. One study observed an 8-fold excess of lung cancer among smoking asbestos workers as compared with smokers in the general population, but the excess was 92-fold when compared to the general population of nonsmokers.[5] This suggests that the combined effect of smoking and asbestos exposure is greater than the simple sum of their separate effects. The relation of this statistical interaction to the pathogenesis of lung cancer is uncertain. However it seems clear that, because of the important enhancement of risk by one cause complementing the other, the increased risk of lung cancer in groups exposed to asbestos may be primarily concentrated among those who also smoke.[6]

Epidemiologic methods used to study groups of workers are:

1. Descriptive studies that involve the determination of the incidence, prevalence, and mortality rates for diseases in large population groups

according to basic group characteristics such as age, sex, race, and geographic area
2. Cross-sectional studies that examine the relationships between disease and other characteristics or variables of interest as they exist in a defined population at one particular time
3. Incidence or cohort studies that look more directly at attributes or factors related to the development of disease.[7]

Data recorded by the occupational health professionals about the workers' health and injury problems permits the calculation of:

1. Prevalence rate: the number of persons with a disease divided by the total number in the group
2. Incidence rate: the number of persons developing the disease divided by the total number of people at risk times the unit of time. Incidence describes the rate of development of a disease in a group over a period of time.[8]

The Nurse's Contribution to Occupational Ecology

The contribution of nurses to occupational ecology is evidenced by:

1. The kind and amount of data they record in workers' individual health records concerning the causes of the injury or illness. For example does a nurse record whether a worker was wearing personal protective equipment and what substance(s) the worker was working with and when the first sign or symptom developed?
2. The number of referrals they make to the safety professional, the industrial hygienist, and/or management that result in changes in work practices or in special environmental studies to determine the amount of the toxic substance in the work environment.
3. The amount of time nurses spend in the work area making inspections, either alone or with the safety and health personnel, checking housekeeping and sanitation, and gathering data about work practices and the environment to help in solving health problems.
4. The ease, knowledge, and ability with which they respond to questions from management, workers, and others concerning the OSHA Standards and the hazards of production associated with the establishment.
5. How well the safety professionals and the industrial hygienists of the industry and of the workmen's compensation insurance company know the nurses and how often they discuss problems with them.

Participation in the many and varied activities that are basic to environmental monitoring gives occupational health nursing its speciality classification. The expert occupational health nurse understands the concept of occupational ecology, is able to identify the special contributions of the industrial hygienist and safety professional, and works cooperatively with them as well as independently as the nurse member of the occupational health team.

References

1. WHO. *Environmental Sanitation*, Technical Rep. No. 10. Geneva, 1950.
2. Du Val, M. K. "The Provider, the Government, and the Consumer," *Daedalus*, Vol. 106, No. 1, Winter 1977, p. 185.
3. Egdahl, R. H., and Walsh, D. C. (Eds.). *Health Services and Health Hazards: The Employee's Need to Know*. New York: Springer-Verlag, 1978, p. 5.
4. Selikoff, I. J. "Cancer Risk of Asbestos Exposure," in *Origins of Human Cancer*. New York: Cold Spring Harbor Laboratory, 1977, pp. 1765–1784.
5. Selikoff, I. J., Hammond, E. C., and Churg, J. "Asbestos Exposure, Smoking and Neoplasia," *Journal of the American Medical Association*, Vol. 204, 1968, pp. 106–112.
6. Levine, R. J. (Ed.). *Asbestos: An Information Resource*, National Cancer Institute. Washington, D.C.: GPO, 1978, p. 33.
7. Friedman, G. D. *Primer of Epidemiology*. New York: McGraw-Hill, 1974, p. 1.
8. MacMahon, B., and Pugh, T. F. *Epidemiology, Principles and Methods*. Boston: Little, Brown, 1970.

PART III

Health Surveillance

Part III of this book deals with the role of occupational health nurses in the assessment of workers' health and in those health promotional activities that aim to maintain and to improve the workers' health. The second of the four sets of correlative activities that are the parameters of a comprehensive occupational safety and health program for workers is:

HEALTH SURVEILLANCE

Physical assessment of workers to determine the workers' state of health and to identify as early as possible any potential health problems

Health promotion initiatives to maintain and to improve the workers' health

The nurse as a member of the occupational safety and health team:

- Participates in the health surveillance program that includes the assessment and recording of the health status of persons at time of job placement and at specific times thereafter
- Participates in planning, conducting, and evaluating the many activities that contribute to the maintenance of the health of the workers.

CHAPTER 6

Health Assessment

A health assessment is a systematic evaluation of a person's state of health or ill health. To be most effective, an industrial health assessment program must be flexible. It should provide sufficient options so that the person performing the assessment can select the procedures necessary to assemble the information for making decisions in regard to job placement, job transfer, and health maintenance. Job descriptions, job requirements, and legal implications, as well as the worker's age and sex, are all factors that influence decisions made by the personnel in charge of the department responsible for health maintenance among workers in an industrial plant, and by personnel responsible for employment policies and placement.

The health and/or physical assessments that are made as a part of an occupational health program are given various designations. The AMA's publication *Guiding Principles of Medical Examinations in Industry* suggests original, periodic, and special evaluations. The OSHA Standards identify preplacement and periodic evaluations. For many years workers were of the opinion that the purpose of these evaluations was to assure the selection of the physically perfect and the rejection of all others. In some industries this may have been true, but the experience of occupational health personnel and the management of the companies providing the examination agree that "proper placement of workers with due regard for the variations in physical demands required by different jobs, and for the safety and health limitations involved in disabilities, can result in improved job performance, less absenteeism, decreased likelihood of injury, less hazards to the health and safety of others, lessened chance of aggravation of disorders, and, doubtless, a longer productive life span."[1] Examinations for the purpose of assisting in job placement are, therefore, practical individualized applications of the principles of preventive medicine.

There is great value in having stated company policies concerning health assessments that are jointly developed and promoted by management, the union, and the health personnel. These statements should be concerned with the requirement of a health assessment as one of the procedures in the job placement process. A second policy statement listing what periods of absence from work and what health problems require that a person have a health assessment by the occupational health unit staff before returning to work is also of value. Policies concerning periodic and health surveillance examinations are the basis for scheduling an assessment, and the recommendations of the occupational health personnel provide management and workers the information needed for protection of the workers' health.

Legal Aspects

The Civil Rights Act of 1964, the Equal Employment Opportunity Act of 1972, and the Rehabilitation Act of 1973 all influence placement and employment policies. The regulation published in the May 4, 1977, *Federal Register*, effective as of June 3, 1977, is officially known as the rule on nondiscrimination for "handicaps" in programs and activities receiving or benefiting from federal financial assistance. This is the United States policy and the national commitment to end discrimination on the basis of handicap. In many establishments the employment policy is that the only health reasons for not accepting a person for employment are a communicable disease, an incapacitating injury or disease, or mental illness.

The federal Fair Employment Practice Act (FEPA) and the Equal Employment Opportunity Commission (EEOC) may challenge the employers concerning their preplacement examinations to demonstrate that the factor tested for is necessary for adequate performance and that the test used is a reliable determinant of that factor. To require that every applicant for employment have the physical qualifications of an athlete rules out a valuable portion of the employable population. Only a few physical abilities are needed to do any given job. It is not necessary to have a person who has the all-around physical qualifications for membership on an Olympic team to perform a job which basically requries normal vision and the use of one good hand. Actually almost everyone is physically substandard in some detail. The term *handicapped* is one of degree. It should be specifically related to static or dynamic defects when used to discuss employability.

Static defects are physical impairments which have reached an end point and are not progressive and will not of themselves grow worse. An amputated hand or muscles of a leg atrophied by poliomyelitis are examples of this type of defect. Persons with such defects are employable when appropriate placement guidelines are used. Many industries employ people with static defects. The productive output of these workers, their absence record, their injury frequency and severity rates, and their labor turnover are as good as or better than the corresponding data for unimpaired workers, provided they are assigned to work for which they are fit. Dynamic defects are those which are progressive and changing. Active tuberculosis or myocardial damage with cardiac decompensation is a dynamic condition. Persons with dynamic defects are usually not employable.

Kinds of Health Assessments

Preplacement Assessments

Original or preplacement evaluations are made for the purpose of determining and recording the physical condition of prospective workers and assigning them to suitable jobs in which their disabilities if any will not affect their personal efficiency, safety, or health, or the safety of others. The aim is to match the worker to the job and the job to the worker. This assessment is made by a physician or nurse to establish the health status of the individual, to assure the compatibility of the person with the physical demands of the specific job applied for, and to put on record base-line health data including a risk factor profile for use in subsequent evaluations.

The person doing the assessment should know the physical requirements of the job, so job descriptions that include physical fitness requirements are essential for the assessment process. These descriptions are usually developed by the safety professional or personnel department representatives. When there is an occupational health team, the physician as well as the industrial hygienist, may be involved. Occupational health nurses who have had specialized education including ergonomics sometimes work with the team to devleop the job requirement statements. Basic principles of ergonomics must be understood by those who develop job requirements. Human factors engineering concepts must be applied to the design of tools and job layouts and be taken into consideration when jobs are studied as the basis for establishing safe and healthful work practices as well as for job placement human factor requirements.

Research into behavioral, psychological, and motivational factors that have been undertaken as a result of the Occupational Safety and Health Act promise new approaches and better understanding of adverse behavioral and neurological functioning and the changes that can occur from exposure to chemical and physical agents. In the future the new insights from such research will be helpful in assessing risk factors, and the test batteries used in the research may prove to be of use in testing worker response to perceptual, psychomotor, and cognitive tasks.

Job placement depends upon knowledge of the demands that the job will make on the worker and the physiological attributes that the worker brings to the job. Tasks are defined, but the physiological expenditures required are just beginning to be studied by occupational physiologists. Time and motion studies do not give the total picture, and more study is required before we truly understand the physiological work cycle.

The preplacement assessment includes:

1. A detailed personal and family health history, including reproductive history for both men and women, and a smoking history

2. A detailed work history, including length of employment in each job, nature and duration of exposures to hazardous conditions, and experience with wearing protective equipment
3. A physical examination
4. Laboratory studies of urine and blood and, occasionally, tissue
5. X-ray examination of the chest and, occasionally, the back
6. Hearing and vision tests and functional lung and neurological tests.

The laboratory, X-ray, and functional tests should be selectively performed to provide the data needed for job placement and for medical surveillance of workers whose jobs involve occupationally related risk factors.

Any physical defect or abnormality discovered at this assessment should be discussed with the applicant or employee. If the condition would interfere with proper performance of the job or might jeopardize the health or safety of fellow employees, the applicant or employee should not be asssigned to the position until the condition has been corrected. If correction is not possible the applicant may be assigned to another position where the condition would not interfere with proper job performance. However a condition which threatens the health of others, such as tuberculosis, may be a barrier to any employment until corrected.

Progressive conditions (for example diabetes or cerebral arteriosclerosis) create placement problems. Applicants with such conditions can be employed for appropriate jobs, but the health service personnel should consider the prognosis and recommend assignments only to positions in which there is a good chance that the health problem will not interfere with performance and that the worker's condition will not be aggravated. This is an individual problem and requires that health professionals recognize that the decision to employ or to assign to a specific position is not theirs alone, for in the placement procedure the health status of the individual is only one of several factors to be considered.

Periodic Assessments

Periodic health assessments are done at intervals during a person's employment to determine whether any adverse health effects have occurred as a result of environmental conditions and if so what corrective measures should be taken. They may be done on a voluntary or required basis. Mandatory evaluations are those provided for workers exposed to processes or materials that are definite health hazards, especially workers whose job activities cause them to be responsible for the safety of others, for example truck drivers or crane operators. The periodic evaluation has as its purpose the early detection of the hypersusceptible person. The voluntary and periodic assessment has as its purpose the finding of chronic illness problems at a time when a person is free of symptoms. Special examinations are many and have various purposes, including determining ability to return to work following illness, fitness for duty, executive health, and preretirement or termination-of-employment assessments.

Fitness-for-Work Assessments

The health assessment that may be performed most often is that done at the time a person returns to work following illness or injury. The purpose of this assessment and/or the health interview is to reassess the fitness of the person and his or her compatibility with the demands of the job. The so-called fitness-for-work or duty assessments are requested by management. Usually such an evaluation is scheduled for workers with emotional problems that seriously interfere with their ability to work or for those on extended leave that do not follow their physician's medical orders.

Health professionals find these evaluations a frustrating experience because the person does not want to have the assessment performed and the occupational health unit physician may come to a different conclusion than the worker's own physician. All too often the person's private physician has little or no understanding of the person's job, and most workers are not good at explaining the energy demands of their work—hence the issuance of the return-to-light-work slips that employees present, most of which are not indicated and many of which cannot be honored as no light work is available. On the other hand, if a worker has an illness that is progressive in nature, the data from an occupational health physical examination and knowledge of the requirement of the job may prevent this worker from being put under too great stress or being kept away from work unnecessarily. The evaluator's recommendation may be termination of employment, including early retirement or disability retirement.

Examinations for Executives

Executives' health examination programs reflect industry's investment in its top-level personnel and its willingness to provide special health programs for them. Executives may elect to go to their own physician or to a special clinic for a complete health assessment. Many industries include executive health assessments as an integral part of their occupational health service. These evaluations are performed by the occupational health physician and the nurse. If a patient's history indicates the existence of a condition that needs to be diagnosed, the X-ray examination may include more than the usual evaluation—a GI series, for example, or a gallbladder X ray.

Increasingly, special exercise programs are being offered at work for management personnel. Aimed primarily at the prevention of cardiovascular diseases, these programs are for those who are overweight, have elevated cholesterol and triglyceride levels, take little or no exercise, and have stressful jobs. Top-line staff with elevated blood pressure are offered the opportunity to enroll and to exercise during the work day.

Those who enter the exercise programs, which are usually supervised by exercise physiologists, are given special medical examinations and are monitored during their exercise routines. The programs are carried on in a specially designed exercise room that is near to the occupational health unit. The facilities include a locker room with shower, sauna, and toilet. The program is planned around different exercise stations: rowing, treadmill, medicine ball, and so on. Each individual has a personal exercise card on which to record resting pulse rate before starting each session and again after completing the station. This introduction to a physical fitness program is included here to explain the need for a complete physical examination before a person begins such an exercise routine. It is recommended that this examination include an electrocardiogram, preferably an exercise electrocardiogram performed when the person is at or near the level to be reached in the program.

The use of community resources for an exercise program for workers is possible. Arrangements can be made with the YMCA or with some other place in the community where there are exercise facilities, someone to supervise them, and a pool. Some smaller industries have established policies that include costs and who pays, who can be enrolled, and the time schedule for the exercise sessions. A hospital in a southern state has a cooperative program with the local Y, with half of the cost being paid by the hospital and half by the worker involved. Sessions are scheduled three times a week, and the workers attend on their own time. The coordinator of the program is the occupational health nurse. Before workers are assigned to the program they have a stress electrocardiogram done.

Final Assessments

Retirement and termination-of-employment health evaluations are of special importance for workers who have had work-connected exposure to toxic substances and/or physical hazards. These assessments should put on record the levels of health and disease, as well as hearing and pulmonary functioning data, so these can be assessed against levels at the time of employment and/or thereafter. The long-delayed incidence of cancer after exposure makes termination-of-employment examinations of special importance to the person, to management, and to researchers trying to establish the cause and effect of low-level occupational exposures to toxic substances. In addition the OSHA Standards require such evaluations as well as the retention of health assessment records for specified periods of time, some for as long as 30 years.

Health Surveillance for Well Adults

In an article in the March 17, 1977, issue of the *New England Journal of Medicine,* Lester Breslow and Anne R. Somers outlined a lifetime monitoring program that is regarded as a reasonable and practical way of maintaining good health in well adults.[2] These authors recommend:

1. For persons aged 18–24, one examination during these years. This examination is likely to be done by the health personnel in an occupational health program, that is, by the physician and the nurse, as the person's preplacement health assessment, which is a condition of employment.

2. For persons aged 25–39, two examinations, one at age 30 and another at age 35. In addition to a complete physical examination the authors suggest that tests, as appropriate, be done for high blood pressure, anemia, and cholesterol level and for cervical and breast cancer. They suggest that the person be informed about why it is important to do self-examination of breasts, skin, testes, neck, and mouth for signs of tumors or tissue change and that the person be taught how to perform them. Counseling concerning nutrition, excessive smoking, and alcoholic intake and about marital, parental, and work stresses at this time is also suggested when indicated.

3. For persons aged 40–59, an examination every 5 years. The recommendation here is for activities to detect chronic disease. At age 50 the person should begin having blood pressure and weight taken annually. Counseling about changing nutritional needs and menopausal problems is indicated as a form of anticipatory guidance.

4. For persons aged 60–74, an examination every 2 years. People in this group should have a complete physical examination with special attention to such chronic conditions as high blood pressure, cancer, glaucoma, diabetes, and poor circulation in the lower extremities. Counseling concerning life-style changes and retirement may be needed. The administration of flu shots is suggested as an additional important activity that can be carried on at the same time.

This time schedule and the compositions of the physical examinations are suggested for well adults whose work environment is such as not to require them to be in an occupational health surveillance program. It is also pointed out that if people become ill, then of necessity their own physician does a physical examination.

The health monitoring program outlined by Breslow and Somers is designed not so much to find disease as to prevent it. Hence much emphasis is given to history taking and to teaching the persons. The need for the persons to understand and carry out the instructions of the health professional makes it imperative that nurse and physician communicate their recommendations in terms meaningful to the persons so they will comply.

Screening

A screening assessment is done to detect chronic illness at a time when a person is free of frank evidence of illness and to involve the worker in health maintenance activities. "The object of screening for disease is to discover those among the apparently well who are in fact suffering from disease."[3]

Screening was defined by the Commission on Chronic Illness in 1951 as the presumptive identification of unrecognized disease or defect by the application of tests, examination, or other procedures which can be applied rapidly. Screening tests sort out apparently well persons who probably have a disease from those who probably do not. A screening test is not intended to be diagnostic. Persons with positive or suspicious findings must be referred to a physician for diagnosis and necessary treatment.[4]

Screening is used profitably for early detection of occupational diseases. For example periodic examinations of urine and/or blood can be scheduled when results are significantly different from base-line data: elevated blood leads and proteinuria, decrease in red blood cell counts, and changes in forced vital capacity.

Screening is generally carried on today to determine the presence of the following conditions: (a) pulmonary tuberculosis; (b) visual defects; (c) chronic glaucoma; (d) hearing loss; (e) venereal disease; (f) diabetes; (g) cancer of skin, mouth, breast, cervix, or rectum; (h) hypertension; or (i) anemia, principally sickle cell anemia. Screening procedures are also utilized during health assessments conducted by occupational health professionals to establish the levels of vision, hearing, and respiratory functions of individual workers. The level of functioning at the time of preplacement evaluation furnishes the base-line data against which subsequent evaluation results are compared to identify workers showing evidence of functional change. The procedures utilized are, by their nature, screening only. When the results give evidence of less than optimal functioning, it is necessary to determine why this is so and what additional procedures should be carried out to establish the validity of the screening test results and/or to make a definitive diagnosis.

Three types of screening are done: (a) mass screening, large scale screening of whole population groups; (b) selective screening, the screening of selected high-risk groups in the population; and (c) multiphasic screening, the application of two or more screening tests in combination to large groups of people.

Health Assessment

Multiphasic Screening

Early in the 1960s automated electronic testing systems were developed. These tested, recorded, and in some systems analyzed the data from individuals against a set of norms. These testing systems were first used in hospitals and community health facilities. Some of the larger occupational health units added these capabilities to their own laboratories. Many more occupational health services collect samples and send them to commercial laboratories for analysis. Increasingly, as OSHA Standards describe medical surveillance, there will be need to do tests for a variety of reasons. Hence multiphasic testing will be used by more and more by occupational health services. In a special article "Organization and Operation of Occupational Health Programs," Henry Howe discusses the options in equipment and in in-house capabilities versus commercial laboratories for the analysis.[5]

Screening for Vision

There is more to occupational visual testing programs than having workers read from a wall chart. Reading the wall chart tests only central distance vision and not always too accurately. There are many binocular screening devices on the market including: Telebinocular, made by Keystone View Company; the Ortho-Rater of the Bausch and Lomb Optical Company; the Sight-Screener of the American Optical Company; and the Titmus Vision Tester of the Titmus Optical Company, Inc. The National Society for the Prevention of Blindness (NSPB) has published *Eyes in Industry: Guide to Better Industrial Vision Testing*, which is of special value to those who are planning or evaluating such a program. For color discrimination the pseudoisochromatic plates are the most accurate. These are available in book form, and some of the stereoscopic instruments have color-testing capabilities.

The five visual skills usually screened are for:

1. Distance vision without glasses. Test first without glasses, if they are worn, and then with glasses.
2. Near vision without, then with, glasses.
3. Muscle balance, near and far.
4. Stereopsis.
5. Color discrimination.[6]

The visual requirement of the various jobs can and should be stated in terms of these basic visual skills. This information should be included in the job description for which a person is being examined and should be available to the person doing the screening examination. In addition to the testing for the five visual skills during the physical examination, the eyes are examined with an opthalmoscope, and the tension of the eye is measured by the tonometer.

Screening for Hearing

Audiometric testing is a method of measuring a person's hearing ability. An audiogram is obtained by presenting pure tones at variable levels of intensity until each tone is barely heard. The audiogram is made with the person in a test room or booth where the noise level does not exceed 50 decibels. In addition to the audiogram the ear drum and the external ear are examined and the condition recorded in the worker's health file, as are the results of the audiogram. The audiogram should be made at a time when the person has not been exposed to noise for at least 12 hours.

The accuracy of the audiometer should be checked at least weekly, and some experts recommend daily testing. The date, the test audiogram, and the name of the tester, should be recorded and maintained as part of the occupational health unit's administrative record system. The person who performs the audiogram should hold a current certified audiometric technician certificate or a credential of at least equal significance. When the number of audiometric examinations to be done is small, it is recommended that they be performed at a local hearing or speech center rather than at either the industrial establishment or a physician's office without the necessary testing booth.

Screening for Ventilatory Capacity

The assessment of ventilatory capacity is especially important for workers who may be exposed to substances hazardous to respiratory health. This assessment consists of three major parts. The first is a medical and occupational history. The occupational history is of little value unless it contains specific information. It is essential that the person taking the history obtain answers to the following questions:

1. What job did the person have before the present one?
2. Did the person ever work in a mine? If yes, for how long? Where? What was mined? What jobs did the person perform?
3. Has the person ever worked in a textile industry?
4. What is the person's smoking history? Does the worker now smoke? If yes, how much and for how long?
5. Did the worker ever have to wear a respirator? If yes, for what reason and for how long?

It is of no value to just record yes-or-no answers. Find out, for example, whether the person ever worked in a cotton mill. If the answer is yes, find out what the jobs were and how long the worker held them.

The second part of this assessment is the taking of X rays. X-ray films of the chest should preserve the lung markings, and these markings should be easily seen. In some industries the chest X rays are taken by the nurse. It is essential that the person who takes and processes the X-ray films follow correct techniques in taking and developing the films. Interpretation of the films should be done by an experienced physician. When the number of films to be taken is great, it is best to have a qualified radiological technician on the staff. When the number is small, however, it is more economical and the results are better if the workers are sent to a local hospital or clinic to have their X rays taken and evaluated by prepared personnel. The importance of the chest X ray to the health assessment program is evidenced by the requirement in the OSHA Asbestos Standard 1919.1001, which specifies that the records of all medical examinations and all X rays shall be retained for at least 30 years.

The third essential part of a medical surveillance for occupational respiratory disease is an assessment of ventilatory capacity. Spirometry is not a difficult technique to learn, but no person should attempt it without understanding the process, knowing what is involved, and being taught the correct technique. (The Cotton Dust Standard of OSHA requires that the person performing the spirometry have completed a NIOSH-approved course.)

The one capacity that is measured by spirometry is the vital capacity. This is the sum of the inspiratory reserve volume, tidal volume, and expiratory reserve volume which is the maximal amount of air that can be expelled from the lungs following a maximal inspiration. When making a plan to perform spirometry it should be remembered that lung volumes are performed at ambient temperature and pressure saturated with water vapor (ATPS) hence final records of all lung volumes and capacities should be corrected to body temperature and pressure (BTP). This is recorded in liters (metric system of measurement). It is important that the temperature in the room and the barometric pressure be recorded each time testing is performed. Tables listing conversion factors from ambient pressure and temperature and body temperature and pressure are available in chemistry and physics reference books. Height, age, sex, race, and the position of the worker during the test (i.e., sitting, or standing) should also be recorded since normal values vary with these factors.

Two parameters are obtained from an analysis of the forced vital capacity tracing. The first is the "forced" vital capacity (FVC, the total amount of air expelled in this maneuver). The second is the volume of air expelled in the first second of this forced expiration. This is called the "forced expiratory volume in one second" (FEV_1).

It is essential that proper instruction and coaching be done by the nurse who is administering the test. The mouthpiece must be placed behind the teeth. The person being tested must be told not to bite the tubing, but to seal the lips around it. The individual must be coached vigorously to perform his best effort. It has been said that "if the subject is not exasperated by the thoroughness of the test, or if the coach has any voice left at the end of the day, then the test has not been done properly." It should be emphasized that the test is not uncomfortable and is very easily performed by the subject.[7]

Reporting Health Assessment Findings

To protect those who have had a health assessment from disclosure of personal health and illness information to nonhealth personnel, many occupational health units use a code system for reporting the results of health assessments to the employment officer. Staffs of both departments, that is, the occupational health unit and the department responsible for selecting employees, must have a common understanding of the job categories to which candidates are usually assigned:

- Class I: physically fit for any job.
- Class II: physically fit for any job but has minor or remediable defects.
- Class III: physically fit for modified work only, in accordance with noted restrictions. Any one of these restrictions may be used to modify work demands of the person whose physical or emotional deficits preclude total interchangeability among all jobs.
- Class IV: physically unqualified for any job applied for.
- Class V: temporary deferment. This classification usually indicates a candidate that manifests an acute illness of short duration which will subside within a few days, when final assessment can be made, or one who has been injured and will be unemployable for a known period of time.[8]

Health Assessment Records

The function of the health assessment record is to permit the ready accessibility of facts about the health status of the individual for the purpose of job placement and health maintenance. The health assessment findings must be completely recorded in order to permit meaningful follow-up and to protect the value of the records for medicolegal reference in cases of alleged occupational injury or disease. Incomplete records are of little value. They provide protection for neither the professionals who perform the procedure nor the worker who was examined nor the employer, who is ultimately responsible. Unless complete data based on examination before placement are available, comparisons with data gathered subsequent to the

Health Assessment

worker's return to work after illness or injury, or with that from periodic examinations, is not possible.

The results of the health assessment procedures must be recorded on a physical evaluation form that permits easy comparison of current and past data. This record is an integral part of an individual's health record and is stored in the worker's file along with all other records of that individual's illness and injury. The record should be signed and dated by the person doing the health assessment. If the employee has had a conference concerning some health problem and recommendations were made, this should be noted, and the plan for the follow-up should be recorded.

Data processing of health assessment information is now an accepted practice in many occupational health programs. Ready availability of the information is necessary and should be built into the system if the data processing is to be more than a means of gathering data for annual reports.

All information about a person's state of health should be considered confidential. The prospective employees and/or employees found to have health problems that require therapy are referred to their family physicians or to specialists for care. The person who does the assessment rates the fitness of the person for the job. This rating should be recorded on the health assessment form, using a rating system like that just described. The health professional uses the rating, without disclosing the details of the medical findings, to communicate with the employment personnel when discussing the applicant's fitness for work.

The OSHA Standards state for how long records are to be maintained for regulated substances, for example, the Vinyl Chloride Standard 1910.1017 states "(iii) Medical records shall be maintained for the duration of the employment of each employee plus 20 years, or 30 years, whichever is longer. (3) In the event that the employer ceases to do business and there is no successor to receive and retain his records for the prescribed period, these records shall be transmitted by registered mail to the Director (of NIOSH) and to each employee individually notified in writing of this transfer." Similar requirements are made in each of the OSHA Standards. As for retention of records, the suggestions are that the records be retained for the duration of employment in the case of exposure(s) with only acute effects; for the duration of employment plus 30 years for exposure to known or suspected carcinogens, and for the duration of employment plus 5 years for the remaining substances. Because 5 years may prove to be too brief a period for such substances as pneumoconiotic agents, it is suggested that no health assessment record be destroyed for at least 10 years after the end of employment, even for those workers whose exposure has been minimal and to substances considered to be nontoxic. Questions about how long to keep records and who has access to information in occupational health unit records have no simple answers.

There are conflicting points of view and conflicting interests, that is, views about protecting the worker and views about protecting the industry. There is the freedom-of-information point of view and the point of view which holds that confidentiality of the record must be maintained. Some of the OSHA Standards have specific requirements. It is suggested that each company have a policy about health record retention that has been developed by the legal representative and the physician so that it is in line with the legal requirements. When a question arises as to whether records can be destroyed, the policy and current advice from governmental agencies should be followed.

Nursing Activities in Health Assessment Programs

Occupational health nurses are doing many of the health assessments of workers. Numerous reports of how they are doing physical examinations, written by nurses, by physicians, and by management personnel, may be found in the literature. Almost all indicate that when the nurse has had special preparation and when a physician is available to take referrals, the nurse can successfully perform the health assessments of workers. The National Commission for the Study of Nursing and Nursing Education in its summary report makes this recommendation: "From the standpoint of many, it makes sense to have the nurse take over as many functions from the physician as she can capably handle."[9]

Occupational health nurses were prepared to do health assessments long before the advent of OSHA. Nurses at the New York Telephone Company were enrolled at company expense in a special training program at Downstate Medical School in 1966, and they now function as nurse clinicians. Some nurses indicate that the preplacement evaluation they do consists of a personal and family health history; some use a standard questionnaire; others interview but also take and record height, weight, blood pressure, and pulse and see that urinalysis, hematocrit, vision screening, audiometry, and chest X ray are performed. Electrocardiograms are performed on applicants over the age of 40 and when indicated by a positive history of cardiac disease. Observations of the musculoskeletal system are done by having the person do a selected list of movements.

This type of nurse-conducted health assessment is often done by occupational health nurses when the workers' jobs do not include heavy labor, exposure to toxic substances, or operating moving equipment. This type of assessment is also used for workers in clerical or other office jobs except that the hearing examination is not performed. In many establishments and for almost as long as health assessments have been performed, nurses have been doing all of these procedures with the physician doing the physical examination. This continues to be the practice in many occupational health units.

With the development of the nurse practitioner programs, nurses have been taught to examine the body systems and to make decisions concerning the health status of the child and the adult. The training is very similar to that given in medical schools and includes the physical appraisal skills of inspection, palpation, percussion, and auscultation. It is pointed out that for nurses to become expert at doing physical assessments they must learn the signs and symptoms of abnormal, as well as the degrees of normal, physiological and neurological functioning.

Performing the mechanics of physical appraisal is a relatively simple task. Relating the findings to decision making (and in occupational health, the issue is whether the person can work with safety to self and others) requires that nurses know what is normal for the adult and what is normal for each individual. In addition nurses must be knowledgeable about the demands of the position and the potential hazards of the environment to which each person is or will be assigned. This requires training and experience. Nurses must also have access to physicians who will take referrals and who will discuss workers' problems with workers and with the nurses when required. In so doing physicians help the nurses acquire new knowledge and insights which they in turn utilize to improve their service to workers.

Occupational health nurses must have an understanding of the toxicology of any substance to which workers have potential exposure. Most importantly, they must know the signs and symptoms of acute and chronic exposure to those substances and what primary and follow-up care are to be provided if health problems develop.

Expert occupational health nurses must have information about administrative and engineering controls and especially what personal protective equipment employees may have to wear. The nurses also require certain supports. They must have an adequate amount of time, adequate working space, and necessary equipment that is well maintained and calibrated. Above all they must be permitted to accept continuing educational opportunities so that they can not only maintain but improve their level of competence.

In establishing a health assessment program, management and the physician must decide whether the nurse is to take on an extended role and do the physical examinations. The nurse or nurses must also be involved in the decision. If the answer is yes, then the nurse's job description must reflect the added responsibilities. Before nurses take on the added responsibility, however, they should receive the necessary preparation for it. Nurses may need to take a leave of absence to get the required training. In the past this preparation was offered as a certificate program. Increasingly it is coming to be offered for graduate credit.

Both management and the physician must recognize that the OSHA

Standards indicate that the health appraisal procedures shall be performed by or under the supervision of a physician at no cost to the employee. Hence physicians who provide medical direction for occupational health units and nurses who perform the examinations must coordinate these activities and have respect for each other's efforts. Nurses, in effect, do the examinations, and physicians review the nurses' reports. Nurses sign the health appraisal records because they performed the examinations. The industry must be able to produce evidence of supervision by a physician to meet the requirements of the OSHA Standards, as these apply if nurses are to be responsible for the conduct of the health assessment examinations of the workers.

References

1. AMA, Department of Environmental, Public, and Occupational Health. *Guiding Principles of Medical Examinations in Industry*. Chicago, 1973, p. 1.
2. Breslow, L., and Somers, A. R. "Lifetime Health Monitoring Program," *New England Journal of Medicine*, Vol. 296, No. 11, Mar. 17, 1977, pp. 601–608.
3. Wilson, J. M. G., and Junger, C. *Principles and Practices of Screening for Disease*. Geneva: WHO, 1968, p. 2.
4. Commission on Chronic Illness. *Chronic Illness in the United States*, Vol. 1, *Prevention of Chronic Illness*. Cambridge, Mass.: Harvard University Press, 1951, p. 45.
5. Howe, H. "Organization and Operation of Occupational Health Programs," *Journal of Occupational Medicine*, Aug. 1975, pp. 528–540. This article is also Pt. 3 of a 3-pt. update with the same title, published by OHI. The first two parts were published in the June and July 1975 issues of the journal.
6. NSPB. *Eyes in Industry: A Guide to Better Industrial Vision Testing*. New York, 1973.
7. Make, B. "Medical Surveillance for Occupational Respiratory Disease," *Journal of Occupational Medicine*, Vol. 17, No. 8, Aug. 1975, pp. 519–522.
8. Felton, J. *Organization and Operation of an Occupational Health Program*, Repr. from the *Journal of Occupational Medicine*, Jan.-Mar. 1964. Chicago: OHI, p. 8.
9. Lysaught, J. P. *The National Study of Nursing and Nursing Education and Its Relationship to the Concept of the Physician's Assistant*. Rochester, N.Y.: National Commission for the Study of Nursing and Nursing Education, 1971.

Selected Readings

Alexander, R. W., Maida, A. S., and Walker, R. J. "The Validity of Preemployment Medical Evaluations," *Journal of Occupational Medicine*, Vol. 17, No. 11, Nov. 1975, pp. 687–692.

AMA, Council on Occupational Health and Council on Mental Health. *Evaluating*

Mental Health Factors in Medical Examinations for Critical Jobs in Industry. Chicago, 1965.

Bernauer, E. M., and Bonanno, J. "Development of Physical Profiles for Specific Jobs," *Journal of Occupational Medicine,* Vol. 17, No. 1, Jan. 1975, pp. 27–33.

Cathcart, L. M. "A Four Year Study of Executive Health Risk," *Journal of Occupational Medicine,* Vol. 19, No. 5, May 1977, pp. 354–357.

Cipolla, J. A., and Collings, G. H. "Nurse Clinicians in Industry," *AJN,* Vol. 71, No. 9, Aug. 1971, pp. 1530–1534.

Coe, J. "The Physician's Role in Sickness Absence Certification: A Reconsideration," *Journal of Occupational Medicine,* Vol. 17, No. 11, Nov. 1975, pp. 722–724.

Collen, M. F., Garfield, S. R., Richart, R. H., Duncan, J. H., and Feldman, R. "Cost Analysis of Alternative Health Examination Modes," *Archives Internal Medicine,* Vol. 137, No. 1, Jan. 1977, pp. 73–79.

"Committee on Nursing, Medicine and Nursing in the 1970s—A Position Statement," *Journal of the AMA,* Vol. 213, No. 11, Sept. 14, 1970, pp. 1887–1883.

Cooper, K. *Aerobics.* New York: Bantam, 1976.

Cooper, W. C. "Indicators of Susceptibility to Industrial Chemicals," *Journal of Occupational Medicine,* Vol. 15, No. 4, Apr. 1973, pp. 355–359.

DHEW, Committee to Study Extended Roles for Nurses. *Extending the Scope of Nursing Practice.* Washington, D.C.: GPO, 1972.

Energy Technology Committee. "Guidelines for Use of Routine X-ray Examination in Occupational Medicine," *Journal of Occupational Medicine,* Vol. 21, No. 7, July 1979, pp. 599–602.

Everett, M. D. "Strategies for Increasing Employees' Level of Exercise and Physical Fitness," *Journal of Occupational Medicine,* Vol. 21, No. 7, July 1979, pp. 463–467.

Gamble, J., and Spirtas, R. "Job Classification and Utilization of Complete Work Histories in Occupational Epidemiology," *Journal of Occupational Medicine,* Vol. 18, No. 6, June 1976, pp. 399–404.

Garb, S. *Laboratory Tests in Common Use* 6th Ed. New York: Springer, 1976.

Goetz, A. A., Duff, E. F., and Bernstein, J. E. "Health Risk Appraisal: The Estimation of Risk," *Public Health Reports,* Vol. 95, No. 2, March-April 1980, pp. 119–126.

Haskell, W. L., Blair, S. N. "The Physical Activity Component of Health Promotion in Occupational Settings," *Public Health Reports,* Vol. 95, No. 2, March-April 1980, pp. 109–118.

Henriques, C. C., Vergadamo, V. G., and Kahane, M. D. "Performance of Adult Health Appraisal Examinations Utilizing Nurse Practitioners, Physicians Teams and Paramedical Personnel," *American Journal of Public Health,* Vol. 64, No. 1, Jan. 1974, pp. 47–53.

Howe, H. F. "Application of Automated Multiphasic Health Testing in Clinical Medicine," *Journal of the AMA,* Vol. 219, No. 7, Feb. 1972, pp. 885–889.

Lerner, S. "Pre-employment Examination and Job Placement of the Pregnant Woman," *Occupational Health Nursing,* Vol. 24, No. 9, Sept. 1976, pp. 15–18.

McQuade, W. "Those Annual Physicals Are Worth the Trouble," *Fortune*, Vol. 77, No. 1, Jan. 1977, pp. 164–173.

Occupational Medical Practice Committee. "Scope of Occupational Health Programs and Occupational Medical Practice," *Journal of Occupational Medicine*, Vol. 21, No. 7, July 1979, pp. 497–499.

Pell, S. "The Identification of Risk Factors in Employed Populations." *Transactions of the New York Academy of Science*, Vol. 26, No. 4, Apr. 1974, pp. 341–356.

Pyle, L. A. "The Use of a Pregnancy Test in Preplacement Medical Evaluations," *Journal of Occupational Medicine*, Vol. 12, No. 1, Jan. 1970, pp. 26–29.

Sana, J. M., and Judge, R. D. (eds.). *Physical Appraisal Methods in Nursing Practice*. Boston: Little, Brown, 1975.

Schussler, T., Kaminer, A., and Pomper, I. H. "The Preplacement Examination," *Journal of Occupational Medicine*, Vol. 17, No. 4, Apr. 1975, pp. 254–257.

Snook, H., and Ciriello, V. "Maximum Weights and Work Loads Acceptable to Female Workers," *Journal of Occupational Medicine*, Vol. 16, No. 8, Aug. 1974, pp. 527–534.

Stokinger, H. E., and Scheel, L. D. "Hypersusceptibility and Genetic Problems in Occupational Medicine—A Consensus Report, *Journal of Occupational Medicine*, Vol. 15, No. 7, July 1973, pp. 564–573.

Tabershaw, I. R. "How is the Acceptability of Risks to the Health of the Workers to be Determined?" *Journal of Occupational Medicine*, Vol. 18, No. 10, Oct. 1976, pp. 674–676.

Yarvote, P. M., McDonagh, T. J., Goldman, M. E., and Zuckerman, J. "Organization and Evaluation of a Physical Fitness Program in Industry," *Journal of Occupational Medicine*, Vol. 16, No. 9, Sept. 1974, pp. 589–598.

CHAPTER 7

Medical Surveillance

"The worker is a monitor of his work exposure, integrating the occupational exposure with similar or related exposures outside the work area and reacting to these according to his/her individual state of health and susceptibility."[1] Hence there must be frequent and meaningful interaction between the worker and the health professional to assure that ill effects do not occur. Environmental monitoring is the keystone of an effective occupational health program, but environmental monitoring alone can lead to a false sense of security. Poor work practices and inadequate personal hygiene can result in worker exposure, as can unpredictable breakdowns in operational controls. Medical surveillance provides the safety factor.

Surveillance is "a close watch kept over a person or group."[2] Health surveillance in an occupational setting encompasses those activities and judgments that are necessary to keep a close watch on the health of workers so that there can be early identification of individuals who have adverse physiological or psychological responses from exposure to toxic substances in their work setting. The concern for worker health expressed in the present and proposed U.S. Occupational Safety and Health Standards is based on recognition of the potential for harm presented by the toxicity of substances used in industrial processes and to which workers are exposed.

The aims of a medical surveillance program whether required by the OSHA Standards or provided voluntarily by the employer on the advice of the occupational health physician are the same. Such programs are designed to find evidence of health effects from job-related exposures early enough to identify the person who is susceptible and to identify damage to worker health before it becomes irreversible. Base-line data about a person's state of health at time of job placement into an area where there is a potential hazard to health is the first step. Such data are generated by health and work histories, physical examinations, X rays, blood and urine tests, pulmonary function, vision and hearing acuity tests, and so on. Periodic examination, health histories, or health screening procedures are scheduled at intervals determined on the basis of the age of the worker, the toxicity of the substance, and the degree of exposure.

Although the Occupational Safety and Health Act has projected medical surveillance into the forefront of occupational health, the content is not new. Periodic assessment of worker health as an occupational activity has been a part of effective comprehensive occupational health programs since long before the advent of OSHA. Similar activities had been carried on in state and federal occupational and hygiene programs as an integral part of field studies on industrial populations to determine health effects of industrial exposures.

Standards Completion Program

When the Occupational Safety and Health Act creating NIOSH and OSHA became law in 1970, workplace exposure limits for some substances had already been recommended by voluntary groups. But these limits, which OSHA was required to adopt as standards, were only permissible exposure levels. In an effort to make these standards more comprehensive, NIOSH and OSHA initiated a joint Standards Completion Program (SCP) to develop more comprehensive standards to assure worker protection. This joint effort to complete the technical criteria was finished in mid-1977. Recommended procedures for 400 chemicals studied under the program now include:

- Informing the employee of potential hazards
- Monitoring, engineering, and hazard control mechanisms
- Establishing effective monitoring techniques and intervals
- Establishing medical surveillance and testing programs
- Evaluating fire and other injury hazards.[3]

The recommendations of the SCP have not been promulgated to standards by OSHA. They could be; and if they are, OSHA will follow the required procedures and announce what changes in the current standards are to be made. These changes will appear in the *Federal Register*.

The Standards Completion Program generated much interest in routine environmental monitoring and medical surveillance activities. Such activities are routinely carried on at some work sites where workers have the potential of exposure to the substances covered by the SCP, although they are not required by law. All criteria for recommended standards prepared by NIOSH for OSHA and published as NIOSH Criteria Documents have a section on medical surveillance.

Medical Surveillance for Women at Work

According to an American College of Obstetricians and Gynecologists (ACOG) research report prepared under contract from the National Institute for Occupational Health, three noteworthy trends have emerged dur-

Medical Surveillance 91

ing the past two decades: (a) the shift of millions of women to employment outside the home, (b) the expectations of equal employment opportunity, and (c) growth of knowledge about environmental health hazards.[4] This report, prepared primarily to help the practicing obstetrician assemble and interpret the information necessary for appropriate clinical recommendations to patients who are pregnant workers, is most useful to occupational health physicians and nurses. The woman and the fetus that she brings to work with her can be at risk in certain work environments. With more women entering employment in industrial concerns, occupational health professionals will need increasingly to: (a) provide information for the pregnant worker's obstetrician, and (b) be able to discuss job placement and job hazards with women workers.

The report suggests four recommendations that could be made by the physician after each visit: (a) The woman may continue to work without any change in job or work behavior; (b) she may continue to work but working modifications are desirable; (c) she may continue to work only after certain modifications in the environment of her particular work are made, and occupational health personnel must assure that modifications will contribute to the worker's safety and health; and (d) the woman and her obstetrician may decide that she should not work,[5] and again the occupational health personnel may be involved to interpret the worker's rights under insurance programs and job security policies. These will vary depending on union contracts, company policies, and the terms in the insurance contract.

Criteria

The health standards promulgated by OSHA since 1972 prescribe the type and frequency of medical examinations and other tests which shall be made by the employer, or at the employer's cost, to employees exposed to occupational hazards in order to determine whether the health of employees is adversely affected by such exposure. The extent and nature of the preplacement examination and the frequency and extent of subsequent examinations are determined by the relative toxicity and degree of hazard for each agent for which federal standards have been set by OSHA.

The first of the standards promulgated by OSHA including medical surveillance was the Asbestos Standard Code of Federal Regulation (CFR) 1910.1001. The extent of a medical surveillance program for workers exposed to asbestos dust is legally determined by the requirements as stated in the standard:

The employer shall provide or make available to the worker within 30 calendar days following the first employment in an occupation exposed to airborne concentrations of asbestos fibers a comprehensive medical examination, which shall include, as a minimum, a chest roentgenogram (posterior-anterior 14 × 17 inches), a history to elicit symptomatology of respiratory disease, and pulmonary function tests to include forced vital capacity (FVC) and forced expiratory volume at 1 second ($FEV_{1.0}$).

On or before January 1, 1973, and at least annually thereafter, every employer shall provide or make available, comprehensive medical examinations to each of his employees engaged in occupations exposed to airborne concentrations of asbestos fibers.

Such annual examinations shall include, as a minimum, a chest roentgenogram (posterior-anterior 14 × 17 inches), a history to elicit symptomatology of respiratory disease and pulmonary function tests to include forced vital capacity (FVC) and forced expiratory volume at 1 second ($FEV_{1.0}$).[6]

See Appendix D for OSHA Standard 1910.1017 Vinyl Chloride. The medical surveillance program as required in Section K and Appendix A focuses on the body systems at risk: liver, spleen, kidney, skin, and connective tissues. The Asbestos Standard focuses primarily on the respiratory system.

Criteria Documentation

The development and periodic revision of criteria documents as a basis for standards for occupational exposure to chemical and physical hazards in the work place is a major legislatively mandated activity of NIOSH. Criteria documents are publications prepared after a critical evaluation of all known scientific information on a particular subject.

The purpose of these documents is to establish recommended occupational health standards. In addition to permissible levels of exposure in the occupational environment, they include recommendations for medical surveillance, personal protective equipment, work practices, and sanitation. Information in criteria documents can also be used for informing the workers of the hazards; for labeling and posting; for monitoring and surveillance; and for record keeping. By law this information is intended to serve as the technical basis for standards to be promulgated by OSHA.[7]

Criteria for standards had been prepared by NIOSH for approximately 100 substances by the end of 1979. Criteria documents for each are for sale from the GPO. Many industrial hygienists and occupational health physicians have copies of the appropriate criteria document in their files, for they find the NIOSH Criteria Documents that deal with the substances used in the industry where they work to be most helpful. They are used as the basis for program planning. The health professionals often recommend to management that the industry aim to meet the criteria for the recommended standard although this is lower than that required by law. They do so because of the prevention factors used by NIOSH as the basis for establishing the criteria. Nurses will find criteria documents to be a most helpful resource as they participate in the planning and the conduct of medical surveillance and worker-training activities.

Protocols

Fundamental to an effective occupational health program is a well-planned health surveillance program that is comprehensive enough to determine a person's state of health and fitness for the job that he or she is seeking or presently responsible for. The protocol must meet the special requirements of the OSHA Standards and should state what procedures are to be done and what deviations from normal are considered to be significant. A well-planned health surveillance program is one that is:

1. Comprehensive enough to protect the workers when jobs place them at risk and that does not overload the occupational health unit staff with physical assessments and other procedures whose usefulness and frequency are not proven
2. Based on recognition that it is rare for workers to be potentially exposed to a single substance only
3. Based on the facts that the state of the art of surveillance presently is incapable in all but rare instances of measuring any impact on the one cause–one effect relationship between an agent and reaction to it and that it is almost impossible to realistically assess the multiple-cause–perhaps-more-than-one-effect condition
4. Designed to deal with the interaction of occupational and nonoccupational factors.

The Nurse's Responsibilities in Medical Surveillance Programs

In the development of the health unit's protocols for health surveillance, nurses work with physicians to identify:

1. Procedures that are to be performed and how frequently
    a. Health history only
    b. Health history and physical examination
    c. Health history and screening tests
    d. Health history, physical examination, and special tests
2. The level of deviation from normal that is considered to indicate that corrective action must be taken
    a. The level of deviation that requires the transfer of the worker from a particular job
    b. The level of deviation that requires referral to a physician for further work-up or for treatment
3. The jobs and the names of all the workers holding such jobs and the

areas of the establishment that are to be included in a medical surveillance program.

Nurses work with the industrial hygienist or those responsible for environmental monitoring to:

1. Identify the areas in the work environment that must be monitored and for what reasons
2. Set up a coordinated medical surveillance and environmental monitoring schedule
3. List the workers to be offered the medical surveillance programs as required by OSHA or that the members of the occupational health team have established as needed on the basis either of NIOSH's proposed standards or of their own evaluation of the hazard
4. Coordinate the scheduling so that workers who are involved in more than one medical surveillance program because of the variety of the potential hazards associated with their jobs are not required to have duplicate examinations or tests.

When there are policy guidelines that have the understanding and support of management, the union leadership, and the workers, nurses can manage a program and should be given the responsibility. They can work up the schedule of appointments and arrange with the laboratory for the necessary work to be done. They can draw the blood and arrange for the collection of urine and stool samples. They can do the audiometric tests and the respiratory function tests. They can test for muscle strength and examine the skin. They can take the health and work history. Interviewing is a goal-directed method of communication; it is how histories are taken. When nurses take health histories they know what information must be sought and the use to which it is to be put. The medical guidelines of the OSHA Standards and those that were developed for proposed standards provide specific information that can be used to formulate health interview questions. These documents identify what body systems are at greatest risk if a person were to be exposed to a harmful substance. Often health histories are completed by the workers, who answer questions on a printed form. Nurses check for completeness and to assure that the questions and answers are understood.

It must be pointed out that, although occupational health nurses often do both the technical and the clerical parts of the medical surveillance program, there is only so much one person can do. When nurses use time to do clerical and screening-test activities, they have that much less time to devote to the professional and administrative activities essential to the smooth functioning of a medical surveillance program and of the total occupational health program. Therefore when the number of health assessments and screening tests to be performed is great, it may be wise use of staff time to employ paraprofessional aides to do the clerical work and to perform, for example, the hearing and vision tests.

Nurse practitioners who have had special training can and are doing physical examinations. It is essential that they, like other nurses, have access to a physician with whom they can discuss problems. Nurses' contributions to medical surveillance are furthered when they are responsible for helping workers understand:

1. Why the examination is being offered
2. What will be involved
3. The results of the tests and of the examination, the recommendations made on the basis of the examinations, and the potential hazards of the job.

Occupational health nurses most meaningful contributions are made to the medical surveillance program when they are involved in those activities that are directed to the workers' right to know and the workers' willingness to participate. For a medical surveillance program to be effective, someone, and it should be the nurse, needs to explain the toxicology of the substance or substances and why they, the workers, are presently enrolled in the medical surveillance program. This information needs to be couched in terms that are meaningful to the workers. Nurses should plan with individual workers for their participation and arrange their appointments so that they fit into workers' travel and work schedules.

The primary goal of occupational health nurses in medical surveillance programs is to assist workers to attain and maintain optimal physical, psychological, and social functioning. Nurses' activities, in addition to those of an educational and motivational nature, include those that require professional judgment as this relates to the workers' health and the environmental monitoring data. Nurses make observations, conduct examinations, perform interviews, and record the information they obtain, including the condition of a worker's skin; the color and condition of mucous membranes; signs of problems like clubbing of fingers or changes in the person's coordination and equilibrium; history of headaches; and problems with memory, reproduction, joint functioning, and muscular strength. Occupational health nurses have the opportunity to know workers over long periods of time, sometimes from the date of their employment to their retirement. Any evidence of change should be noted and brought to the attention of the physician and the industrial hygienist, and the cause should be looked for. In addition to helping workers understand why the medical surveillance program is necessary and why they should take part, nurses help workers understand the results of the program and follow any recommendations that are made.

The Reference Library

The occupational health unit staff should have access to copies of the OSHA Standards that apply to the substances in use in the establishment and copies of any other governmental publications that deal with the health and safety aspects of any and all substances used in the process of production. Nurses will find that one of the most useful items is a ready reference file that includes the pertinent information for each of the toxic substances that are in use and to which workers have potential exposure. The OSHA Standards direct that when a medical examination is required the industry must send information about the exposure and a copy of the Standards appendix that deals with medical surveillance to the physician who is to do the examination.

One of the reasons for this is that physicians in the community cannot be expected to be knowledgeable about all of the chemical substances used in industry, and in many instances their medical libraries lack the needed reference books. The medical surveillance guidelines in the OSHA Standards and the book *Occupational Diseases: A Guide to Their Recognition and Control,* developed by NIOSH and published by the GPO, provide much of the information needed by the physician. In addition data generated by the Standards Completion Program have been incorporated into the book *Chemical Hazards of the Work Place* by N. H. Proctor and James P. Hughes, published in 1978 by Lippincott. These sources will be of value to occupational health nurses. They can use them to increase their understanding of how toxic substances cause harm to workers. They also provide the basis for the health surveillance protocols that nurses and physicians develop for occupational health unit programs and which nurses will follow as they coordinate the activities of the health assessment of the workers. The protocols also provide a framework for the therapeutic care nurses provide for those who have been injured or become ill from exposure, and for the health teaching nurses do to give workers the information necessary for their informed participation.

References

1. Messite, J. *Medical Monitoring—Is it Important?* Lecture given at New York University Medical Center, June 1979.

2. Stein, J. (ed.). *The Random House Dictionary of the English Language*, Unabridged ed. New York: Random House, 1977, p. 1432.
3. NIOSH. *Criteria Documentation and Standard Development*. Washington, D.C.: GPO, 1978, p. 1.
4. American College of Obstetricians and Gynecologists. *Guidelines on Pregnancy and Work*. Washington, D.C.: GPO, 1977, p. iii.
5. Ibid., pp. 12–13.
6. 1910.1001 Asbestos 39 FR 23502 June 1974. Amended at 41 FR 11505 Mar. 19, 1976. *OSHA Safety and Health Standards General Industry Standards (29 CFR 1910)*. Washington, D.C.: GPO, 1977.
7. NIOSH, op. cit., p. 4.

Selected Readings

Boggs, R. F., and Powell, C. H. "NIOSH/OSHA Development of Supplemental Health Standards," *Transactions of the 37th Annual Meeting of the ACGIH*, May 31–June 6 1975, pp. 157–158.

DHEW. *Baseline for Setting Health Goals and Standards*, HRA 76-640. Washington, D.C.: GPO, 1976.

Dixon, E. M. "Medical Surveillance in Industry," *Journal of Occupational Medicine*, Vol. 15, No. 10, Oct. 1973, pp. 796–798.

NIOSH. *Occupational Safety and Health Symposium 1976*, GPO: 017-033-00249-5. Washington, D.C., 1977.

NIOSH. *A Conceptual Framework for Occupational Health Surveillance*, Pub. No. 78-135. Washington, D.C.: GPO, 1978.

Perkins, J. L., and Rose, V. E. "Occupational Health Priorities for Health Standards: The Current NIOSH Approach," *American Journal of Public Health*, Vol. 69, No. 5, May 1979, pp. 444–447.

Rose, V. E. *Reliability and Utilization of Occupational Disease Data*, NIOSH Pub. No. 77-189. Washington, D.C.: GPO, 1977.

WHO. *Environmental and Health Monitoring in Occupational Health*, Technical Rep. No. 535. Geneva, 1973.

CHAPTER **8**

Occupational Health Maintenance, Conservation, and Promotion

Three words sometimes used interchangeably but which have separate and distinct meanings are used to describe OSH activities undertaken to keep workers well: maintenance, conservation, and promotion. *Maintenance* means upkeep. A more useful definition states that maintenance is "designed or adequate to maintain a living body in a stable condition without providing reserve for growth, functional change, or healing efforts."[1] *Conservation* is "the process whereby something is preserved or saved from loss, injury, decay, or waste."[2] *Promotion* is used in this chapter to mean remaining in a safe or sound state as by deliberate, planned, intelligent care. In reality, health conservation and health maintenance activities are health promotional activities.

The fact that medical surveillance requirements are included in the OSHA Standards enacted since 1972 means that management must make these services available for employees whose work environment contains any of the OSHA–regulated substances in concentrations at or above the action level. The characteristics of occupational health maintenance, conservation, and promotion apply with the added proviso that the program must be offered if the industry is to be in compliance. The OSHA Standards outline what activities are to be carried on and at what frequencies, and they stipulate how long the records must be kept.

This chapter deals with characteristics of occupational safety and health activities that nurses must be able to plan, carry on, and evaluate. The special-emphasis programs most often initiated in industrial establishments are:

1. Vision conservation programs
2. Hearing conservation programs
3. Respiratory disease surveillance programs
4. Dermatitis control programs
5. Programs to control substances hazardous to workers' progeny
6. Immunization programs
7. Medical surveillance programs associated with compliance to OSHA Standards.

All of these programs required the development and adoption of a detailed plan of action. All too often an activity is undertaken without planning, and all too often such undertakings are not successful. The plan should have a measurable objective based on a stated need, and it should include what is to be done by whom and in what period of time. The following key requirements are critical to the achievement of the objectives of the seven special-emphasis programs just listed: all must

1. Have as their purpose the conservation or promotion of the workers' health status and be predicated on an awareness of the hazards of the work environment
2. Have the active participation of the employees and all members of the occupational safety and health team
3. Be planned to meet the special needs of the workers and of the specific industry and to include the identification of who and how many workers are at risk
4. State what behavior workers should develop as a result of participation
5. Outline the activities that need to be undertaken, at what time, and by whom
6. Include overall objectives and the statement of policy that shows the approval and active support of management and the union
7. Provide for educating the worker as to why certain work practices must be followed
8. Provide for educating the supervisors as to the intent of the program and why and how they must participate in certain parts of it to assure that the workers follow prescribed work practices including the wearing of protective personal equipment
9. Require constant vigilance from supervisory and health care personnel, because conserving workers' hearing and vision and protecting their skin, respiratory tract, and offspring from work-connected hazards are not one-time activities nor are they responsibilitites that can be assigned to any one person
10. Be evaluated periodically, evaluation including a critical look at what was involved, what the costs were, and whether the outcome was worth the cost and these aspects looked at against what was planned.

All of the planning for the special emphasis programs has as its purpose the prevention of illness or injury from work-connected causes. In addition to the need to plan together, all members of the occupational health team must work together to achieve the desired results. The nurse can play a significant role in the planning and evaluation processes and in the conduct of the programs as well as helping workers understand why they should participate and how they can do so.

Vision Conservation Program

Although the cause-and-effect relationship between an industrial accident and blindness is easy to establish, such accidents are impossible to undo. The eye can be damaged by a single agent or by a combination of agents. Injuries include lacerations, contusions, and burns—chemical or thermal. Foreign bodies are the most common cause of discomfort. Some may be loose; others may be imbedded in the eye's covering; and some may penetrate into the globe. Because of the specialized nature of eye care it is essential that the establishment employ a consulting ophthalmologist who will consult with the occupational health care professionals, work with the nurse and the physician in developing protocols for the care of workers with eye injuries, and accept referrals of workers with special eye problems.

A well-planned vision conservation program provides for two types of activities: (a) prevention of eye injuries, including job placement procedures, and (b) optimal care for eye injuries and illnesses, including care, treatment, and rehabilitation. Programs should be designed to fit the special needs of the workers and the particular industry and should include:

1. Identification of the eye hazards in the environment. This is usually accomplished by careful study of all the jobs and identification of any hazard connected with them.

2. Establishment of visual requirements for performing the various jobs. Sometimes this can be done by the same professional who identified the hazards. In any case it is best accomplished by an expert who understands human factors engineering. Lighting requirements for various industrial operations are set forth in the ANSI booklet *Practices for Industrial Lighting* (ANSI/IES RP 7-1973). Adequate lighting without glare is an essential factor of the work environment in modern factories. Color is also an important aspect of lighting. Assistance with problems in this area is available from the utility company and from the Illuminating Engineering Society, which provices recommendations on amount of light necessary for various types of industrial operations.

3. Establishment of an eye protection policy. Management should concur in the development of a policy which may be all-inclusive, as a universal safety goggle rule that requires everyone to wear eye protection at all times, with the safety eye wear being supplied by management. Or a policy may require that eye protection be worn only in selected areas of the establishment. Accident prevention specialists believe that 90% of all eye injuries and loss-of-sight accidents could have been prevented by the conscientious use of safety wear.[3] The Wise Owl Club of America, with almost 67,000 members,[4] has a national program to prevent loss of sight due to

accidents in industry, off the job, and in schools. Membership is limited to persons whose eyesight is saved because the person was wearing eye protection during an accident that would have caused loss of sight were it not for protective eye wear.[5] The Wise Owl Club is a most effective method of interesting workers in prevention; if a worker's sight is saved because of the use of protective eye equipment, the person should be recommended for membership. Two other policies are suggested as basic to a vision conservation program: (a) Because of the increased risk to eyes, the NSPB strongly "advises that the use of contact lenses of any type by industrial employees while at work should be prohibited except in rare cases,"[6] and (b) it is also a good idea to have a rule that only a doctor or a nurse be allowed to remove a foreign body from a worker's eye and to see that this rule is rigidly enforced.

4. Screening. Screening is done to assess a worker's level of visual acuity at the time of job placement and at appropriate times thereafter. Most binocular testing devices have special features that allow for the tailoring of tests to the established norms for the various tasks workers are called upon to perform. Glaucoma screening is also important and should be done at the time of each health assessment, especially for workers 35 years of age or over. Vision screening should be specific to the industry and the job the worker is to do. Matching the worker's visual acuity to the job often reduces the possibility of accidents or costly errors.

5. Treatment. Specific instructions for the care of the worker who has sustained an eye injury should be stated in the health unit protocols. The essential element in the care of any eye injury involving a chemical is the immediate first aid that either the worker or first-aid personnel must provide at the site of the accident. That is, within 15 seconds and for at least 5 minutes the eye must be flushed with uncontaminated water. This may come from any source—drinking fountain, hose, bucket, or best of all, a special eyewash fountain. The injured person should be brought to the health unit as soon as possible following the immediate first-aid treatment. Upon arrival the nurse again irrigates the eye, usually with normal saline solution and for 15 minutes. A local anesthetic will help to relieve pain. After the irrigation the nurse may use a fluorescein buffered solution to stain the cornea and outline any area of injury. The solution is dropped in the eye, or a sterile individual applicator is used, and then the eye is flushed with normal saline solution. If a stain remains, the cornea has been damaged. This useful test makes it much easier for the nurse to decide whether to send the worker to the ophthalmologist immediately and is well within the limits of nursing diagnosis. All information concerning the injury, the extent of the damage, and the treatment given is recorded on the worker's health record. The visual acuity is checked and recorded. It is

suggested that a diagram of the eye be applied to the record and used for recording the area of damage.

The care given by the nurse in the health unit is for the purpose of protecting and conserving the worker's sight. Every procedure the nurse performs must contribute to the prevention of further damage. He or she should always wash his or her hands before taking care of a person with an eye injury. All equipment and solutions, except tap water, should be sterile. An eye dropper should never be put back into the stock bottle after use. The use of eye cups is not recommended. All solutions used in treatment should be made up in small quantities and kept separate from other medications. Great care should be exercised so as not to contaminate the stock bottles. Fluorescein is easily contaminated and must be checked frequently, a good reason for using the individually wrapped, sterile fluorescein applicators. In addition the nurse teaches workers to keep their hands away from their eyes and to use only a clean handkerchief or towel or a disposable tissue when wiping around an injured or sore eye. The treatment room should be equipped with a comfortable treatment chair with a head rest, adequate lighting, appropriate medications and solutions, and an "eye tray" kept well supplied and in readiness.

6. Rehabilitation. Finally, vision conservation programs include placement of those workers who are blind, have sight in only one eye, or have diminished vision in jobs they can do safely. Sometimes such placement is temporary, but it may also be for the rest of the person's working life. Sending a person back to work with an eye patch in place or wearing dark glasses following the instillation of medication must be done with caution, and the worker must understand and follow safe working practices. Loss of sight can be most devastating, and rehabilitation requires the services of many specialists. The person will have to acquire new skills, new means of getting about, and a new self-image that incorporates acceptance of this loss.

The basis for effective planning for any visual conservation program is to identify the authoritative sources of information and to secure copies of their publications to use as references. NSPB publishes at least four items of special value for those involved in planning such a program: (a) The Wise Owl Club of America, (b) Organization of a Glaucoma Screening Program, (c) The Occupational Health Nurse and Eye Care, (d) Eyes in Industry: A Guide to Better Industrial Vision Testing. Another useful source of information is the publication *Guiding Principles and Procedures for Industrial Nurses in Care of Eye Injuries*, which is put out by the AMA's Council on Occupational Health.

Hearing Conservation Programs

The keystone in hearing conservation programs is control of noise at its source. Activities associated with conservation of workers' hearing acuity and which must be taken into consideration when planning and implementing a program include:

1. Identification of areas where a noise hazard exists
2. Surveys of such areas to measure the noise levels and the duration of exposure during a typical workday
3. Identification of the workers at risk
4. Audiometric testing by qualified personnel during the workers' preplacement health assessment and at appropriate times, places, and frequencies thereafter
5. Fitting workers with ear defenders and teaching them why and when the defenders must be worn and how to care for them
6. Providing anticipatory guidance that stresses the need for workers to have clean hands when inserting the defenders (to prevent dermatitis) and the advisability of reporting all ear, nose, and throat infections to the health unit.

A hearing conservation program that includes the wearing of defenders sometimes falters because some of the workers fail to wear the appliances. If ear defenders are necessary, then all workers whose environment is too noisy must be helped to know why they must conform. The nurse, the first-line supervisor, the safety professional, and the union representative must all have a similar understanding of the intent of the hearing conservation program and must, in their own roles, reinforce employees for adaptive behavior and penalize those who exhibit nonadaptive behavior. To this end the nurse can have a purposeful conversation with nonconforming employees to find out if the defenders fit properly, what wearing them means to workers, and whether some health problem is aggravated by the wearing of defenders. For example if 20 workers are involved in a hearing conservation program and all but 5 follow instructions, the nurse must try to find out why these 5 do not cooperate and help them find a way to overcome their hang-ups. When ear protection is required, the burden of finding a way to get workers to wear the equipment rests with the first-line supervisors and the occupational health personnel. Often the worker who does not take part in a health promotion program does not believe that people who are promoting it truly care about what they are promoting. When teaching is not reinforced by supervision and follow-up, the worker gets two messages: "They want me to wear ear defenders," and "They don't care whether I do or don't."

Two sources of additional information for those planning or carrying on a hearing conservation program are:

1. Salmon, V., Mills, J. S., and Petersen, A. C. *Industrial Noise Control Manual*. NIOSH. Washington, D.C.: GPO, 1975. (GPO Stock No. 017-033-00073, $3.25)
2. AAOO, Committee on Conservation of Hearing, Subcommittee on Noise. *Guide for Conservation of Hearing in Noise*, Rev. Ed. Dallas, Tex.: AAOO Research Center, 1969.

Nurses are reminded that a literature search is an important step in planning. It is also pointed out that nurses and others who have been involved in a successful program should prepare an article based on their experience and submit it for publication, for only in this way can others benefit. The journals contain many useful articles, for example B. J. Dye, "Hearing Conservation Education Program," *Occupational Health Nursing*, Vol. 27, No. 1, Jan. 1979, pp. 12–14. Those who are to do audiometric testing should have as minimum preparation the audiometric technician training program developed by the American Academy of Ophthalmology and Otolaryngology (AAOO) and the American Association of Industrial Nurses (AAIN). Check with the American Association of Occupational Health Nurses (AAOHN) office in New York for additional information.

Respiratory Disease Prevention Programs

Many industrial exposures can and do cause both acute and chronic respiratory disorders. An effective ventilatory disease prevention program that aims to maintain, preserve, and promote the respiratory health of workers includes obtaining a health, smoking, and occupational history; obtaining chest X rays; and assessing ventilatory capacity. The procedures and techniques for carrying out these procedures are discussed in some detail in Chapter 6 because of the importance of doing these activities at the time of preplacement assessment.

An important aspect of a respiratory disease prevention program is to determine any change that may have occurred in the worker's lung volumes, since changes in most of the lung volumes measured by spirometry (i.e., tidal volume, inspiratory reserve volume, and expiratory reserve volume) are present in advanced disease but are often absent early in the course of the disease. The sensitivity of spirometry is greatly enhanced by careful examination of the forced maximal expiration portion of the maneuver (see p. 81).

It is usually recommended that five vital capacity maneuvers be carried out. To check if the subject is giving the utmost effort, compare the vital capacities to see if the largest two tracings are within 5% of each other. It is the usual practice to accept the first two tracings of the five as "practice" runs because the worker needs a few trials to become familiar with the equipment and the procedure. In an industrial setting the usual practice is to use the largest FVC and the largest FEV_1 of the last three maneuvers as the values that represent the person's vital capacity at that point in time. In all industries where respiratory diseases are expected, it is essential that spirometry be a part of preemployment testing. Such screening can identify employees with preexisting respiratory impairment. These base-line values permit subsequent test results to be compared so that appropriate intervention can be carried out if there is evidence of change in the vital capacity.

OSHA Requirements

OSHA has set maximum exposure standards for many airborne toxic materials. If employee exposure to these substances exceeds the standard, the law requires that feasible engineering controls and/or administrative controls be installed or instituted to reduce employee exposure to acceptable levels. If these controls do not prove feasible or while they are being installed or instituted, the employer is required to provide appropriate respiratory protection for the employees. Respiratory protection is also required when working in oxygen-deficient atmospheres, that is, where oxygen content in the breathable air is insufficient. Respiratory protection may also be necessary for routine but infrequent operations, for nonroutine operations in which an employee is exposed briefly to high concentrations of a hazardous substance, for example during maintenance or repair activities or during emergency conditions.

Providing respiratory protective equipment to employees, however, is only one aspect of the employer's responsibility pertaining to the use of respiratory protective equipment as a control measure. A respiratory protection program must be implemented. The program is "established" by management, and an individual is designated to head the program. This person develops the standard operating procedure, which describes the following program aspects:

1. The basis for selection of a specific type of respiratory protective equipment
2. Provision for medical screening of each employee assigned to wear respiratory equipment to determine if the worker is physically or psychologically able to wear a respirator
3. Provisions for assigning respiratory protective equipment to employees for their exclusive use, where practical

4. Provisions for testing for the proper fit of the respiratory protective equipment
5. Provisions for regularly cleaning and disinfecting the respiratory protective equipment
6. Provisions for proper storage of respiratory protective equipment
7. Provisions for periodic inspection and repair of respiratory protective equipment
8. A periodic evaluation by the administrator of the program to assure its continued functioning and effectiveness
9. An employee training program in which employees can become familiar with the respiratory protective equipment and be trained in the proper use and the limitations of the equipment.

This program must be instituted as a control measure only after it has been determined that: (a) employee exposure to chemical agents exceeds established limits (OSHA Standards) and (b) engineering controls to alleviate the exposure are not feasible or (c) while engineering controls are being implemented. However even if you do not have operations in which employee exposure to a substance will exceed the standards, a respirator protection program should be developed to address any infrequent but necessary use of respirators.

Dermatitis Control Programs

Unlike vision, hearing, and respiratory disease prevention programs, which focus on the workers who are at risk, an occupational dermatitis control program should be designed to be applicable for all the employees. A second difference is that, if and when a worker does develop a skin problem, a personalized plan needs to be developed. Such a plan must take into consideration the person's life-style, job, and total health condition. Helping workers to understand the function of the skin and how to maintain its health and integrity should be incorporated into the health education program. These educational programs should be conducted often enough to assure that new workers have a chance to learn from them and to reinforce their learning by association with those who have participated in earlier sessions. The nurse who formulates a personalized plan for the worker who develops a work-connected skin problem needs to know what substances the worker uses at job, home, and play and what can be done to protect the skin from exposure to these substances. How to wash and dry hands and the importance of clean work clothes need to be stressed.

Workers who are diabetic, those who have allergies, and those who already have a skin problem—adolescent acne or psoriasis, for example—should be in a control program that brings them into the health unit for periodic examination of the skin and a review of their diet, personal hygiene practices, and health history. Ideally, the protocols for care of workers with skin problems should be developed with consultation from the dermatologist and the occupational health physician. When recording information about skin conditions, the nurse should carefully select the term that best describes the condition of the skin. A list of such terms and their meanings can be incorporated into the policy and procedure manual along with the protocols for care. Two sections of the book *Occupational Diseases: A Guide to Their Recognition*, NIOSH Pub. No. 77-181, available from the GPO, are pertinent as the nurse works at developing and carrying on a dermatitis control program: the chapters "Routes of Entry" and "Dermatosis." Another useful source is Arndt's *Manual of Dermatologic Therapeutics with Essentials of Diagnosis*, 2nd Ed., published by Little, Brown in 1978.

Programs to Protect Workers' Progeny

A topic of fairly recent concern and one that health professionals must deal with is the effect of industrial environments on workers' offspring. Approximately 3% of all newborns have a congenital anomaly requiring medical attention, and approximately one-third of these conditions can be considered life threatening.[7]

Teratogens are agents which produce structural abnormalities. They are capable of damaging the embryo by disturbing the maternal homeostasis or by direct action on embryonic tissues or organs. The first trimester, particularly the first eight week period of embryonic organogenesis, is the time of greatest susceptibility to environmental influences and the majority of teratological effects are induced during this period. The drug, thalidomide, furnished a documented example of a substance that produces its effects solely during this critical period. . . .

Mutagens are compounds causing heritable alteration in DNA. They can damage egg and sperm cells prior to fertilization, as well as the embryo. A chemical substance or physical agent may act directly on the germ cells so that fertilization does not take place or it may cause such severe anomalies in the zygote as to result in an early, at times unrecognized abortion. There are relatively few reports of parental exposures related to either outcome, although the risk is recognized. It is during this pre-conception period that both paternal and maternal exposure to mutagenic agents must be considered, for either—together or independently—may result in the inhibition of fertilization of the production of abnormal embryos.[8]

The occupational health professionals, that is, physicians and nurses, are instrumental in formulating company policies as these relate to the employment or job transfer of those employees, both male and female, who plan on parenting children and whose jobs expose them to a toxic agent. The health professionals must be aware of the legal implications, the social and economic issues, and the employer's liability for damage to the parent, fetus, or child. In a paper presented at the National Safety Congress in 1978, L. Warshaw said, "Awards to adult workers are limited by workers' compensation, but suit can be brought on behalf of a child. . . . Case law is ambivalent about the legal status of a stillborn fetus within the wrongful death status but recovery for prenatal injuries suffered at any time after conception by a child who was born alive is permitted under Common Law."[9]

Immunization Programs

In the AMA's publication *Scope and Objectives*, seven activities are suggested for an occupational health program, one of which is "immunization." The extent of an immunization program depends upon several factors: the age distribution of the work force, the health status of the community of which the industry is a part, the amount of travel and to what parts of the world the employees may need to travel, and the environment to which the workers are exposed.

Prophylaxis is the term applied to measures designed to preserve health and prevent the spread of disease, and it usually refers to immunization. The use of immunization to prevent disease caused by bacteriologic agents has a long and successful history. Smallpox and tetanus, for example, have long been controlled by vaccines that create an immunity in vaccinated persons. Vaccinations for smallpox are no longer recommended because the disease has been virtually eliminated the world over.

For Influenza

The principles followed in an occupational health immunization program are the same as those followed in comparable community health programs. For example flu vaccine is recommended for workers with chronic respiratory disease or heart disease and for those who are older. The philosophy and policies of the company, the state medical society, and the occupational health physician are all involved in the decision as to whether workers in a particular establishment will be given flu vaccine. This may be done at no cost to the employee or for a fee. The staff may also recommend that workers go to their own family physician or to a city health department clinic for this inoculation. Nurses need to have ready access to information from the USPHS Center for Disease Control (CDC) when flu vaccine is advised. They need to confer with the physician and management on how they are to proceed. It is a good idea for nurses, before asking for a policy statement, to work out a tentative plan they believe will be effective if a program is to be undertaken. When a policy statement has been issued, nurses develop the program, order the necessary vaccine and syringes, announce the program, and carry it out.

For Travelers

The travel that workers must do can be a challenge to nurses, for they must be prepared to get workers and sometimes their families ready to go to distant lands, often on very short notice. This consists of protecting them against diseases they may encounter and usually consists of inoculations, instructions on how to protect their health from water supplies that may not be as safe as they are used to, and explanations of sanitation practices that must be understood lest their differences not be appreciated.

For Tetanus

Tetanus is a toxemia due to an endotoxin produced by *Clostridium tetani*. It results from contamination of a wound that is not exposed to oxygen, often a penetrating wound. In humans the incubation period is between 5 and 10 days, which allows for spore germination, growth, and toxin production, with the development of symptoms of toxemia.[10] Nurses working for heavy industry and construction where trauma injuries are possible recognize the need and the value of a universal tetanus immunization program based on a policy that states who is eligible and how the program is to be administered. It is suggested that the health histories taken at the time of employment include information about when each person last had a tetanus shot. When an applicant is found not to have had the first three inoculations, the nurse explains the program and secures the worker's cooperation in obtaining them. The nurse gives the first injection of an adult-type toxoid and sets up appointments for the second and third injections not less than 4 weeks apart and for a reinforcing injection about 8–12 months later. If and when a booster is required because of injury and time since the last shot, this information is recorded on the worker's immunization record.

Compliance with OSHA Standards

The intent of the requirements for medical surveillance were discussed in Chapter 7. It can be anticipated that, as OSHA promulgates new health standards, each one will require that the employer provide medical surveillance and worker-training activities. The OSHA Health Standards currently in force require medical surveillance, environmental monitoring, and worker-training activities. They also require that a respirator program include all the facts discussed on page 105. There must be evidence that these programs are in place and available to the workers, and such evidence must be available to the OSHA compliance officer upon request (see

App. D for the requirements if workers are exposed to vinyl chloride at or above the "action level"). The record-keeping requirements are also stated in the standards (see (m) "Records" and (n) "Reports," of App. D). The Occupational Safety and Health Act of 1970 has determined, and increasingly in the future will determine, what must be done for workers whose jobs involve working with toxic substances. There must be evidence that the management of the establishment has a plan that includes all required activities and that this plan is known to the workers and is being carried out for the protection of worker health.

The three sources of information that are of help in planning and conducting such a program are the relevant OSHA standard, the NIOSH Criteria Document dealing with the substance, and the book, previously cited, *Occupational Diseases: A Guide to Their Recognition*. For those health professionals who work in establishments where one or more of the carcinogens are in use, there is urgent need to be involved in protecting worker health. Two particularly useful publications are the DHEW/NIOSH *Carcinogens Regulations and Control*, GPO No. 017-033-00259-2, $2.10, and the DHEW/NIOSH *Working with Carcinogens*, GPO No. 017-033-00258-4, $1.90, both published in 1977.

References

1. Gove, P. B. (Ed.). *Webster's Third New International Dictionary*. Springfield, Mass.: Merriam, 1966, p. 1362.
2. Ibid., p. 483.
3. NSPB. *The Wise Owl Club of America*. New York, 1979, p. 2.
4. Personal communication from J. O'Neill of the NSPB, Sept. 1979.
5. O'Neill, J. E. "Use of Contact Lenses in Industrial Environment," *Sight-Saving Review*, Vol. 47, No. 3, Fall 1979, pp. 131–134.
6. Ibid., p. 132.
7. Messite, J. *Reproduction and Work*, paper presented at the New York Academy of Sciences, Feb. 21, 1979.
8. Ibid.
9. Warshaw, L. "Non-Medical Issues Presented by the Pregnant Worker," *Journal of Occupational Medicine*, Vol. 21, No. 2, Feb. 1979.
10. American Academy of Pediatrics. *Report of the Committee on Infectious Diseases*, 18th Ed. Evanston, Ill., 1979, pp. 284–287.

PART **IV**

Primary Care

Workers do get sick and some are injured because of hazards in the work setting. The occupational health nurses' role as providers of primary care is the focus of Part IV of this book. The third of the four sets of correlative activities that are the parameters of a comprehensive occupational safety and health program for workers is:

PRIMARY CARE

Identification of occupational or general health problems by medical and/or nursing diagnosis to determine care required

Management and continued care of the individual as an ambulatory consumer or referral for specialized care and rehabilitation

The nurse as a member of the occupational safety and health team:

- Participates in the formulation of the occupational health unit's protocols that determine the extent of the primary care and the medical surveillance program
- Provides primary care for workers who have been injured or become ill at work
- Counsels and/or provides crisis intervention for workers experiencing interpersonal, family, and/or work-related problems that interfere with or have the potential for interfering with ability to carry on regular work.

CHAPTER 9

Occupational Primary Care

As members of occupational health teams, nurses provide primary care for the workers who have been injured or become ill at work. "Primary care consists of either or both of two types of care: (1) care the consumer received at the point of contact with the health care system; and (2) the continued care of the individual as an ambulatory consumer. Primary care is two dimensional in that it includes (1) the identification, management, and/or referral of health problems; and (2) the maintenance of the consumer's health by means of preventive and promotional health care actions."[1]

The extent to which occupational health nurses provide primary care to workers depends upon three factors. First, there is a requirement in the workmen's compensation law that the employer is to provide medical care for employees who have work-connected injuries and illnesses. In many establishments this is the reason for employing a nurse. Treatment of illness or injury in an occupational health unit extends from first care for a major problem that requires safe handling and quick transfer to a hospital to complete ambulatory care for minor injuries and illnesses.

The second factor that influences the nurse's involvement in primary care is the legal definitions of nursing practice and medical practice in the state in which a nurse works. All states have laws that define and delegate areas of professional responsibility. The medical practice acts assign to the physician the legal responsibility and ultimate accountability in matters involving medical care. The nurse practice acts assign responsibility and acocuntability for nursing care and set the boundaries within which a nurse performs both dependent and independent nursing functions. As professional persons nurses are responsible for their own actions or inactions. The standard of conduct that should be expected of occupational health nurses is the same as that expected of any prudent professional with the degree of expertise which corresponds to the educational preparation required for licensure as a professional nurse.

The third and most influential factor is the working relationship established between a nurse and the physician. Ideally this relationship permits the physician to be responsible for the medical aspects of the program and for the nurse to be responsible for providing most of the services. The physician provides written directives for the care of injured or ill workers. These directives are incorporated into the occupational health unit protocols and should be so written that they permit the nurse, who functions as the physician's agent, to provide the primary care that is required. It is important that the employer specify at the time of engaging a physician that he or she is to be available for consultation with the nurse about how to proceed when special circumstances arise. A collaborative doctor-nurse relationship is essential to an effective occupational health program.

Sometimes it is difficult to distinguish occupational from nonoccupational diseases. Few workers present with specific pathogenic, clinical, or laboratory findings. The bronchitis associated with byssinosis (brown lung) can be accurately diagnosed only when an employee's occupational history indicates that, at some time, cotton dust has been present in his or her work environment. The importance of the history of exposure has double value in that the condition may then be considered to be covered under workmen's compensation, but of equal importance, environmental control of the exposure can be implemented.

The major form of primary prevention is the control or elimination of a known toxic substance from the work environment. Establishing the cause-and-effect relationship between an exposure and an occupational illness is difficult at times, but it is essential if the aim of the occupational health care, namely the protection of worker health, is to be achieved. The essence of primary care is a combination of diverse services and knowledge and/or information about them. Access to primary care is not merely access to a series of therapies for injuries and simple or chronic illnesses; it also involves access to preventive medicine and to public health measures. Beyond access to them there must also be access to knowledge about health and illness, information about treatment services, and understanding of why and how to use both.

Too many people regard health services as something that a professional provides for them. The patient or client—and in occupational health, the worker—is viewed as passive, the health professional as active. But the great health problems of our era—those that are self- or environmentally-produced—do not lend themselves to a laying on of hands.[2] These must be dealt with primarily by the client or worker, and to deal with them, he or she needs knowledge about them. The health professional rendering primary care must be both teacher and therapist.

There are almost as many definitions of *primary care* as there are speakers and writers who deal with the subject. Some attempt to define it in terms of the knowledge and skill of the provider. Some explain it in terms of the severity or the incurability of the patient's illness or disability. Others include in their definition the prevention of disease and the enhancement of health. Still others think of primary care as consisting only of the first contact an ill or injured person has with a care provider. However that first contact is more often than not with a provider working in a secondary or tertiary care establishment. The skier with an obviously broken leg needs the services of the ski patrol, an emergency room and X-ray equipment, and an orthopedic surgeon. The worker who has been splashed by an acid spill needs immediate first aid; in reality he needs to be put into the drench shower and to flush his eyes at the eye fountain. Recovery depends on the first-aid care that fellow workers help him to get and on the accessibility of wash fountains; the worker may or may not have to go to the hospital for care. Occupational health nurses continue the care started at the site of injury; their assessment determines what additional care is required. Their teaching of first aid and what to do if a chemical gets onto the skin or into the eyes is a part of primary care as practiced in occupational health.

Primary care as provided by nurses in occupational settings has the following characteristics:

1. It is given primarily for conditions that have a work-connected cause or for those that can be aggravated by work.
2. When given for non-work-caused health problems the conditions are usually self-limiting or of a stable chronic illness nature that respond well to a recognized treatment plan.
3. In addition to cure as a purpose the care provided has the aim of helping the person be able to function on the job, whether the problem is arthritis, a heart condition, or a second-degree burn.
4. The care provided reflects the nurse's recognition of the need
   a. To involve the environmental specialists—safety professionals and industrial hygienists—in the data-gathering process to establish causes of illness or injury and to assure that any environmental hazard is corrected as a means of primary prevention.
   b. To refer and to stay involved until the referral results in a treatment plan that others will carry out or in guidance as to how the nurse should proceed to treat the patient.

The protocols a nurse follows when providing primary care are developed jointly by physician and nurse. They reflect the amount of autonomy and decision making regarding diagnosis that both agree are within a nurse's ability to perform. Alternative means of treatment are delineated. Contraindications are listed. The availability of the physician is specified. Decisions to refer workers to the physician are made by the nurse. The care plan includes directing a worker to come back at any time if a dressing needs to be changed and/or if he has any questions or is worried. The proximity between the nurse and the worker makes close surveillance of the health problems possible.

The Occupational Nurse–Physician Relationship

More has been said about the occupational health nurse's need for medical direction than about any other doctor-nurse relationship. Guides for writing standing orders for occupational health nurses have been prepared by local, state, and national medical and nursing organizations. In 1955 the Council on Industrial Health of the AMA published *Guiding Principles for Industrial Nurses*. This statement, a revision of the council's earlier publication *Standing Orders for Nurses in Industry*, and other similar statements have focused on the occupational health nurse's need for medical direction. Yet only when the nurse works with, not for, the physician, does a safe and adequate working relationship exist. However such a relationship is often difficult to establish because it is only in the large establishment that the physician will work full time. The usual pattern is for the nurse to be a full-time employee and for the physician to work part time or as a consultant who does not come into the health unit routinely.

Unlike the hospital nurse, the occupational health nurse sees the injured or ill worker first, exercises clinical nursing judgment, and provides primary care. It is this handling of health problems before the doctor sees the employee that has caused, and continues to cause, some concern. There may be a significant delay between the time the nurse provides the initial care and the time the employee is seen by a physician. For many injuries the total care is provided by the nurse. This may include redressings and treatments over a period of time for as long as the healing process is progressing normally.

Loosely drawn-up medical orders, labled standing orders and signed by a physician who has little or no contact with the workers, the nurse, or the industry, do not give the nurse liberty to practice medicine. Signed medical orders are important, but they should never be considered a substitute for proper medical management. If the nurse has any doubt or the worker gives any indication of concern, then the nurse should have the option of referring the worker to the physician for care and/or of discussing with the physician the care the nurse will give. The ideal working relationship between the nurse and the physician is one in which both respect the abilities of the other, work together, and confer on what is to be done.

The term *protocol* is associated with the nurse practitioner movement. It is a written document that includes a statement of the condition in medical terms, (e.g., second-degree burns), the usual diagnostic procedures to be followed, and the critical elements of therapeutic management. The major difference between protocols and medical orders for the occupational health nurse is that protocols are much more detailed and include instructions for the continued care that ends in discharge from therapy. When protocols are prepared jointly by the nurse and the doctor, each learns how the other functions; and once developed, the resulting protocols become the modus operandi of the unit (see pages 136–137 for examples of a health unit protocol).

A collaborative relationship between occupational health nurse and physician can be established only when the physician comes into the establishment often enough to carry out the medical responsibility for the continuing care of injured workers. The ideal occupational health nurse–physician relationship is not a destination to be reached but a road to be traveled. The team relationship develops as physician and nurse work together and learn to trust each other. Each must feel secure in his or her professional ability; each must have respect for the other's profession as well as a conviction that the skills and understanding of both are required if workers are to receive optimal care. The scope of both medicine and nursing changes with each advance in knowledge. Yet despite changing and overlapping responsibilities, the nurse is still responsible for nursing care, the physician for medical and surgical care. It is imperative that nurse and physician understand that nurses are liable and responsible for the decisions they make and the procedures they perform.

In summary, the relationship of working with, not for, involves the following concepts. The doctor is legally responsible for the conduct of the medical aspects of the occupational health program. To fulfill this responsibility the doctor needs to come into the plant to work directly with the nurse. The nurse needs to be able to make a nursing diagnosis to determine a worker's needs for care, then proceed to treat those she can treat effectively and safely, referring others to the physician or to selected medical specialists. The nursing care plan she makes aims for safe and prompt handling of the problem by personnel in the hospital emergency room or the physician's office. Nurse and physician must be satisfied that the treatment the nurse provides is in the best interests of the worker and is legally and ethically sound. If the nurse goes beyond her area of competence, she may be guilty of practicing medicine or of nursing malpractice. If the nurse does not or cannot function as an expert nurse practitioner, the occupational health program will fall short of its maximum potential.

Nursing Diagnosis

As a basis for giving care, nurses make nursing care plans, but before they can do this they must make a nursing diagnosis. The diagnosis is in turn based on their observation of a patient, the data they gather from interviewing the patient, tests they may perform, and their evaluation of this data.

A nurse's first observation is likely to be concerned with a patient's consciousness and breathing. Are the respirations rapid and shallow or deep and labored? What is the color and condition of the skin? Is there any evidence of bleeding, internal or external? Of shock? Are any of the muscles contracting involuntarily? Does the patient appear to be acutely ill? How extensive do the injuries appear to be, that is, are tendons or nerves involved? Is there any swelling or redness or malalignment of extremities?

Then, if the situation is not an emergency requiring that the patient be sent immediately to the hospital, the nurse checks temperature, pulse, respirations, blood pressure, and muscle control and performs screening tests, for example, a urine test for sugar. When indicated, the nurse also performs an electrocardiogram, takes an X ray, or takes blood to test for carboxyhemoglobin.

While gathering the facts and putting them together, the nurse evaluates them and considers the questions What does this mean? Where have I seen this combination before? What are the possibilities? Is this a major or minor illness? Does any occupational factor play a part? Using the gathered facts and her own judgment, the nurse decides what the problem is and what needs to be done. Making a nursing diagnosis is as much a part of nursing and as important to successful functioning as the medical diagnosis is to the practice of medicine. Each nursing technique and procedure should be carried out, not automatically, but according to the needs of each situation and each worker, who is at that moment the nurse's patient. The occupational health nurse observes, asks questions, tests, and decides what needs to be done.

When faced with a worker who complains of headache, for example, the nurse will ask, "How long have you had this? Where do you work? Do you have frequent headaches? Show me where it bothers you?" While talking to the worker the nurse observes the person's color and general appearance. Does the patient look tired? Is the worker's breathing labored? The nurse checks the person's temperature, pulse, respirations, and blood pressure. The answers to the questions, the observations made by the nurse, and the results of the tests may add up to what seems to be a simple headache possibly caused by too late hours the night before and little or no breakfast. Or it may add up to the conclusion that the patient is ill and is in no condition to work. In the first case the worker is given aspirin or, if allergic to this drug, Tylenol, and the nurse suggests a stop at the cafeteria for a light lunch. In the latter case the worker is put at rest and plans are made to transport the worker to the hospital, to a doctor's office, or to a health maintenance organization (HMO) to which he may belong.

If it appears that the headache may be the result of carbon monoxide build-up in the work area, the nurse alerts the first-line supervisor of this possibilty and calls in the safety professional and/or the industrial hygienist. Prevention of a similar overexposure to others takes precedence, as the worker with the carbon monoxide caused headache is now out of the area. This worker may or may not be sent back to work, having been cautioned to not smoke and given aspirin if discomfort continues after having breathed oxygen under controlled conditions in the health unit.

The ability to make a nursing diagnosis and to take appropriate action develops with training and experience and is a significant factor in the occupational health nurse's involvement in primary care. One who merely knows how to carry out nursing procedures and does not understand the principles underlying the procedures cannot make a nursing diagnosis. More is involved than the usual data gathering about a patient; the nurse must know how to obtain data about the work place exposure and know the possible toxic effects of substances used in production.

Records

The nurse records information about the worker's health problem so that the relationship between a complex situation or a single stress agent, and the worker's response can be established. As part of the record-keeping responsibility the nurse completes the OSHA forms as required. It is important that this data be available for OSHA and for management, since it becomes the basis for corrective action. The nurse also completes the worker's compensation form so that the worker's rights are protected. The employee's records should be set up so that the person's problems can be identified by the several health professionals who work with the employee and so that progress or lack of it in terms of health promotion can be identified. See Chapter 20 for a more detailed discussion of record keeping and the role of the nurse.

References

1. ANA, Council of Primary Health Care Nurse Practitioners. *Operational Guidelines*. Kansas City, Mo., 1977, p. 1.
2. Rogers, D. E. "The Challenge of Primary Care," *Daedalus*, Vol. 106, No. 1, Winter 1977, p. 91.

Selected Readings

Ardell, D. "From Ombibus Tinkering to High-level Wellness: The Movement toward Holistic Health Planning," *American Journal of Health Planning*, Vol. 1, No. 2, Oct. 1976, pp. 15–33.

Brown, M. L. "The Implication of Research for Occupational Health Nursing Practice," *Occupational Health Nursing*, Vol. 24, No. 1, Jan. 1976, pp. 10–12.

Egdahl, R. H., and Walsh, D. C. *Industry and H.M.O.'s: A Natural Alliance*. New York: Springer-Verlag, 1978.

Egdahl, R. H., and Walsh, D. C. *Containing Health Benefits Costs: The Self-insurance Option*. New York: Springer-Verlag, 1979.

McMichael, A. J. "An Epidemiologic Perspective on the Identification of Workers at Risk," *Occupational Health Nursing*, Vol. 23, No. 1, Jan. 1975, pp. 7–10.

Rogers, D. E. "The Challenge of Primary Care," *Daedalus*, Vol. 106, No. 1, Winter 1977, pp. 81–103.

Terris, M. "Approaches to an Epidemiology of Health," *American Journal of Public Health*, Vol. 65, No. 10, Oct. 1975, pp. 1037–1045.

CHAPTER 10

First-Aiders in an Occupational Setting

First aid is the immediate care given to a person who has been injured or has suddenly been taken ill. Such care, when provided by a prepared health professional in an occupational health unit, is called primary care. The health professional is held responsible for his or her actions to the extent that this person has had preparation for giving first aid. Hence the physician is held to a standard of care expected of a physician, the nurse to that expected of a professional nurse. In an effort to remove the fear of malpractice suits arising from the rendering of emergency care, many state legislatures have enacted various laws giving statutory immunity from suit. These Good Samaritan laws protect the physician who, for example, stops at the site of an automobile accident to offer aid to the victims. The physician does not have at that time or site the support services or equipment that he would have at his usual place of practice; can give only first aid, not primary care; and is protected by the Good Samaritan legislation.

OSHA requires that a first-aider be employed (29 CFR Subpart K, 1918.51). This is the minimum coverage as set forth in the regulations for the small establishments that cannot justify the employment of health professionals. It is not required if a full-time nurse is employed.

Depending on its size and type, an industry may need to employ a corps of workers also trained as first-aiders even though it also has an occupational health unit staffed by professionals. This is especially true in plants where chemicals are manufactured or used. Another situation which requires employment of trained first-aiders occurs when an industry is spread out over a wide area and workers are located a long way from the health center. Lives and vision are saved by instant and adequate first-aid care. The person who has a heart attack while at work has a much better chance of surviving if someone who really knows how to give cardiopulmonary resuscitation is readily available. The worker who has had a chemical splashed into an eye or the worker caught in an environment that does not support life needs instant expert first aid, and this can be given by well-prepared nonprofessional personnel. A corps of prepared first-aiders who are recognized as the first line of defense can quickly swing into action when necessary. It is important for them to recognize that they must work cooperatively with the occupational health nurse or nurses to the end that workers get effective first aid when required.

When the health unit staff consists of only one nurse, it is wise for her to have one or more trained first-aid workers to call into the health unit for back-up should a true emergency arise. The need for this type of help must be interpreted to management and arrangements made for when and how the nurse can call for this person's help. There may need to be an item in the occupational health unit budget to cover the salary of a first-aider called away from his or her usual job to work in the health unit. For example a nurse dealing with a very anxious, upset person aims to help the person reduce the feeling of panic as quickly as possible. To do this the nurse needs to stay with the person, which is easier to do if there is a person trained in first aid to provide the first-aid care for others who may have been injured.

Another wise use of trained first-aid personnel is to have one assigned to the health unit for certain periods each month. During these times the nurse schedules counseling sessions with workers and is free to work with them while the first-aider staffs the health unit. To be successful this type of planning requires that both the nurse and the person with first-aid training recognize what each can do, have respect for each other's competence, and be willing to work together until trust is established and they learn to support each other. Similarly a first-aid worker can be assigned to work part time in a health unit so that the nurse can be out in the work areas doing walk-throughs or participating in planned health and safety training for employees.

Special protocols will be required for the first-aid person working in the health unit. These should be written to guide the first-aider and determine what he or she is to do. A special treatment tray should be set up for use by first-aid personnel in the absence of the nurse. First-aid records should be established that will permit the person giving first aid for minor injuries to record this. Only when the care given by first-aiders is recorded can an assessment be made of what if any are the safety and health problems that arise during the hours covered by the first-aid personnel. A record of what problems the first-aider is called upon to deal with and how the person makes the decision to do what needs to be done should be reviewed by the nurse, who discusses the situation with the first-aider and when indicated, calls in the injured or ill worker for evaluation by the nurse and/or physician.

Training

The American Red Cross (ARC) and the Bureau of Mines of the U.S. Department of the Interior have long experience in training people to give first-aid care to workers. In 1950 the Detroit Industrial First Aid Advisory Committee published the *First Aid Guide for the Small Business or Industry*. It was up-dated in 1977 and is based in part on the ARC's and the American Heart Association's first-aid manuals but with the procedures modified by experts on the committee to fit the special needs of an industry. This reference book is recommended as the manual of choice for the industrial first-aider, especially when this person is responsible for care when no health professional is on duty. (See page 302 for availability of this publication.)

Many occupational health nurses hold ARC instructor certificates and conduct first-aid training courses. Others arrange for the workers to attend training sessions conducted by the ARC or other agencies in the community. The teaching of cardiopulmonary resuscitation (CPR) is frequently a responsibility that the occupational health nurse assumes. Many also teach the Heimlich maneuver.

Both the nurse and the first-aid personnel need to know about the local emergency medical services (EMS), and the phone number should be posted so that no one need spend time looking for it if and when the EMS is required. Inviting key personnel into the establishment from the emergency medical service and/or the ambulance service can mean that those people will be better able to respond if and when their service is required, since they have seen the area and the routes of entry and egress.

In a Disaster Situation

During a disaster, as at no other time, it is essential that the first-aider and the occupational safety and health professionals be able to work together smoothly. This requires that each:

1. Know her or his own and the others' roles in the fulfillment of the objectives of the disaster plan
2. Know the special skills and abilities of the others
3. Know the others by sight so that if confusion reigns they can spot each other and be able to communicate effectively
4. Know the disaster plan and be able to function accordingly.

The old saying that an ounce of prevention is worth a pound of cure is the basis of any disaster control plan. One of the objectives of a safety and loss control program is to prevent explosions and major fires. However such human-caused and natural disasters as floods and hurricanes do strike. It is essential that communities have a disaster plan that people know about and in which they know how to fulfill their roles in order to control loss of life and property. An occupational health department disaster plan should be a part of the overall industrial health plan, which in turn, is a part of the community's plan.

The occupational health disaster plan will need to deal with the special hazards, if any, of the industrial process. Plans made ahead of time with the local hospital for special handling of persons who have been injured or made ill from very toxic substances can prevent contamination of the hospital emergency room, which could put it out of service until decontamination could be accomplished. This can be prevented by having a prior agreement with the hospital whereby the person or persons are not taken into the emergency room but into a room set-apart that will be maintained by the industry. This is very important if there is any possibility that those injured in a disaster can be contaminated by a radioactive substance.

The storage of supplies is an important part of a disaster plan. Supplies should be rotated through the normal supply so as not to be left in storage beyond the safe shelf life of medications and other materials needed to handle care for the injured.

The AMA publication *Guide to Developing an Industrial Disaster Medical Service* provides information about the key issues to be dealt with in making such a plan and in its implementation if and when this is required.

Selected Readings

AMA, Council on Occupational Health. *Guide to Developing an Industrial Disaster Medical Service*. Chicago, 1967.

ARC. *Advanced First Aid and Emergency Care*. Garden City, N. Y.: Doubleday, 1973.

ARC. *Standard First Aid and Personal Safety*. Garden City, N.Y.: Doubleday, 1973.

Braker, W., and Mossman, A. L. *Effects of Exposure to Toxic Gases—First Aid and Medical Treatment*, 2nd Ed. Lyndhurst, N.J.: Matheson Gas Products, 1979.

Comprehensive Health Planning Council of Southeastern Michigan, Detroit First Aid Advisory Committee. *First Aid Guide for the Small Business or Industry*. Detroit, 1977.

DHEW. *The Ship's Medicine Chest and Medical Aid at Sea*, Pub. No. HSA 78-2024, GPO: 017-029-0026-6. Washington, D.C., 1978.

Emergency Care and Transportation of the Sick and Injured. Menasha, Wi.: Banta, 1971.

Warner, C. G. *Emergency Care Assessment and Intervention*. St. Louis: Mosby, 1978.

CHAPTER 11

Occupational Illnesses and Injuries

Occupational Illness

The term *occupational disease* is used to identify any illness or any abnormal condition or disorder other than one resulting from an occupational injury, caused by exposure to environmental factors associated with employment. It includes acute and chronic illness or disease which may be caused by inhalation, absorption, ingestion, or direct contact. Of particular concern is the increased incidence of cancer and the part that work exposure plays in the causation or aggravation of chronic illnesses.

Except for occupational dermatoses, the occupational health nurse seldom sees a classic case of occupational disease. This is because so many years must elapse between exposure to a hazardous substance and the appearance of the chronic illness that is also an occupational disease. This can be 20 years, as for example asbestosis and the asbestos-caused lung cancer of workers who have been exposed to asbestos, and for angiosarcoma in workers who have been exposed to vinyl chloride.

That is not to say, however, that occupational diseases do not occur in much less time. Chrome ulcers do develop; workers exposed to lead and mercury do have increased body burdens, and occasionally neurological symptoms and signs will be manifested. Employees who work with methyl butyl ketones have developed peripheral neuropathy. Exposure to arsenic can cause workers to develop mild tracheobronchitis, and ulceration to perforation of the nasal septum has been reported from exposures to chromates and arsenicals. Spills and other accidents expose workers to irritating chemicals with the result that some develop an acute respiratory illness, and the distress of pulmonary edema may necessitate their hospitalization.

Historical Overview

Commenting on occupational health in the early part of the century, T. Hatch said: "Control of occupational diseases has been effective more or less in direct proportion to the specificity of the separate disease etiologies, that is, in proportion to the certainty with which the causative agent was known and could be located and measured in the environment and the equal certainty with which the disease was recognized and its level could be measured in man."[1] At that time, the objective in occupational health programs was to prevent frank cases of specific occupational disease which took the form of unquestioned illness and which could terminate in serious disability or death. Hatch was referring to the cases of "phossy jaw" that occurred as a result of the absorption of yellow phosphorus by workers in the match industry and the cases of lead poisoning in battery workers and brass foundry workers that were common in the early part of this century.

The author of *Alice in Wonderland*, as a commentary on the hazards associated with working in the hat industry, made the rabbit mad, had him exhibit symptoms of mercury poisoning, and dressed him in a tall fur felt hat. Mercury poisoning was common among people who were employed in making felt hats. The felt was made from rabbit fur treated by a mercury process, and workers were exposed to high levels of mercury as they converted the felt into hats. In the early 1940s an epidemiologic study of mercury intoxication as an occupational disease was conducted by the USPHS Bureau of Industrial Hygiene in cooperation with the Bureau of Industrial Hygiene of the Connecticut State Department of Health. This study proved the relationship between mercury in the work environment and the health problems of employees in the several Connecticut establishments that made men's felt hats. Symptoms included feelings of inadequacy and fear, tremors, changes in handwriting, and high blood levels of mercury. This study illustrates very nicely the teamwork that goes on between industrial hygienists and physicians of the federal and state health agencies and between employers and the unions. See the selected readings at the end of this chapter for reports and books that describe other epidemiologic studies that match with certainty environmental exposure levels with the level of workers' ill health.

Recently we have become more aware that certain industrial work environments contribute heavily to the cancer death rate. However the first direct connection between an occupational exposure and risk of specific type of cancer was that between chimney sweeping and cancer of the scrotum, pointed out by Percivall Pott in 1775.[2] He recognized this association because he saw the disease in several chimney sweeps but little or none of it in persons engaged in other occupations. In 1895 the German surgeon Rehn published his perceptions on bladder cancer among dye workers and pointed out the association between the high frequency of the disease and the dye exposure of the workers. Joseph Wagner, speaking at the Conference on Occupational Carcinogenesis held by the New York Academy of Sciences in March of 1975, reminded the audience that this year was the 200th anniversary of the discovery of occupational carcinogenesis by Percivall Pott. He went on to say, "Today as we enter into the second two hundred years since Percivall Pott, the problems of occupational carcinogenesis are greater, more visible yet more subtle, and more pervasive than they were in the past."[3]

What goes on in industry has an impact on the community. We live in a chemical age and have done so since World War I. Humans continually and increasingly create most of their environment. Past director of the National Institutes of Health (NIH) Robert S. Stone recently stated that "most known environmental carcinogens are a result of our increased agricultural and industrial technology."[4] Indeed it has been established that over 700 new chemicals are introduced into industry each year, most without any prior testing to evaluate the potential for carcinogenesis. Furthermore it has been estimated by the WHO that 75–85% of all cancers are related to our environment.[5] During this period of rapid change, the causes of death have also shifted; in the technically advanced countries, communicable and infectious diseases have been replaced by cancer as the principal cause of death.

Chemical Hazards

Portals of Entry

Only when potentially hazardous substances are present in sufficient quantity and in a form that can be taken into the body does a chemical hazard exist. There are three main portals of entry for toxic substances:

1. The mouth. Substances that enter the body via the mouth are absorbed through the gastrointestinal tract. Of the three routes, oral ingestion is of the least importance in occupational health, provided that good personal hygiene and sanitation programs are established and enforced. This means no eating and no smoking allowed in the work area; handwashing before eating; showers and clean work clothes when necessary; and separate clean eating and smoking areas. The importance of these practices must be incorporated into health education program planning and into the work habits of the supervisors, who must understand and accept the responsibility of requiring workers to conform.

2. The lungs. Inhalation is the route of greatest concern in occupational health. The OSHA Standards spell out the requirements of a respirator program. These include a health assessment of the workers' respiratory systems, the fitting of the proper respirator for the exposure, and training to assure that employees understand why and when the respirator must be worn, how to wear it, and how to care for it. The adult lung has an enormous tissue interface. This large surface, together with the extensive blood capillary network, makes possible an extremely rapid rate of absorption of gaseous substances.

3. The skin. Certain substances are absorbed through the intact epi-

dermis. The notation *skin* in the OSHA Standards for a toxic substance refers to the potential contribution to the overall exposure by the cutaneous route, including mucous membranes and the eye, either by airborne, or more particularly, by direct contact with the substance. Calling attention to all body surface areas capable of absorbing toxic substances is intended to suggest appropriate preventive measures so that the threshold limit is not invalidated. Good work and health practices include the provision and use of handwashing and shower facilities, clean work areas, and sometimes, special protective clothing and equipment.

Registry of Toxic Effects

Section 20(a)(6) of the Occupational Safety and Health Act requires that NIOSH publish annually a list of all known toxic substances and the concentration at which toxicity is known to occur. First published in 1971, *The Toxic Substance List* contained information on approximately 8,000 substances. The present publication is entitled *Registry of Toxic Effects of Chemical Substances*. The book is revised annually by NIOSH and is printed by the GPO, from which it is available. It can also be obtained on microfiche which is updated quarterly.

The 1977 edition contains listings of 26,478 different chemical substances along with their associated toxicity data. Of these approximately 4,700 are new chemical compounds which did not appear in the 1976 edition. The registry includes all data on positive findings in studies of humans and the lethality, mutagenicity, teratogenecity, and carcinogenicity in vertebrate animals exposed to specific toxic substances at a specific dose level.

The Registry enables the occupational health professional to:

1. Locate toxicity data, chemical name, and synonyms for compounds when only a trade name or common name is known
2. Obtain information about relative toxicity of an offending substance
3. Locate quickly the relevant U.S. Environmental Health Standards for a particular compound
4. Identify toxic compounds through the physical description and definition for each compound
5. Determine quickly the relative acuteness of toxicity in cases of accidental exposure
6. Identify potential chemical hazards in the work place
7. Anticipate hazards that may be created by use of a substance
8. Identify possible toxic effects of substances on the basis of their chemical structure.

Hazards

Health hazards are identified as chemical, physical, and infectious agents which cause injury as well as mental and organic disease. A pharmacological classification of the chemical agents and the related physiological effects of exposure to them is included here to indicate the wide scope of the medical effects occupational exposures may have. It is intended as a guide for the development of medical surveillance programs and primary care activities of an occupational health service. It permits an assessment of the scope and number of protocols that must be developed if a nurse is to provide safe and optimum care for workers who are injured or who become ill from work-related causes. The classification has eight categories:

1. Asphyxiants
2. Irritants
3. Narcotics or anesthetics
4. Systemic toxins
5. Pneumoconiotic agents
6. Dermatitis-producing agents
7. Cancer-producing agents
8. Mutagenic and teratogenic agents.[6]

Asphyxiants

Agents that interfere with the supply or utilization of oxygen are asphyxiants. These may be simple asphyxiants which displace oxygen (e.g., gases such as helium, methane, or carbon dioxide) or chemical asphyxiants such as carbon monoxide or cyanide. Carbon monoxide poisoning results from a combination of the gas and hemoglobin to form a compound, carboxyhemaglobin, which cannot transport oxygen to the tissues.

Irritants

Biological or chemical agents that elicit an inflammatory response of the surface tissues of the lungs or gastrointestinal tract constitute the irritant category. The lung's response varies from coughing caused by inhalation of such gases as chlorine or ammonia fumes, to pulmonary edema from exposure to ozone and phosgene.

Narcotics or Anesthetics

Any of the agents that blunt the senses and produce euphoria, stupor, coma, or death constitute the narcotics and anesthetic category. Examples are the alcohols and most solvents.

Systemic Toxins

Agents that produce change and damage to visceral organs are known as systemic toxins. The heavy metals such as lead and mercury are general protoplasmic toxins that produce adverse changes that may lead ultimately to death of tissues. Carbon disulfide and nitrobenzene cause nervous tissue damage. Carbon tetrachloride and chlorinated hydrocarbon are liver and/or kidney toxins, and benzene is a bone-marrow toxin.

Pneumoconiotic Agents

Dusts are pneumoconiotic agents. The heavier the dust exposure, the more likely it is that it will have an adverse effect on a worker's respiratory system. Coal miners often develop bronchitis. Pneumoconiosis is the accumulation of dust in the lungs and the tissue reaction to its presence, for example silicosis with silicotic nodules, coal worker's pneumoconiosis with coal macules from carbon and silica, and asbestosis with interstitial fibrosis.

Dermatitis-producing Agents

Direct causes of occupational dermatitis may be grouped into five major categories:

1. Mechanical agents: Friction and pressure may result in injury to the skin.
2. Physical agents: Heat, cold, sunlight, and radiation all can cause damage to the skin.
3. Biological agents: Included in this group are bacteria, fungi, and parasites
4. Botanical agents: Plant poisons are a frequent cause of dermatitis.
5. Chemical agents: Included in this group are primary irritants and sensitizers. The primary irritants include acids and alkalis. These agents react on contact. Some are likely to affect most people, and many will affect all individuals. It is estimated that four out of five cases of industrial dermatosis are due to primary irritants.

Unlike the primary irritants, the sensitizers affect only a small number of persons exposed to them. These chemicals have little or no effect upon the initial contact. However, certain individuals suffer a change in body chemistry following a subsequent contact, and serious symptoms may develop. Dermatitis is the most common occupational disease. The skin is the largest organ of the body and is vulnerable to many insults from the environment. Predisposing factors in dermatitis include skin pigmentation; for example dark skins are less susceptible to skin irritants than light skins.

Age is also a factor; young workers seem to be particularly susceptible to acnelike lesions. Preexisting skin diseases are believed to predispose the worker to the occupational dermatoses.

Cancer-producing Agents

Cancer is a term used to identify a certain type of disease. It is not one specific disease but many diseases each with its own history and characteristics. Cancer is characterized by uncontrolled growth of abnormal cells. NIOSH has identified well over 1500 carcinogens, substances that are suspect because of evidence that they have produced mutagenesis, teratogenesis, or carcinogenesis in biologic systems ranging from cell cultures to man. A carcinogen may be a physical agent, like ionizing radiation (such as X-rays) or a nonionizing radiation (such as ultraviolet light). It can be a particle like asbestos. It can be a chemical agent such as calcium chromate.

The link between scrotal cancer and the exposures of the London chimney sweeps to the hydrocarbon in the soot was recognized in 1775. In 1974 the connection between vinyl chloride and angiosarcoma of the liver was established. One cannot usually tell the cause of a human cancer. A case of lung cancer from the chemicals in cigarette smoke may be identical with a cancer from an occupational exposure. Mesotheliomas caused by asbestos is an exception. It has been estimated that 80 percent of all human cancers are caused by factors in the environment and are at least theoretically preventable. It is estimated that approximately 5 percent of the cancers can be attributed directly to occupational exposures. These are preventable, hence the need to establish the cause and effect relationship.

Lung cancer accounts for about 14% of all cancer cases and for 22% of all cancer deaths. Cigarette smoking is the predominant cause in both sexes,[7] but increased risk of lung cancer has also been reported in asbestos workers, coke oven workers, uranium miners, workers in certain metal smelting and refining plants, and in workers in some branches of the chemical industry. Generally incidence has been found to be proportional to the dose or duration of exposure to the carcinogen. Variation in individual susceptibility is possibly due to either genetic or immune factors.[8]

Teratogens. Agents that produce structural abnormalities. The thalidomide catastrophe made the general public aware of the fact that a pregnant woman's exposure to a toxic substance can endanger her unborn child.

Dr. J. Warkany, speaking at the Conference on Women and the Workplace held in Washington, D.C., June 17–19, 1976 said:

There is ample proof that adverse environmental factors can deform human embryos and fetuses. These proven factors are not numerous and they are very heterogeneous. Environmental teratogens in man include iodine deficiency (which caused endemic cretinism), carbon monoxide, X-rays, toxoplasmosis, rubella, and organic mercury, which caused Minamata disease.[9]

Mutagens. Compounds that cause heritable alterations in the DNA and damage the embryo.

In this century, man has sought to use chemicals to raise the quality of life. Among these chemicals are those that by their usage alone touch many aspects of life in this country: drugs, pesticides, food additives, industrial chemicals, etc. "With hindsight, it is now not too surprising that some of these substances have had unintentional results. Some widely used chemicals have been shown to induce adverse, chronic effects such as carcinogenic and mutagenic responses."[10]

The finding that some man-made chemicals presently in widespread use in the population are mutagenic in subhuman experimental systems suggests that such chemicals constitute a potential genetic hazard for man. The risk poses itself to both present and future generations: to the former, as the production of genetic lesions in somatic cells, possibly leading to cancer; while to the latter, as the production of transmissible gene mutations and alterations in chromosome structure and number.

"Unfortunately, comprehensive data on the incidence, variety, distribution, and etiology of actual gene mutations and chromosomal aberrations has not been compiled. Estimates on the occurrence of true genetic disease in the population would indicate that 12 million people carry defective genes or chromosomes that manifested themselves with birth defects."[11]

Seldom will all of these agents be found in any one work establishment, although nurses who work in chemical manufacturing industries soon learn that the work environment contains a wide variety of hazardous materials which, if not controlled by engineering methods and safe work practices, can affect workers' health. A nurse must be prepared to provide care for workers made acutely ill from such hazards as well as be able to spot the possible relationship between symptoms workers identify and hazards associated with their jobs. The book *Occupational Diseases: A Guide to Their Recognition* was used as the basis for this section. Available from the GPO, it is one nurses will find useful as a handy desk reference.

Nonchemical Hazards

Physical conditions in the work area can also cause harm. In Chapter 3 references were made to:

1. Abnormalities of air pressure
2. Abnormalities of temperature and humidity
3. Noise
4. Chronic friction

Occupational Illnesses and Injuries

5. Environmental stress
6. Occupational radiation (radioactive substances, ultraviolet and infrared rays, microwaves, and lasers).

Abnormalities of Air Pressure

Nurses working at construction sites, especially those which utilize compressed-air shafts, caissons, or hyperbaric chambers, must be aware of hazards associated with too rapid decompression following use of such equipment. The danger is that nitrogen bubbles may form in the bloodstream and body tissues. Workers on jobs in the building of bridges or tunnels may develop caisson disease, commonly called "the bends."

People who work at high altitudes, particulary aviators, can be exposed to low atmospheric pressure and consequently, may be subject to blackouts or loss of consciousness as a result of lowered oxygen pressure.

Abnormalities of Temperature and Humidity

The body regulates its internal temperature within narrow limits. All too often, "hot" jobs also involve heavy work. Workers exposed to furnaces, as in the manufacturing of steel, or to the sun, as in dam-building operations in desert areas, may develop heat cramps, heat exhaustion, or heat stroke. Workers exposed to cold and dampness may develop frostbite, especially of the feet and hands.

Noise

The words *sound* and *noise* are used interchangeably, but generally sound is used to describe useful communication or something pleasant like music, while noise is used to describe discord or unwanted sound. The sensation of sound or noise is produced when sound waves reach a responsive ear. The men and women who work on the flight lines of airports where jet planes land and take off are exposed to the noise of the jet engines. Those who work at making tin cans and those who work in coal mines and in textile mills weaving cloth also have a noise hazard. Their prolonged exposure (time and level of noise) causes many of these workers to develop a hearing loss.

Chronic Friction

Vibration, produced by repeated motion and pressure, causes friction, which may, if extreme, cause serious or permanent damage. Workers who operate pneumatic tools or ride tractors or large earth-moving machines are frequently exposed to high levels of vibration. Reports indicate that they develop changes in bone structure, and some reports have identified more widespread systemic effects. In less serious cases, blisters and callouses may form on the hands, and the involved muscles may be painful for several days. Compressed-air drill operators sometimes develop "white fingers" associated with Raynaud's phenomenon. It is estimated that eight million workers in the United States are exposed to occupational vibration. Most of these people are engaged in transportation, farming, and construction work.

Environmental Stress

The word *stress* is used by both psychologists and physiologists in their consideration of workers' health. Some jobs produce a state of worker stress so great as to impair task performance and cause ill health. "For the individual to experience stress as an undesirable state, three conditions are necessary: a basic susceptibility to stressors in general; exposure to a significant change in environment or interpersonal relations; and interpretations of the change as a stressor and that it is dangerous and threatening."[12] Stress as a life experience is as inevitable as pain or anxiety; yet complete freedom from stress is death.

A simple concept for interpreting stress is that stress is a positive or a constructive force depending on whether one handles it or it handles one. "Within the context of ergonomics, work stress is defined as any action of an external vector upon the human body, while work strain manifests itself as a physiological response to the application of stress."[13] Stress and strain do not necessarily happen together. The person who works in a very hot environment may experience heat stress; the resulting sweating is referred to as heat strain.

Occupational Radiation

The National Council on Radiation Protection Measurements defines *harmful effects* as "any body injury, disease or impairment, except when such condition is transitory, infrequent, or of short duration and does not endanger persons so affected."[14] Health problems associated with radiation include both burns that laboratory workers or technicians can get from X-rays and eye damage from exposure to laser beams. Glassblowers sometimes develop ultraviolet conjunctivitis, better known as "flash." The bone sarcoma that radium dial painters used to develop is well known as an occupational disease which is, fortunately, now controlled by engineering and good work practices.

Recognition of the increased risk of exposure to ionizing radiation and the development of cancer, including leukemia, among workers in the nuclear power plants, research laboratories, and laboratories making radioactive isotopes has resulted in the development of special environmental and medical surveillance programs. "The safety standard established by the Federal Radiation Council stipulates that occupational exposure of the whole body and the most radiosensitive organs of the body (the bone marrow, lens of the eye, and the gonads) should not deliver a cumulative dose (in rems [roentgen equivalent man]) exceeding five times the age of the worker (in years) beyond age 18. A worker aged 28, for example, would be allowed a cumulative total dose of up to 50 rems."[15]

Occupational Injuries

An *occupational injury* is any condition major or minor, such as a cut, fracture, sprain, or amputation, which results from a work accident or from exposure involving a single incident in the work environment. It is relatively easy to establish the cause-and-effect relationship in a case of occupational injury compared to one of occupational illness. For example if a worker dropped a carboy of perchloric acid, was not burned, and hence, having no obvious injury, did not see a health professional at the time and only later developed chest pain and presented himself at the hospital emergency room, valuable time could be lost because the occupational cause might not be considered.

The provision of care for workers injured at work is an essential service of an occupational health unit. An appreciation of the extent of the problem—the number and type of injuries that can be expected—determines the size of the professional staff and the amount and type of medical and treatment supplies required. Most of the injuries will be minor; many require no more care than that specified by the OSHA definition of first aid. That is, for OSHA recording purposes, it is not necessary to record those injuries that do not require more than one-time treatment or subsequent observation of minor scratches, cuts, burns, splinters, and so forth, which do not ordinarily require medical care even though such care may have been provided by a physician or other health professional. Although the nurse is not required to record such injuries on the OSHA Log, the basic data about what happened, when, where, and how, and the result, whether it be a scratch, loose foreign body in the eye, or first-degree burn, should be recorded in the worker's individual record along with the information locating the injury as to body part and what care was provided.

Occupational illness and injury data collected by the OSHA Logs and reported by the Bureau of Labor Statistics reveals that:

- Job-related injuries and illnesses continued at virtually the same rate in 1977 as in the previous year—9.3 injuries and illnesses per 100 full-time workers as compared with 9.2 in 1976.
- Approximately 5.3 million work-related injuries occurred during 1977, an in-

crease of 300,000 from the 5.0 million level of 1976. Exposure hours increased at approximately the same rate.
- Nearly 162,000 recognized occupational illnesses were estimated for 1977 compared with 168,000 for 1976.[16]

The NSC, on the basis of preliminary data, estimated in April of 1979 that there were 13,000 deaths from work accidents in 1978. Wage loss, medical expenses, and administrative and claim settlement costs of insurance for work accidents in 1978 amounted to $10.8 billion.[17]

The causes of occupational injuries were listed in Chapter 5. Types of injuries include lacerations, contusions, fractures, burns, sprains, and tenosynovitis as a result of repeated motion. The complications of infection, nerve and tendon involvement, and embedded foreign bodies must be dealt with. Amputations can and do occur. Eye injuries require special care and great nursing skill so that no additional damage is done.

The occupational health unit protocols should spell out the care to be provided for injured and/or ill workers and should include the follow-up care they are to receive from the nurse. Major emergencies require that planning and training be done beforehand and that the staff maintain their level of competence and skill.

Nursing Care

The basis for nursing care of workers injured or made ill from a work-place hazard is a nursing evaluation of a person's need for care. Nurses must get answers to the following questions:

1. What signs and symptoms of illness or injury does the worker demonstrate or explain to the nurse and what does the nurse observe?
2. What was the worker doing? What happened?
3. What was the worker's degree of exposure?
4. How long has the worker felt as she or he does now?

Nurses also need to have access to the following data:

1. What systemic effects can be anticipated if someone has been exposed to the substance involved in the episode that brings the worker to the health unit?
2. Can the substance cause tissue damage?
3. Can the substance have a delayed effect?
4. Does the worker have a history of chronic illness? If yes, what medical care plan is being followed?

The nursing diagnosis is the basis for the primary care nurses then provide. This may be to arrange for transfer to the hospital. It may be to arrange for the person to be seen by the occupational health physician, dermatologist, or other specialist. It may be to clean and dress burns on worker's ankles caused when, for example, a carboy of perchloric acid was dropped off the back of the truck by another worker during unloading. The nurse's care will include anticipatory guidance as to what both workers are to do if they develop chest pain or have difficulty breathing after going home or during the night. Perchloric acid can cause irritation of the respiratory tract; hence the need to alert exposed workers.

The information gathered to make the nursing diagnosis is recorded, as is the nursing care provided. The safety professional is told of the accident, and she or he or the nurse will alert the janitor as to how to clean up and to dispose of the broken glass but not before the safety professional or the foreman determines if the area where the accident occurred is safe to enter. Nursing care of people involved in an occupational accident that involves a chemical exposure of necessity requires that some one be concerned about the other workers so that they are not harmed.

To give effective nursing care it is necessary for nurses to know what materials are used in the plant and what by-products result from the manufacturing process that might be toxic and hence hazardous to health. Nurses can work with safety professionals, industrial hygienists, and someone from purchasing to develop a list of these substances. All the pertinent data can be recorded on individual safety data sheets or incorporated into a toxicology chart that summarizes the information for all the substances used. Information that needs to be readily available includes:

1. The name of the substance
2. The chemical formula for the substance
3. The pharmacological classification of the substance
4. The OSHA TWA and/or the TLV of the substance
5. The areas in the establishment where the substance is used
6. The mode of entry of the substance into the body
7. The symptoms of acute and chronic exposure
8. The emergency care for acute symptoms, and primary care protocols for definitive handling of an illness episode
9. The special precautions to be taken, if indicated, upon an affected worker's return to work.

Knowing where the person works as well as the potential hazards of that area and the signs and symptoms the substances can produce gives nurses clues to use in making a nursing diagnosis, especially when providing care for an unconscious worker or one showing evidence of acute respiratory distress. The history that the occupational health nurse takes includes asking the workers questions about when the first symptoms were noticed, what the symptoms were, and whether they have become more or less severe since first noticed. Nurses also ask: what happened and were there any breaks in techniques or changes in the usual operating procedures? The data generated by such questions can be most helpful, especially if the substance to which a worker was exposed involves the respiratory tract, the skin, or the nervous system and if there is evidence that the cause might be work-connected.

Acute exposure to chemicals that are respiratory irritants requires that the nurse be aware of those which may have a delayed effect so that the care provided makes certain that workers and a significant number of others know what to do if an emergency should develop after a worker has gone home. If a worker is sent to a hospital it is wise to alert the hospital and the physician to the actions of the substance that the person was exposed to. The OSHA Standards require that the employer make medical guidelines information available to the physician to whom a worker made ill from an overexposure is sent for care. In addition all other pertinent information is made available to the doctor, including the amount of the substance, what the worker was doing upon becoming ill, what body systems are at risk from the overexposure, and any other information in the worker's health records regarding that person's level of functioning prior to exposure.

Another kind of delayed reaction can arise when a welder or a fellow employee is exposed to the ultraviolet light from the welder's torch. Hours after the exposure, a very painful eye condition may develop that brings the uncomfortable, sometimes very anxious, worker back to the health unit or to the emergency room of a hospital.

The functions of the nurse in the provision of primary care for workers who have been injured or made ill from work-connected causes include:

1. Participation in the formulation and updating of the unit's treatment protocols
2. Participation in the development of the policies that spell out:
   a. Extent of care to be provided
   b. What hospital or treatment centers are to be used
   c. What physicians are to be called as referral sources when specialized care is required, and who can make the referral
3. Provide care that is appropriate, safe, and humanistic
4. Provide and coordinate the continuing care to assure the recovery of the worker
5. Record the facts so as to protect the rights of the worker and of the employer.

The toxic hazards workers may be exposed to determine what protocols nurses need to develop for use if and when workers require first-time care. When such care must be provided by a first-aid worker, it is essential that this person be given special training to assure that the care provided is safe. Some of the factors that need to be taken into consideration when developing the scope of first-time care that must be planned for include:

1. The toxic substances and the mechanical hazards associated with the production process
2. The age and sex of the people in the work force
3. The distance to the nearest hospital
4. The amount of time during the workday that the health unit is staffed by health professionals
5. The medical-nursing climate of the community
6. The extent of the nurse's responsibility for giving care
7. The ability of the nurse to make a nursing diagnosis and provide care as an expert nurse practitioner.

Rehabilitation

Rehabilitation must be started as soon as possible after a person has been injured. The process is also important when workers become ill with chronic diseases like arthritis or diabetes. When major surgery is required for cancer of the breast or colon the hospital nurses who provide nursing care for these people need to be aware of what work these persons do and incorporate planning for their return to work into the nursing care plans. The rehabilitative process requires that very specialized services be utilized to help the injured and ill person attain the highest possible level of functioning of which he or she is capable. Major surgery for cancer and treatment of chronic illnesses create a very real need for special planning if the person is to return to work. These services, in addition to medical and surgical care, may include fitting the person with a prosthesis and teaching him or her to use it or how to be mobile in a wheelchair or specially fitted automobile. It may involve making arrangements for the person to learn new skills. One of the essential activities is helping him or her deal with a loss of function or change in appearance.

Equally important, and often hard to maintain, is people's confidence in their ability to handle what must be done to support a family throughout the period of rehabilitation. Serious industrial injuries may result in paraplegia or quadriplegia. Burns may cause extensive scarring and limitation of motion; accidents may result in amputation or blindness. Workers who become very sensitive to substances in the work environment may have to change jobs, and this sometimes involves retraining.

Back injuries require very special handling lest victims become "cripples." Some workers have very low pain thresholds, and some whose job and self image are less than satisfactory may retreat into illness as an unconscious means of coping. Consequently behavior modification experts and industrial psychiatrists are sometimes involved in helping to rehabilitate injured employees. When the cause is accepted as work-connected, workmen's compensation insurance frequently pays for the rehabilitation services.

In less serious injuries occupational health nurses with special training in physiotherapy techniques may be involved in treating workers with sprains, bursitis, tenosynovitis, and loss of function following fractures. A few large industries employ physiotherapists and have an equipped physical therapy department. Others send employees needing such therapy to a local hospital or private facility in the community.

Nurses become involved in rehabilitation when they provide first-time care for seriously injured workers. Helping workers understand what is happening to them and why is important. Remember that even very seriously injured people can hear. It is essential that nothing be said that can be misinterpreted or that gives the worker the idea that the case is hopeless. One nurse who was preparing a worker for transfer to a hospital following a very serious penetrating injury to his right eye covered both eyes and immobilized the man's head with sandbags for the trip to the hospital. The foreman asked the nurse how serious the injury was as the stretcher was placed in the ambulance. Her answer and the fact that the man did not know why *both* his eyes had been bandaged resulted in hysterical blindness which lasted for months following the accident. The patient withstood the surgery for the removal of his right eye but insisted that he could not see with the other eye. He kept repeating, "The nurse said it was very serious." Had she provided a few words of explanation—"John, I'm covering both eyes so as to keep you from moving your eyes on the way to the hospital"—and given a less cryptic answer to the foreman's questions, she might have started this man on his way to recovery and saved him from months of anxiety and expensive therapy.

Rehabilitation as seen in industry, is often the end result of the cooperative efforts of many people. It is the restoration of the handicapped to the fullest physical, mental, social, vocational, and economic usefulness of which they are capable. This is necessarily a complex process involving all segments of society. No single program, official or voluntary, is complete in itself. Actual services are usually provided to civilians by voluntary or other nonofficial programs. Federal programs offer chiefly financial support, except to veterans. State programs may provide hospital care. However the final phases of rehabilitation involving job training and work adjustment are generally carried out at private nonprofit rehabilitation centers. Frequently occupational health departments provide rehabilitation services for their own employees.

Many states support rehabilitation services in designated state hospitals. General hospitals are making increasing efforts to develop some phases of rehabilitation, sometimes under county or city auspices, sometimes independently. Services are offered for ambulatory patients as well as those confined to the hospital. Rehabilitation centers have grown to meet the needs of patients after convalescence. These are people who may be physically able to do certain jobs but who lack the training and speed to carry on competitively. Different types of therapy—physical, occupational, speech, and hearing—as well as vocational training and work adjustment or temporary sheltered employment may be provided.

Several insurance companies carry on active rehabilitation programs for workers with compensable conditions. State compensation acts often provide for payment for restorative services for workers with compensable injuries. The United Mine Workers Welfare and Retirement Fund provides rehabilitation services for disabled miners.

Rehabilitation is a program of many disciplines including medicine. The person with a heart condition benefits from rehabilitation as much as the worker who has had a traumatic amputation of a leg. Rehabilitation is a method of approach to total care of the sick or injured. To be fully effective, rehabilitation requires an organized program with four phases, one or more of which apply to every sick or injured worker. The first is medical diagnosis; the second is medical and surgical care. In these two phases, treating the whole person is most important, for mental care is as important as physical care—sometimes more important. The third phase consists of vocational counseling and training by vocational and educational experts. This is a broad category and includes training the severely handicapped in the activities of daily living as well as helping the less severely handicapped to learn new skills. Physical, occupational, and educational therapy constitute the fourth phase, although these activities also contribute to every step of rehabilitation. Often in the late phases of the program people are given work adjustment tasks or sheltered employment before going into competitive employment.

The occupational health service personnel play end-position roles in rehabilitation. They frequently give the initial professional first-time care. While giving first-aid to a seriously injured worker or to a very ill person, nurses must be careful of what they say about a person's prognosis. They must not make statements people may take to mean they are going to be blind or never able to work again. All occupational health personnel should see that the care given injured or ill workers is the best and that everything is done to assure early rehabilitation. In a modern occupational health program, rehabilitation and prevention go hand in hand.

References

1. Hatch, T. "Changing Objectives in Occupational Health," *Industrial Hygiene Journal*, Vol. 23, Jan.–Feb. 1962, pp. 1–7.
2. Wagner, J. K. "Occupational Carcinogenesis: The Two Hundred Years Since Percivall Pott," in *Occupational Carcinogenesis*. New York: New York Academy of Sciences, 1977, p. 1.
3. Ibid., p. 2.
4. Stone, R. S. *The Role of an N.I.H. Program in Carcinogenesis and Cancer Prevention*, paper presented at the Second Annual Carcinogenesis Collaborative Conference, San Antonio, Tex., 1973.
5. WHO, *Prevention of Cancer*. Technical Rep. Series 276. Geneva, 1976.
6. Messite, J. Adapted from classification prepared for publication (in preparation).
7. Fraumeni, J. F. *Persons at High Risk of Cancer*. New York: Academic, 1975, p. 223.
8. Ibid., p. 168.
9. Warkany, J., "Toxic Substances and Congenital Malformations." *Proceedings: Women and the Workplace*. Washington, D.C. Society for Occupational and Environmental Health, 1977, p. 28.
10. Bingham, E. "Introduction." Ibid., p. 6.
11. DHEW NIH, Pub. No. 75-370. *What Are the Facts About Genetic Disease?* Washington, D.C., GPO, 1974, p. 6.
12. Selye, H. *The Stress of Life*. New York: McGraw-Hill, 1956.
13. Dohrenwend, B. S., and Dohrenwend, B. P. (eds.). *Stressful Life Events*. New York: Wiley, 1974.
14. National Council on Radiation Protection and Measurements. *Basic Radiation Protection Criteria*, Rep. No. 39. Washington, D.C., 1971, p. 3.
15. Stannard, J. N. "Problems of Ionizing Radiation," one of three articles on "What Every Physician Should Know about Radiation," in NIOSH, *Occupational Safety and Health Symposium 1976*, GPO: 017-033-00249-5. Washington, D.C., 1977, pp. 22–45.
16. DOL, Bureau of Labor Statistics. *Results from the 1977 Survey of Occupational Injuries and Illnesses*, Program Bulletin No. 38. Washington, D.C.: GPO, 1978.
17. Hoskin, A. F. "For 1978 Preliminary Accident Report," *National Safety News*, Vol. 119, No. 4, Apr. 1979, pp. 90–91.

Selected Readings

Adams, R. M. *Occupational Contact Dermatitis*. Philadelphia: Lippincott, 1978.

Billmaire, D., Yee, H. I., Craft, B., William, N., Epstein, S., and Fontaine, R. "Peripheral Neuropathy in a Coated Fabric Plant." *Journal of Occupational Medicine*, Vol. 16, No. 10, Oct. 1975, pp. 189–195.

Buell, G. "Some Biochemical Aspects of Cadmium Toxicology," *Journal of Occupational Medicine*, Vol. 17, No. 3, Mar. 1975, pp. 189–195.

Burton, G. G., Gee, G. N., and Hodgkin, J. E. *Respiratory Care.* Philadelphia: Lippincott, 1977.
Casarett, L. J., and Doull, J. *Toxicology, the Basic Science of Poisons.* New York: Macmillan, 1975.
Creek, J. L., and Johnson, M. N. "Angiosarcoma of Liver in the Manufacturer of Polyvinyl Chloride," *Journal of Occupational Medicine,* Vol. 16, No. 4, Apr. 1974, pp. 150–151.
Damme, C. "Diagnosing Occupational Disease: A New Standard of Care?" *Journal of Occupational Medicine,* Vol. 20, No. 4, Apr. 1978, p. 251.
Jablan, S., "Radiation," Chap. 10 in NCI, *Persons at High Risk of Cancer.* New York: Academic, 1972.
Key, M. M., Kerr, L. E., and Bundy, M. *Pulmonary Reactions to Coal Dust.* New York: Academic Press, 1971.
Lloyd, J. W. "Long-term Mortality Study of Steelworkers: Respiratory Cancer in Coke Plant Workers," *Journal of Occupational Medicine,* Vol. 13, No. 2, Feb. 1971, p. 56.
McCormick, E. *Human Factors Engineering,* 3rd Ed. New York: McGraw-Hill, 1970.
McMichael, A. J., Gerber, U. S., Gamble, J. F., and Lednar, W. M. "Chronic Respiratory Symptoms and Job Type, within the Rubber Industry," *Journal of Occupational Medicine,* Vol. 18, No. 9, Sept. 1976, p. 611.
NIOSH. *Occupational Diseases: A Guide to Their Recognition,* Pub. No. 77-181. Washington, D.C.: GPO, 1977.
NIOSH. *A Guide to the Work-relatedness of Disease.* Pub. No. 79-116. Washington, D.C.: GPO, 1979.
NSPB. *The Occupational Health Nurse and Eye Care.* New York, 1972.
Roglieri, J. L. "Multiple Expanded Roles for Nurses in Urban Emergency Rooms," *Archives of Internal Medicine,* Vol. 135, No. 10, Oct. 1975, pp. 1401–1404.
Rummerfield, P. S., and Rummerfield, M. J. "What You Should Know about Radiation Hazards," *AJN,* Vol. 70, No. 4, Apr. 1970, pp. 780–786.
Schilling, R. S. F. (ed.). *Occupational Health Practices.* London: Butterworth, 1973.
Toxicological and Carcinogenic Health Hazards in the Workplace, Proceedings of the First Annual NIOSH Scientific Symposium. Park Forest South, Ill.: Pathotox, 1978.

CHAPTER 12

Workmen's Compensation Laws

Workmen's compensation laws are designed to provide a quick and fair means for handling problems relating to occupational disability. Six basic objectives underlie activities undertaken to carry out the intent of these laws.

1. Providing sure, prompt, and reasonable income and medical benefits to victims of work-related injuries and illnesses, or income benefits to their dependents, regardless of fault
2. Providing a single remedy for work-related injuries and illnesses with appropriate consideration for employer and employee
3. Relieving public and private charities of financial strain incident to uncompensated industrial illnesses and injuries
4. Reducing or eliminating costly and time-consuming trials, court delays and appeals, and payment of fees to lawyers and witnesses
5. Encouraging maximum employer promotion of safety and rehabilitation through an appropriate experience-rating mechanism
6. Reducing preventable accidents and human suffering through continuing study of causes of accidents and illnesses rather than concealment of fault.[1]

Workmen's compensation laws are federal and state statutes that establish:

1. The extent of the employer's liability
2. The amount of money payable to a worker for loss of wages due to occupational injury and disease
3. The circumstances under which the employer is responsible for the medical care to ill or injured workers and the procedures for providing this care and for payment of compensation.

Federal employees are covered by the Federal Employees' Compensation Act (FECA), which is administered by the Office of Workers' Compensation of the DOL. For cases in which the decision is disputed there is the

Employees' Compensation Appeals Board, a separate entity of the DOL authorized to hear and make decision on appeals from otherwise final determinations made by the Office of Workers' Compensation. Workers in the private sector generally are covered by state workmen's compensation acts; and workers, private or public, in the maritime industry are covered by the U.S. Longshoremen's and Harbor Workers' Compensation Act. There is also the Workers' Compensation Law of the District of Columbia.

History

Prior to the enactment of workmen's compensation laws an injured worker had to prove negligence on the part of the employer in order to recover lost wages or the cost of medical care. That is, the employer was liable for the employee's disability only to the extent that the employer could be proved negligent in a legal action which the employer could defend under the following common-law defenses:

1. *Assumption of risk.* Under this defense it was assumed that a worker was aware of and accepted the risks incident to the job. When the employer used reasonable care in the selection of workers and in providing a suitable work place for them, he was not responsible for injuries or diseases arising out of the risks that were common among similar occupations.
2. *Fellow servant rule.* Under this defense a worker who accepted a position took upon himself or herself the risk of fellow workers' negligent acts. The employer was not responsible for the results of the carelessness of the worker's fellow servants. In the past, the employer could often claim that a worker's injury was the result of an act of another employee. When the evidence supported this the injured worker had no legal recourse except to sue the fellow worker.
3. *Contributory negligence.* Under this defense if an injured worker contributed to her or his own injury through carelessness or negligence, the employer was not held liable.

Thus, before workmen's compensation laws were enacted, to gain redress for loss of earnings and the costs of medical care for an occupational injury or disease, workers had to prove through lengthy and often costly legal procedures that the employer was at fault.

Compensation laws did not develop spontaneously; they were the result of social and economic pressures. The common-law doctrine served the needs of the people at the time it was developed, for people then worked in small groups. Employers knew workers and probably their families as well; the work performed was not mechanized and hazardous. As more and more workers were employed by one employer, the common-law defenses more and more protected the employer but not the employee. Society, through public charity, bore the cost of occupational injuries and diseases. Workers so ill or badly injured that they could not work had no way to feed their families except through public relief or by taking them to a "poor farm."

Early Laws

In 1881 Switzerland became the first country to declare that for accidents occurring in certain types of employment the employer was to be held liable without any proof of fault. The German Industrial Act of 1884, supported by Bismark, is considered to be the first modern compensation law embodying the compulsory insurance principle. England adopted a law based on this compensation principle in 1897 and in 1906 amplified its provisions. The United States passed its first Workmen's Compensation law in 1908. This law protected only designated classes of the public employees. It became the Federal Employees' Compensation Act.

There was strong opposition from employers to workmen's compensation, and several of the early state laws were declared unconstitutional. Wisconsin's law was the first to become effective, in 1911. Between 1911 and 1921, the majority of the states and territories enacted compensation laws. The last state to pass a workmen's compensation act was Mississippi, in 1950. Over the years the laws have been amended, and provisions have been made for increasing the amounts paid for medical care and as compensation for lost wages. Increasingly, occupational illness as well as injuries have been covered by the acts.

Current Laws in the United States

Modern compensation laws are based on the concept that a worker is entitled to reasonable payment for wages lost during a disability arising out of a work-related or occupational injury or illness. In addition the laws provide that the employer is to pay for medical, surgical, and hospital care as well as for rehabilitative services for such injuries and illnesses. These costs are considered to be a legitimate part of the cost of production and, hence, are to be borne by the employer as a cost of doing business, not by the worker as a personal loss.

No state workers' compensation law covers all classes of employees. Agricultural workers, casual workers, domestic servants, and people engaged in nonhazardous employment are in classes sometimes excluded by some states. Certain states provide for exemptions to the law in part or in full if the employer has less than a stipulated number of employees (usually three). However provisions are frequently made for voluntary acceptance of the law by such employers.

All state compensation laws require the employer to buy insurance or to show proof of a financial reserve sufficient to cover the risk. Insurance may be bought through a state fund or from a licensed insurance company. The premium the employer pays is usually based on the average frequency and severity rates of occupational disability for the industry as a whole and on the frequency and severity rates of the particular firm for the 3 years preceding the purchase of insurance coverage.

The Chamber of Commerce of the United States publishes annually a summary of the changes in the state compensation laws. This is a useful publication, especially for anyone responsible for keeping records of compensation cases for employees covered by more than one state law. A copy of the state compensation laws should be on file, and the names, positions, and phone numbers of key people in the compensation administration should be readily available (see page 307 for availability of the Chamber of Commerce publication).

The 1978 edition of the Chamber's *Analysis of Workers' Compensation Laws* reported that all jurisdictions now have unlimited medical care coverage. Indemnity benefits were increased in 1977 in 51 jurisdictions. Of this number, 42 states now provide for annual automatic adjustments of benefits based upon the state average weekly wage. In 43 states, the maximum weekly benefits now equal or exceed 66 ⅔% of the average weekly wage for temporary total disability cases. Of these, 23 pay 100% or more. All jurisdictions now have broad coverage for occupational diseases. Minors are covered by workers' compensation acts in all jurisdictions, and some jurisdictions double compensation or levy penalties if a minor is injured under the conditions stipulated.[2]

Not all state compensation laws are compulsory; a few are elective. That is, an employer or the employees may or may not elect to place themselves under the provisions of the law. Employers who accept the act are generally exempt from damage suits instituted by their employees. When employers reject the law the common-law defenses are usually abrogated. They must also post notices telling their workers and prospective workers of their rejection of the law. When an employee rejects the act and sues an employer who has accepted the state law, the employer usually retains the common-law defenses. In 1976, 88.5% of all wage and salaried employees were covered by workers' compensation.[3]

Premium Rates

Premium rates for workers' compensation insurance are computed actuarily. Accident experience throughout the nation is collected by the National Council on Compensation Insurance. Member companies of the council report experience incurred under workers' compensation policies. This serves as a basis for workers' compensation rate determinations that are made in accordance with a standard nationwide rate-making procedure approved by the National Association of Insurance Commissioners. This procedure is traced to a conference held in 1915 when an agreement on rate making for compensation was established.

Reporting in the *Social Security Bulletin*, the DHEW estimated that employers spent $10.8 billion in 1976 to insure or self-insure their work-injury risks. This was almost $2 billion, or 22.5% more than the 1975 cost of workers' compensation. Medical costs totaled $2.33 billion in 1976, while compensation payments amounted to $5.13 billion—a total of $7.46 billion, or about 75% of all workers' compensation costs.[4]

Administration

Administration of the compensation laws differs among the states. Most states have created, by law, an adminstrative board or commission, and a few administer their law through the courts. The appointed commissioner, or commission, has the power to interpret the law, to hold hearings on compensation cases of questionable validity, and to adjudicate such claims.

A compensation hearing is less formal than a hearing in a court of law. In most cases the reason for the hearing is to establish the relationship of the injury or the disease to the worker's job. An introduction to the problem of determining whether an injury or illness is job related or occupational, with suggestions for those responsible for this aspect of workers' compensation administration, is a NIOSH publication, *A Guide to the Work-Relatedness of Disease*, Pub. No. 79-116.

Not all claims go through a hearing, as the laws provide for the prompt handling of claims for compensation when both the worker and the employer are agreed as to the validity of the claim, the amount of money payable, and to whom. Most claims are settled by a voluntary agreement which is reviewed by the state's compensation authority to ensure that the rights of the worker are protected.

The amount of compensation paid to a worker for loss of wages is usually a percentage of the average weekly wage. It is seldom equal to the average wage because it is generally believed that recovery is more prompt and complete when there is a financial incentive for the worker to return to work. Compensation payments are considered as partial indemnity for lost wages, not as a reward. Such payments may be made to the worker or to the worker's family until the worker is able to return to employment, or for several hundred weeks to life for total disability. Usually a waiting period of a specified number of days of disability must elapse after an injury before compensation indemnity payments are begun. The average waiting period for minor conditions is 3–7 days. In some states a worker who suffers a major disability that requires him or her to be away from work for an extended time is paid compensation that covers the time lost during the waiting period.

Compensation for "Second" Injuries

Most of the state and territorial laws contain provisions regarding payment of compensation for so-called second injuries. These provisions protect both the worker and the employer. They apply when a worker who has suffered an injury has a second accident that results in another such loss. The resulting disability from the two injuries must be greater than two times that of a single such injury. For example a worker who is blind in the right eye takes a job in which he sustains an injury to his left eye and is now totally blind. This, then is a permanent total disability. If the employer had to pay the compensation cost for such total loss, handicapped persons would find it difficult to get gainful employment. To solve this problem, second-injury funds have been established. If a second injury happens to a handicapped person, the employer pays only for the current injury, the remainder of the compensation payments being provided by the second-injury fund.

Second-injury funds are built up in several different ways. In some states a special charge is made against the employer or the employer's insurance company; in others, when a fatal accident happens to a worker who does not have any dependents to whom the compensation may be paid, the employer or the insurance company remits these payments to the second-injury fund. Some states require the insurance carrier or the self-insured company to pay into the fund a percentage of their total yearly compensation payments for one or more classes of disability. Once the fund has grown to a predetermined figure, further payments are not required until the fund has been reduced to a predetermined level.

Some states permit persons with physical handicaps to sign waivers whereby they legally waive their rights to compensation in the event of a subsequent injury or aggravation of the specified condition. A worker with approximately 35% loss of function of her right elbow due to a childhood accident, for example, may be asked to sign a waiver identifying the specific loss. If she later has an occupational injury to her right elbow that results in 100% loss of function, both she and her employer are protected by the waiver. The worker is assured of compensation for the additional loss, but the employer pays only the amount stipulated by law for 65% loss of function.

Reporting

In most states, occupational injuries and diseases are reportable conditions. Each state has its own requirements for reporting injuries, and these requirements vary. The U.S. Bureau of Labor Statistics is the federal agency that collects and compiles occupational injury rates, and the labor department in the state government is the responsible agency at the state level. The compensation authority in each state requires that all compensable conditions be reported to them.

The Williams-Steiger Occupational Safety and Health Act of 1970 mandated a comprehensive method for recording and reporting work accident and illness experience. Members of Congress felt that the American National Standard method of recording and measuring work injury experiences, Z16.1–1967, had grown too sophisticated in its efforts to assure uniformity of reporting and, in so doing, did not accurately reflect the actual occupational accident and illness experience. Therefore, in preparation for the new act, a study group was recruited by ANSI to develop a detailed report. Their recommendations were filed with the Secretary of Labor in August 1970 as proposed national system for uniform recording and reporting of occupational injuries and illnesses. These became the basis of the OSHA reporting system.

The American National Standards Institute

ANSI, founded in 1918, is a federation of leading trade, technical, and professional organizations, governmental agencies, and consumer groups. Its principal function is to act as a clearinghouse for coordinating the work of standards development in the private sector, which is currently carried on by nearly 400 different organizations. Through its procedures, competent, efficient, and timely development of standards is made possible; and a neutral forum is provided to consider and identify needed changes in standards.

In 1975 the American National Standards Z16 Committee (on Standardization of Methods of Recording and Compiling Accident Statistics) began work to make the American National Standard Z16.1–1967 compatible with the OSHA reporting system. It published ANSI Z16.4 in 1977 for uniform record keeping for occupational injuries and illnesses. A copy of this ANSI code is most useful and should be in every occupational health unit's library (see App. C for information about ANSI).

The ANSI Z16.4–1977 code covers the definitions and guidelines necessary to maintain basic occupational illness and injury records and incidence rates suitable for statistical purposes that are compatible with the record-keeping requirements of the Occupational Safety and Health Act of

1970. The three rates that are developed from the OSHA record-keeping requirements are: (a) the incidence rate of total recordable cases (in which all recordable cases are counted), (b) the incidence rate of death cases plus lost workday cases with days away from work (in which all recordable cases that resulted in death, plus lost workday cases with days away from work are counted), and (c) an incidence of lost workdays. This is a measure of severity.

The appendix of Z16.4—published in 1977—has two major sections numbered to match the appropriate section in the OSHA Standards: "(1) Definitions" and "(2) Measurability of Recordable Injury and Illness Experience." This latter includes "Table A1, Tabulation of Scheduled Charges." This is the basis for calculating incidence rates of lost workdays that is an alternative measure of severity.[5]

The National Commission

Congress set up the National Commission on State Workmen's Compensation Laws at the time it enacted the Occupational Safety Health Act of 1970. As noted in Section 27(a)(1) of that act, the Congress found that:

A. The vast majority of American workers, and their families, are dependent on workmen's compensation for their basic economic security in the event such workers suffer disabling injury or death in the course of their employment; and the full protection of American workers from job-related injury or death requires an adequate, prompt, and equitable system of workmen's compensation as well as an effective program of occupational health and safety regulations; and
B. In recent years serious questions have been raised concerning the fairness and adequacy of present workmen's compensation laws in the light of the growth of the economy, the changing nature of the labor force, increases in medical knowledge, changes in the hazards associated with various types of employment, new technology creating new risks to health and safety, and increases in the general level of wages and the cost of living.

This national commission was to undertake a comprehensive study and evaluation of state workers' compensation laws in order to determine if such laws provided an adequate, prompt, and equitable system of compensation. The commission was to make a final report, containing a "detailed statement of the findings and conclusions with such recommendations as it deemed advisable." This report was transmitted by the commission to the President and to the Congress on July 31, 1972.

The report reflects the evaluation of the state workers' compensation laws and the national commission's conclusions that state laws were not being enforced to their fullest potential and that there were many discrepancies in payments, coverage, and rehabilitative services to injured workers. Despite this negative assessment the commission indicated it was convinced that workmen's compensation is a fundamentally sound system and a valued institution in our industrial economy.

The commission stated that there are four basic objectives that should be the basis of a modern workers' compensation program. It also pointed out that to achieve these objectives it is essential that there be an effective system for delivery of benefits and services. The objectives, according to the commission, are:

1. To extend protection to as many workers as feasible and to cover all work-related injuries and diseases
2. To replace a high proportion of a disabled worker's lost earnings by workers' compensation benefits
3. To restore the injured worker's physical condition and earning capacity as promptly as possible
4. To use economic incentives in the program to reduce the number of work-related injuries and diseases.

The constructive criticism rendered by the commission gave new impetus to the further development and growth of workers' compensation laws, and many state laws now enjoy an increasingly prominent role within the social insurance system of the United States.[6]

The Nurse's Responsibilities

It is essential that the occupational health nurses know the benefits of the workers' compensation law in effect in the state they work in. It is also important for them to know how this law is administered. Because the injured or ill worker frequently reports the problem first to a nurse, nurses' records are important. What nurses tell injured or ill workers about rights to compensation is also important, and nurses should clear with management how they counsel workers in this regard.

It is not a nurse's responsibility to determine whether an injury or illness is compensable. The function of nurses is to provide primary care and to record the information the workers give them about injury or illness as well as the information they gather to determine the extent of the problem and the care needed. All such information is important and is used in the decisions made by the workers' compensation authority.

In disputed cases it is the adminstrator of the state law who makes the final decisions at the hearings, and these decisions are appealable generally to the courts. Occupational health nurses need to be familiar with all aspects of the workers' compensation law in order to help workers utilize the mechanisms set up to protect their rights under these laws.

References

1. Chamber of Commerce of the United States. *Analysis of Workers' Compensation Laws*. Washington, D.C., 1978, p. 3.
2. Ibid., p. 4.
3. Ibid.
4. Ibid.
5. ANSI, Z16.4, *Method for Uniform Recordkeeping for Occupational Injuries and Illnesses*. New York; 1977.
6. Ellis, L. "Workmen's Compensation and Occupational Safety: A Review and Evaluation of Current Knowledge," *Journal of Occupational Medicine*, Vol. 18, No. 6, June 1976, pp. 418–425.

CHAPTER 13

Nonoccupational Health Problems of Workers

Workers can and do get sick at work, and some come to work not feeling well. Sooner or later workers with one of the hundreds of disease conditions listed in the medical index will be seen by the staff of the occupational health unit. For every day lost from work because of a compensable injury or disease, many more days are lost by workers because of nonoccupational illness. These illnesses are exactly the same as those that affect people everywhere. They range from very serious conditions such as heart attack, diabetic coma, or rupture of a duodenal ulcer, which completely incapacitate, to such relatively minor conditions as toothache, dysmenorrhea, heat rash, or an upset stomach, which cause discomfort and may or may not interfere with ability to work.

The practice in occupational health is to give first-time care, counseling and guidance, and palliative treatment. These services both make it possible for workers to continue a productive day and contribute to shortening the ensuing disability. Occasionally a worker will come back to work with a burned hand which occurred when a packet of matches caught fire while lighting a cigarette. This is an example of a condition that requires care for two reasons: to prevent infection and to assure that the worker's work does not aggravate the condition.

Men and women in a work force come to the occupational health unit for a variety of reasons. Many of them come for health care for problems that, though not caused by their work, interfere with their ability to work. Others come for advice as to what if anything needs to be done for their problem. The variety of problems that nurses encounter in the course of a week is almost endless. The degree of severity of the problems is equally variable, ranging from simple headache to a major medical emergency such as a heart attack, which will require immediate care by a health professional. The first hours after a myocardial infarction are the most critical. One study report indicated that 63% of the deaths from ischemic heart disease among middle-aged and young men occurred within 1 hour of the onset of symptoms.[1] On the other hand a worker who comes to the health unit because of a mosquito bite will probably simply be advised not to scratch it.

Workers with less serious health conditions are provided care by a nurse. A policy should be developed that states the extent to which the occupational health unit staff is to provide definitive care and for what health problems. For the minor nonwork connected health problems, the staffs of many occupational health units have developed a philosophy that it is useless to recommend that workers see their own doctors, as they have learned that such referrals are frequently not completed. When the problem is self-limiting in nature and is known to respond well to an established regimen of care, and when the physician has established enabling protocols, the staff provides definitive care including prescribing medications, if the worker elects to have them do so.

The safety feature that both ill workers and the nurses have is proximity. Workers may go back to work and still come to the unit daily, if indicated, for reevaluation, and nurses can determine whether the treatment is curing the problem. This permits the nurses to make a specialized referral if it appears that the condition requires a more sophisticated type of treatment than the unit is equipped to handle.

Nurses' responsibility for workers who are seriously ill is to give them first-time care as quickly as possible and to get them under the care of a physician. It is imperative that medical and administrative policies for the handling of medical emergencies be established. The procedure manual and the physicians' standing orders should specify what nurses are to do in such situations. Administrative policy should establish the company's responsibility for transporting ill workers to their homes or a hospital and for notifying their families.

Special Programs to Control Special Problems

Occupational health professionals are involved in programs that aim to identify and control chronic disease problems. Because they know the employees and are known by the employees and because the staff of the O.H. Unit has the ability to do so, these health professionals carry on activities that permit them to identify problems. Sometimes they refer the person with a health problem to his or her physician for care. Increasingly they are offering the person the option of having the health unit staff supervise health care. Such services do not require a wide variety of complicated expensive equipment. Such programs do require direction from someone who understands and believes in prevention. For such programs to be effective there must be prepared staff who have the time and the opportunity to follow up. It is this that keeps the persons who enter into the program following the plan that has been made to meet their special needs and life styles.

Most people who have hypertension have mild to moderate elevation of pressure and respond well to relatively uncomplicated therapy. Pilot programs in which the health team approach has been used have conclusively demonstrated that it is possible to control the vast majority of hypertensive patients. The alternative to the current practice of one-to-one patient-doctor encounter not only increases the number of patients who may be brought under the care of a single physician, but more importantly, the quality of the care is improved emormously. One such ongoing program is the Cornell Work Site High Blood Pressure Control Program. Using a step-by-step protocol as a guideline for treatment, nurses and paraprofessional health workers have been able to provide most of the direct patient care required for long-term follow-up without risking safety or therapeutic efficiency.[2]

Experts continue to stress that many hypertensive persons have not been identified and many more are not being adequately treated. These facts and the fact that occupational health nurses can be and are involved in screening for hypertension and in providing supervision of those who are under medical care make a hypertension program an accepted part of an occupational health service. Several essential decisions need to be made. The first decision—to develop such a program—involves the physician, the nurse, and the representative of management who must collaborate in presenting the project to the workers in terms that say, in effect, "We are concerned about your health; we will provide the services that will help you, the worker, to learn whether you do or do not have high blood pressure and to stay under care." The second decision involves the development, by the doctor, the nurse, and management and worker representatives, of a policy that states the extent of the program and the part the nurse and/or nurses will play in it.

If the decision is to mount a high blood pressure control program, the nurse and the physician would be well advised not to try to reinvent the wheel but to secure copies of the protocols developed by one or more of the ongoing occupational health programs. The book *Hypertension: The Nurse's Role in Ambulatory Care*, edited by Michael Alderman, will prove exceptionally useful. Occupational health nurses who need to update their understanding of hypertension, its diagnosis and treatment, will find it of particular value.

Factors That Influence the Scope of Care

Health Care Costs

Increasing health care costs are a critical problem in the United States, and actions to contain these costs are being taken by a wide variety of agencies. The increase in the costs of health care, which are also felt in occupational health services, are increasingly influencing the practice of occupational health nursing. The proportion of the national resources allocated to the health care industry has increased dramatically. These expenditures have risen from $3.6 billion in the fiscal year 1929 to an estimated $162.6 billion in 1977.[3] As a proportion of the Gross National Product (GNP), the 1929 expenditures represented 8.8%. The per capita expenditures were $29.16 in 1929, $333.57 in 1970; and $736.92 in 1977.[4]

A major cause of this increase in expenditures has been a change in the source of reimbursement for health care services. The creation of the Medicaid and Medicare programs in the mid-1960s and the growth of private health insurance plans have resulted in a substantial decrease in the percentage of out-of-pocket payments. This decrease in direct payments and the corresponding increase in payments by third-party payers has hidden the full impact of spiraling costs from both the consumer and the provider of health care services. However the growing reliance on funds from public sources has brought increasing governmental attention to the problem and provided the impetus for the creation of cost-containment policies at all levels.

Analyses of personal health care expenditures have shown that per capita expenditures for hospital services, the most costly type of care, were over twice the amount expended for any other type of care in 1976.[5] There is also a disparity in third-party coverage in that existing plans provide extensive coverage for nearly all costs associated with hospital care but limit coverage for other types of health care services. Thus the existing payment mechanisms have provided little incentive for using alternative, less costly services and have, in fact, indirectly offered incentives for using the more costly hospital services.

Industry pays a significant percentage of the worker's health insurance costs in that hospital and medical care insurance as well as other types of health insurance are provided by management as fringe benefits. In 1977 the private sector paid 57.9% of the nation's health expenditures, with 42.1% being paid by the public sector.[6]

The Family's Impact on Worker Health

The impact of the family on the behavior of the worker has long been recognized. A person who comes from a home situation where little value is attached to getting places on time may have great difficulty getting to work on time. The worker who has been identified as having diabetes and whose wife is a Christian Science practitioner may have additional problems to handle as he learns about the medical care plan established for him and how to deal with his illness.

When workers are unable to deal constructively with their health problems, the occupational health nurse needs to be aware of and concerned about pressures within the family that contribute to the situation. Helping the worker to recognize the problem and to know what agency can help is a role the nurse must be able to fill. The occupational health nurse may or may not have the freedom to go into the home and provide therapy. A referral for family therapy is indicated when it is found that there are family problems that must be dealt with if a worker's behavior is to become more adaptive. Nurses need to know what services are available from the local agencies and how to help the worker use them. To do family therapy themselves, nurses need special preparation as well as time to get to know the family and vice versa.

The Nurse as the Workers' Health Advocate

The functions of the occupational health nurse as health care provider to workers with nonoccupational health problems include:

1. Knowing the people in the work force who are at risk from the standpoint of nonoccupational health problems and their personal health profiles
2. Planning and conducting health promotion activities that have as their purpose changing workers' behavior
3. Conducting screening programs so as to have data that can be used to make referrals and/or convince workers of the need to change a life-style
4. Reinforcing the teaching and medical regimens as set up for workers by their personal physicians
5. Intervening when changes in behavior or appearance are noticed to determine whether there is a problem and helping workers accept referral for care.

Lowering the incidence of cardiovascular disease and accident by limiting, reducing, or avoiding factors in the coronary-proneness profile is considered a most promising area for the application of predictive medicine. One need only look at the occupational health records of a group of workers who have had heart attacks to be able to identify the problem. Health professionals are knowledgeable people, but it is obvious that they often do not know how to help individuals accept recommendations. Obesity, hypertension, and smoking are identified in the record as conditions and behavior that must be modified. Year after year the same recommendations are made, and nothing happens except that the person gains more weight and smokes more—that is, until the emergency happens—the heart attack. One nurse recalls having said to the vice-president of her company as she took his blood pressure, "Mr. C., you are smoking too much and you are too heavy." He turned to her and said, "Mrs. X., that is none of your business." Her answer: "Sir, I'm sure that it is. My job is to help you stay well and if you don't begin to take care you are going to be incapacitated." Just 2 weeks later, while playing golf, Mr. C. died at age 52.

The needs of workers can be multiple. Occupational health nurses usually work within an adminstrative framework that permits them to deal directly only with those needs that are job-related and to provide services for the employee, not the family. Nevertheless nurses employed to work in occupational health have a great opportunity to be helpful to workers. They can function as their ombudsmen, as their teachers, and as the providers of primary care.

Translated literally, *ombudsman* means "on behalf of man." The ombudsman's role suggested for nurses is that of helping people to know their rights and to use the resources they have available. For workers who have few resources, who in the past have had less-than-satisfactory experience when in need of health care, and who do not have family physicians or dentists, occupational health nurses can be facilitators in obtaining care. They can smooth the way by helping to make appointments and by helping workers understand and accept their need for medical and dental care for themselves and their families. The long-term mangement of nonacute problems requires that someone be available to answer questions, to do health teaching, to provide dietary advice, to provide supervision of the medical care plan, and to watch for changes that require intervention. Occupational health nurse practitioners are increasingly being recognized as the professionals of choice to carry out these functions.

A Typical Day for the Occupational Health Nurse

A young man who has just begun to realize that he may possibly have contracted gonorrhea comes into the unit for confirmation and advice. He has told his supervisor that he had a headache and wanted to see the nurse. Depending on how busy the nurse is and the amount of privacy afforded each worker in the health unit, he may tell her about his concern or he may ask her for two aspirins and leave.

The nurse is called and told that there is a woman in the rest room hemorrhaging. As the nurse turns from answering the call the young woman, who has had a spontaneous abortion, is rushed into the health unit by three very excited, upset fellow workers.

One of the men who works outdoors comes to the health unit dressed in warm work clothes. He tells the nurse, "I feel terrible. I'm so cold." She takes his temperature, listens to his chest, and determines that this is a very sick man who probably has pneumonia. He lives alone in a mobile home miles away from work and travels to and from work in a car pool. All of these facts must be taken into consideration if the nurse is to provide the care this worker really needs.

Another worker comes into the health unit, and in response to the nurse's query, "Tell me how I can help you," pulls up the sleeve of his shirt and reveals an arm bandaged from just above the wrist to the elbow. He had been in a fight the night before, and his opponent had slashed him with a knife. The only care he has received was provided by a friend. He tells the nurse that he could not go to the hospital because the staff there would tell the police and that his assailant was his wife's brother.

On the same day the nurse may see a worker who has a cold, one with an upset stomach, or one with dermatitis on her hands from using a detergent to clean a rug. The worker whose husband is an alcoholic, and the young man who hurt his elbow playing tennis also come to see the nurse. They too need her attention.

To make nursing diagnoses and decisions about care for these and others who suffer illness or injury that is not work related the nurse will:

1. Collect information by questioning and by observing the worker so as to be able to determine the extent of the problem or problems
2. Provide first-time care that will prevent further damage and assure improvement of the patient's condition
3. Help the person with a communicable disease to recognize the need for communication with others who may also have been infected, so as to get them under care
4. Assure that her interventions do not establish her employer's liability
5. Record the facts so that, if a question arises as to the diagnosis, the care given, or the resolution of the problem(s), the data will be available for review
6. Stay involved until her responsibility for care is transferred to someone who is competent to provide the care the person requires
7. Abide by company policy and follow directions outlined in the occupational health manual
8. Make appropriate referrals and help the worker to accept the referral
9. Provide care in such a manner as to assure in so far as possible that the health problem as presented by the worker is not aggravated by work-related activities and so that it becomes a work injury covered by worker's compensation.

The Changing Role of the Nurse

The role of the occupational health nurse is inextricably tied to the scope of occupational medicine. This is being determined by the full-time medical directors who have responsibility for the health and safety of many thousands of workers. Although the fifth basic objective of the AMA's *Scope, Objectives, and Functions of Occupational Health Programs* revised in 1972 is "to encourage and assist in measures for personal health maintenance, including the acquisition of a personal physician whenever possible,"[7] "there is a predictable, albeit a gradual, shift to an inexorable reorganization of what is perceived as the health needs of this nation and of the mechanisms whereby those needs will be satisfied."[8]

Lorning Wood, Director of Medical Care for the Bronx's O.H. unit of the New York Telephone Company, who spoke at the Annual Meeting of the American Occupational Medical Association Health Conference in April 1975, presented the Telephone Company's concept called "health care management" (HCM). The three basic elements of HCM are:

- To deliver just enough care in-house to gain from the employees their authority to let us manage their health
- To document all employee health data confidentially
- To work closely with community care resources in treating those clinical episodes needing their services.[9]

The health care professionals who determine the policy for the Telephone Company based their plans for a HCM program on the fact that health care may be divided into seven parts. These are: health education, preventive measures, early detection, ambulatory treatment, hospitalization, rehabilitation, and after care. The occupational health professionals were well aware that the effectiveness of health care depends upon how well each part of the health care continuum is carried on. They were very aware that the cost of health care is loaded into the latter end of the seven part continuum. They believed that if one wants to reduce costs and improve out-comes the greatest leverage is in the front end of the health care continuum. Hence if the occupational health unit's health professionals were to deliver for the employees the front-end parts which require relatively less than their share of total systems facilities, capital, and organizational structure, the total costs would be less and the total quality of health care better.

The costs of medical care, the emphasis being placed on prevention and early diagnosis, the involvement of individuals in decisions about their care, and the nurse practitioner movement all are influencing and will influence the role that the occupational health nurse will be called upon to play in the provision of care for workers who have stable chronic illness problems and acute self-limiting disease.

References

1. Pace, N. A. "An Approach to Emergency Coronary Care in Industry," *Journal of Occupational Medicine*, Vol. 15, No. 10, Oct. 1973, p. 793.

2. Alderman, M. H. (Ed.) *Hypertension: The Nurse's Role in Ambulatory Care*. New York: Springer, 1977, pp. 120–121.
3. DHEW, Social Security Administration. *Social Security Bulletin*, April 1977–July 1978. Washington, D.C.: GPO, 1978, p. 3.
4. Ibid., Table 6.
5. Ibid., Fig. 15.
6. Ibid., Table 5.
7. AMA, Council on Occupational Health. *Scope, Objectives, and Functions of Occupational Health Programs*. Chicago, 1972, p. 6.
8. Warshaw, L. J. "Patterns and Perspectives," C. O. Sappington Memorial Lecture, *Journal Occupational Medicine*, Vol. 6, No. 8, Aug. 1966, p. 353.
9. Wood, L. U. "The Bronx Study—A Trial of Health Care Management," *Journal of Occupational Medicine*, Vol. 17, No. 10, Oct. 1975, pp. 648–651.

Selected Readings

Alderman, M. H. "Organization for Long-term Management of Hypertension," *Bulletin of The New York Academy of Medicine*, Vol. 52, 1976, pp. 697–717.
AMA, Council on Occupational Health. "The Role of Medicine within a Business Organization," *Journal of the AMA*, Vol. 210, Nov. 24, 1969.
ANA, Council of Primary Health Care Nurse Practitioners. *Operational Guidelines*. Kansas City, 1977.
Capell, P. T., and Case, D. B. *Ambulatory Care Manual for Nurse Practitioners*. Philadelphia: Lippincott, 1976.
Clark, E. M. "A Non-automated Multiphasic Health Testing Program in a Student Health Service," *American Journal of Public Health*, Vol. 63, No. 7, July 1973, pp. 610–618.
Collings, G. H. "Health—A Corporate Dilemma; Health Care Management—A Corporate Solution," *Industry's Changing Role in Health Care Delivery*. R. H. Egdahl (Ed.), in New York: Springer-Verlag, 1977, pp. 16–28.
"Conference on Ethical Issues in Occupational Medicine," Bulletin of the New York Academy of Medicine, Vol. 54, No. 8, Sept. 1978.
Finnerty, F. "The Nurse's Role in Treating Hypertension," *New England Journal of Medicine* Editorial, Vol. 293, No. 7, July 1975, pp. 93–94.
Millis, J. S. "Primary Care: Definition of and Access To. . . ," *Nursing Outlook*, Vol. 25, No. 7, July 1977, pp 443–445.
Perry, H. M., and Smith, U. (Eds.) *Mild Hypertension: To Treat or Not to Treat*. New York: New York Academy of Sciences, 1978.
Scott, J. M. "The Changing Health Care Environment: Its Implications for Nursing," *American Journal of Public Health*, Vol. 64, No. 4, Apr. 1974, pp. 364–369.
Verdesca, A. S. "Hypertension Screening and Follow-up," *Journal of Occupational Medicine*, Vol. 16, No. 6, June 1974, pp. 395–401.

CHAPTER 14

Occupational Mental Health

Occupational mental health, in the narrowest sense, is concerned with psychiatrically ill workers whose symptoms interfere with effective functioning on the job. In a broader sense it is concerned with thoughts, feelings, and behavior, both healthy and unhealthy, as they are experienced by workers and as they relate to performance on a job. Occupational health personnel deal with factors in the work environment which support healthy mental behavior as well as those that may trigger the development of symptoms of emotional disturbance.

In his book *Principles of Preventive Psychiatry* Gerald Caplan refers to the term *preventive psychiatry* as

> that body of professional knowledge, both theoretical and practical, which may be utilized to plan and carry out programs for reducing (1) the incidence of mental disorders of all types in a community ("primary prevention"), (2) the duration of a significant number of those disorders which do occur ("secondary prevention"), and (3) the impairment which may result from those disorders ("tertiary prevention"). [He goes on to say,] My emphasis and comprehensive approach is based on the belief that not only are mentally disordered behavior patterns part of a whole system of ecological responses of a population in its interaction with the environment, but our own operations as preventive psychiatrists are also part of the total community system whereby socially deviant responses and undue individual victimization are kept in check.[1]

Mental Health in the Industrial Setting

When providing primary care occupational health nurses must be aware of the psychological overtones that can be associated with illness and injury. Those who are involved in an accident but not injured may experience a very real crisis either immediately or days or weeks later as feelings of grief or guilt build up to such a point that the person cannot understand or handle the situation. This worker's need for nursing care is as great as the injured worker's. A nurse with a strong preventive orientation will make a point of seeing the others who were involved in a major accident, permitting and encouraging these people to talk about what happened and how they feel about their part in the incident. In so doing that nurse may very well be practicing preventive psychiatry.

Effects of Change in the Work Setting

A trouble-shooting industrial hygiene survey conducted by the Division of Industrial Hygiene of the New York State Department of Labor involved a firm engaged in the manufacture and assembly of dials, indicators, and other small parts. This company had moved into a new building. To consolidate its operations the firm located all finishing operations in a large, well-ventilated room. Soon after the firm relocated, the division was requested to determine the reason for complaints of headache, nausea, dizziness, and malaise by the female workers. No chemical cause was found.

In an effort to reassure the workers and to determine any physical cause, members of the study team had extended conversations with management personnel, first-line supervisors, and the workers. These efforts paid off; the origin and cause subsequently became clear. The concern employed about 40 female workers, mainly of Puerto Rican origin, most of whom lived in the same part of the city and had come to this country fairly recently from the same area of Puerto Rico. In the old plant all of the women employees worked together in one large room. The operations were manual and required little skill or attention. There was a considerable amount of socializing and bantering among the workers. When the plant moved to the new building, where they were cut off from the mainstream of the plant's activities, they could not see what was going on, and they missed the pleasant association with the entire group which had made the day pass quickly. Apparently this condition found expression in symptoms of minor illness.

At a conference with management two alternatives were suggested. It was recommended that, if at all feasible, the 10 workers be relocated in the main workroom. If not feasible it was suggested the firm install a large picture window in the finishing room so that the workers confined to it could see what was going on in the main plant. The company accepted the former recommendation, and the complaints vanished. This example points up the value of talking and of listening to the workers.[2] The need to assure that there is no chemical exposure should be the first activity undertaken; when none is found, "people problems" should be considered. Change in the work environment can be very upsetting to some people. Finding out what the change means to the workers is essential if they are to be helped to adjust.

Psychogenic Illness Episodes

Psychogenic illness has been described as "the collective occurrence of a set of physical symptoms and related beliefs among two or more individuals in the absence of an identifiable pathogen.[3] Little is known about this phenomenon, although efforts are currently being made by behavioral scientists to take a closer look at such responses in the work setting. The episodes, impossible to identify in advance, consist of a sudden mass outbreak of somatic, nonspecific complaints of illness by the workers. In some instances dramatic manifestations such as fainting and strange tactile sensations are reported by a large number of workers. Usually one worker becomes ill, then two, then many more. They relate their symptoms to some physical or chemical hazard in the work environment; occasionally so many workers are involved that plant operations have to be suspended.

The first step after providing care for those who are ill is to have an industrial hygiene survey. If this fails to reveal evidence of environmental toxicity, workers will usually resume work. Recurrences of outbreaks have been known to occur. They can be very disruptive, and there is concern that whatever is causing the problem is being missed. Studies of such outbreaks have revealed certain commonalities. They usually begin with a triggering event like exposure to a solvent or an odor. The work is boring and repetitive, and the incidents frequently occur during a period of peak production when overtime is required. Often poor relationships exist between labor and management. These episodes of disruptive behavior with nonspecific complaints are referred to as occupational psychogenic illness.

Occupational health nurses, physicians, and environmental personnel are seldom exposed to this phenomenon. Reports in the literature indicate that psychogenic illness episodes have, for the most part, occurred in small establishments none of which have employed a nurse.

The potential environmental agents that served as triggers in the documented episodes included solvent odors, noise, and exhaust fumes. In these instances the triggering agents were found to be below levels considered capable of producing adverse effects in humans. Nevertheless, when an environmental agent is suspected, evaluation must be immediate and comprehensive to determine whether a valid relationship exists. If the industrial hygiene survey is negative and organic disease is ruled out, the nurse should review the situation for social, emotional, or psychological factors as potential contributors.

When an episode of psychogenic illness occurs, the nurse should begin to focus on the group as a whole to determine the common variables in the case histories. Should a pattern emerge the nurse is in a key position to forestall a reoccurrence. When a group illness episode of a sudden and dramatic nature and involving many workers occurs, the nurse relies on triage techniques, that is, provides immediate attention for the most seriously ill people. It may be necessary to transport the acutely ill to the nearest hospital, which may require setting up a shuttle ambulance service. Advance notice should be given to the hospital that several people have become suddenly ill and are being sent to them for care. If there is any indication that a toxic substance is involved, this information should also be communicated to the hospital physician, and any medical surveillance information should be sent with the employees so that the necessary tests can be done promptly to establish the degree of exposure. Collaboration with environmental personnel is crucial at this point primarily if a potentially toxic agent is suspect. A nurse who is the only occupational health professional employed must also report the incident to management and recommend an immediate environmental investigation. Rash judgment should be avoided; do not predict or label. Make every effort first to evaluate the work environment to find the cause. One of the critical needs is for the nurse to deal with workers' anxiety, since reports indicate that when psychogenic illness episodes occur anxiety mounts and spreads throughout the establishment.

Since most of the reported episodes of psychogenic illness have occurred in small establishments, it seems evident that larger establishments which support a health unit and a professional health staff are able to deal with such problems before the situation builds to the point of a full-blown episode.

Psychiatric Illness and the Industrial Worker

Workers with diagnosed psychiatric illnesses yet able to function on the job are persons occupational health nurses must be concerned about. Helping such a person to stay on prescribed medications is essential. All too often as soon as such persons begin to feel better they decide they do not need their medicine. This is when new problems often develop. At other times such workers develop obsessive-compulsive rituals that can become so pronounced as to interfere with their ability to work. Equally important is the fact that such a person's behavior may be so disruptive as to generate anxiety in fellow workers that in turn decreases their work effectiveness, making it necessary for the occupational health nurse to intervene. The nurse tries to get the ill worker's trust so as to get the worker to accept referral or to return to his therapist. The nurse calls the ill person's doctor to share information about the person's behavior with the doctor or with his nurse. When the behavior becomes too disruptive, the person's family will have to be persuaded to intervene, and sometimes the ill person may have to be admitted to the hospital for care.

The silent person is also often found in the occupational setting, one who is very depressed and withdrawn. This person may not be recognized as presenting a psychiatric emergency about to happen, but such a person may become so depressed as to drop out of work, and a few commit suicide. When this happens the nurse may find that those who knew the person but tried not to get involved are now caught in the web of guilt that surrounds a suicide. Some of these people, depending on their coping mechanisms, may need help to understand how to deal with these feelings and reactions.

Psychiatric Emergencies

In any work force the possibility exists that someone will become acutely ill and will exhibit bizarre behavior or perform antisocial acts. The need to be prepared to deal with a person who, for example, climbs to some high point and threatens to jump is very real. The worker who becomes very withdrawn or who becomes manic can be very upsetting to others in a work force. The primary care provided by the occupational health nurse is to intervene so as to provide care for the sick person and to make it possible for all the others to return to work. Depending on the environment in which the emergency happens, the nurse may be able to handle the situation by establishing contact with the disturbed person and helping him or her to the health unit. At other times a member of the first-aid team will have to try to reach the person. To assure the safety of the sick person and others, it may be necessary to call for help from the security force or the community police.

The more common emergency that occupational health nurses have to deal with involves the upset, angry person or someone who is hysterical. Sometimes these people do harm to others but more often they just disrupt work and make others feel anxious. The need is to keep cool, to get the disturbed person to a quiet place, and to provide the care that is required. In all such emergencies nurses work with others who are responsible for the safety and the protection of the work force. This is not the time or place for heroics on the part of a nurse. Nurses work cooperatively with management and the police or security force of the company.

Occasionally emotional disequilibrium is precipitated when, for example a worker hears that his home has been destroyed or a family member has been killed, or a worker sees a fellow worker killed, or a worker's work practices contribute to the death or serious injury of another. In such an instance the worker's customary coping mechanisms may be inadequate. The primary care that the nurse must provide is to assess as quickly as possible the strengths of the person and to identify a significant other who can and will get involved in helping the individual who is at crisis.

Behavioral Change Following Exposure to Toxic Substances

A 28-year-old laboratory worker complained of great fatigue and loss of intellectual vigor. His sleep patterns were poor; he had abdominal pain and was depressed. The change in this worker's behavior was so great that he could not comprehend or visualize organic formulas although he was a research chemist. He tended to remain quietly by himself. When his physician had special blood and urine studies done, the urine was found to contain a high level of mercury. This helped to make the diagnosis, as did the environmental investigation of the man's work place—a research laboratory. This investigation revealed that some of the equipment he used contained mercury and that the equipment was malfunctioning, thus leading to high levels of mercury in the work environment.[4]

Again, nurses must know what toxic substances the people in their industries work with and the symptoms caused by overexposure to these substances. For example trichloroethylene is primarily an anesthetic. Acute poisoning due to overexposure to this chemical is characterized by headache, dizziness, giddiness, disturbed gait, and the general picture of drunkenness.[5] This is important for the nurses to know so that they will not overlook environmental exposure as a possible cause of change in workers' behavior. Control measures do not always work; and when behavior changes are noted, it is good practice to have the environment checked to assure that the changes are not the result of toxic effects of chemicals or metals used in the work place.

Drug Abuse

Occupational health nurses often have to deal with people who misuse drugs. Sometimes this is due to not following the orders of the physician who prescribes the drug, for example taking two, not one capsule as ordered. Workers have been known to give some of their tranquilizers to fellow workers and to exchange drugs to see if the other person's medication will help them. Workers who have two jobs sometimes take a drug to keep themselves awake, and then nurses find that they must handle very anxious persons.

History taking can be a disturbing experience for nurses when they realize they are dealing with a drug user or when they observe evidence that a young person applying for work is a mainliner. Some industries have a policy that the use of addictive drugs is a reason for disciplinary action, perhaps firing. The sale of such drugs within the plant is, of course, against the law and is a problem for the plant security personnel to handle.

The people in the work force are the people of the community. Some industries have people on their force who smoke marijuana and others who use hard drugs. The foreman is the person who has the most direct contact with the workers; sometimes he needs information about what to look for and how to handle such a person. Nurses need to be alert to this and to be prepared to offer useful information. One occupational health nurse offered to meet with several foremen so they could exchange information about drugs and drug abuse. This proved to be a very successful approach, as not only did the nurse teach the foremen but the foremen taught each other by citing examples of how they handled workers with drug problems. It was also an example of how the nurses can conduct meaningful health education sessions.

Many young people in the work force are on methadone; as part of their rehabilitation, some industries have accepted them for employment. These workers must report to a methadone clinic every day to receive their dosage. Because of the conflicts between clinic hours and the person's work hours, problems arise and nurses may have to help both the workers and foremen who may not know why these persons are so frequently late for work. One nurse reports that she helped to clear up such a situation by assisting the worker to get his clinic appointment changed from the morning to the late afternoon. Some occupational health units have arranged with methadone clinics to handle distribution of the drug at the unit for their workers who are in the program.

Occupational health nurses may have to learn how to work with the person who is a drug user. Understanding their own feelings about drugs and people who misuse them is essential because nurses' feelings can be a factor in how effective they will be in their efforts to work with such persons.

Return to Work

The return to work of someone who has been hospitalized with a psychiatric illness can cause concern to the others in the work force. They are often afraid they will say or do something to upset the person. A young woman in a clerical pool of a large insurance company's office attempted suicide. She was first reported dead, but she recovered and was able to return to work. The girls in the pool were in a panic. What do we say to her? How do we treat her? They asked these questions of the nurse. At her suggestion the supervisor called a meeting of the girls; the nurse talked to them and gave them a chance to express their concerns.

At the time of the return-to-work physical the nurse got the young woman who was returning to work to accept her suggestion that if she became anxious she would come to the health unit. The nurse promised to be available to see her. She also set up an appointment for the young person to stop in to report on how she was doing. The supervisor also agreed that she would call the nurse if the young woman showed signs of depression.

In this instance, the nurse helped the others to deal with their concern and gave them a better understanding of depression and modern medical care for psychiatric problems. In addition she created a communication channel for receiving information about the behavior of the person with a mental problem so as to be able to intervene quickly if this was indicated. In cases such as this the nurse works with the person who has the problem and with the supervisor who has the responsibility of getting the work done. The nurse's aims are to increase understanding, provide support, and when required, intervene, for it may become necessary to remove the ill person from the work area so as to protect and get the person under care. Equally important, by intervening the nurse frees the others to return to work and lessens their anxiety.

Factors That Increase Nurses' Effectiveness

Consultant Service

"Consultation is the interaction between two professional persons—the consultant, who is a specialist, and the consultee."[6] The availability to nurses of mental health consultants increases nurses' effectiveness in dealing with workers' mental health problems. Consultants attempt to help the nurses in their efforts to help workers solve mental health problems within the framework of the nurses' usual professional functioning. While nurses are receiving professional consulting services, they are also learning new ways to deal with problems and in the future will be better able to handle similar problems in an effective manner.

Privacy

Having a quiet private place where nurses and workers can talk is important, as is the peace of mind it gives nurses to know that someone else will answer the phone and take care of any worker who comes to the unit for a dressing or first aid while they are engaged in counseling. This is a luxury that few occupational health nurses have. Nurses who work alone have to learn how to give individual counseling and, when required, do something for someone else without making the counselee feel deserted. The working relationship between nurse and first-aider suggested in Chapter 10 was proposed to give the nurse freedom to carry out those activities that require special preparation and time free to do it.

Counseling Skills

"Counseling is reality oriented and focuses on solving specific problems arising from situational or inter-personal difficulties. The role of the counselor is to direct actively toward the finding and acceptance of a solution to an immediate difficulty while not intentionally exposing the counselee's feeling or attitudes for the purpose changing them."[7]

Hildegarde E. Peplau has described counseling in nursing as "having to do with helping the patient to remember and to understand fully what is happening to him in the present situation so that the experience can be integrated with rather than disassociated from other experiences in life."[8] It is essential that occupational health nurses, their employers, and the workers to whom they give care not think of counseling by the nurse as giving guidance, and this requires much professional skill. "The therapist's role is to supply clarification and support to enable the person to bring conflictual feelings about the specific problem into conscious awareness and to ventilate them without increasing anxiety, guilt, or fear."[9] When this level of care is needed, the occupational health nurse helps the worker to accept referral to a mental health professional.

Caplan has said, "If you want to work with people, you must get an invitation. Make it easy for people to say, 'Help me:' reduce the threshold so they may come to you." He calls this "creating proximity." "It is based on the fact that, if you are around and if people get to know you and talk to you, it does not matter what about, but if they see you, there is a geographical proximity that by itself lowers the barrier."[10] This is one of the reasons why it is important for occupational health nurses to be out in the work area. It gives them more opportunities to get that invitation from those workers who do not believe their problems are of sufficient importance for them to seek help. Others ask questions to test nurses' interest and willingness to get involved. Nurses understand the importance of maintaining production and will not keep a person away from work unnecessarily; therefore they invite workers to come to the health unit for a purposeful discussion and make definite appointments.

The aim of nurses' counseling is to help workers find acceptable solutions to immediate difficulties. The nurses' role is to help people focus on a problem, identify it, and then select what they might do to solve it. Once they have decided what they might do, the nurse tries to get them to follow that course of action. As counselors occupational health nurses are concerned with workers' intra- and interpersonal problems. Nurses are not psychotherapists. Psychotherapy is a form of treatment for problems of an emotional nature in which a trained person deliberately establishes a professional relationship with a patient with the object of removing, modifying, or retarding existing symptoms and of promoting positive personality growth and development.[11]

The aim of nurses in counseling differs from that of psychotherapists in that nurses do not attempt to explore the generic roots of a problem or to investigate recurring patterns and operations but rather to work specifically on one presenting difficulty. For example a very obese young woman was helped into the health unit at midmorning. She was flushed, perspiring profusely, dyspeptic, and so weak she had to be helped to a chair. Her opening statement was, "I think I am going to die. My heart wants to fly right out of my chest." The nurse began with, "What do you think is causing this?" The woman named an antidepressant recently prescribed by her doctor. She had felt discouraged because she had not had a dramatic weight loss, so that morning she had taken two capsules instead of one and had drunk two cups of strong, black coffee.[12]

The nurse assessed the situation and, after securing an order for a barbiturate and administering it, said, "I have a few minutes right now to spend with you; let's talk about how this situation developed." In the conversation that followed, the nurse discovered the gaps in the worker's information about diet, medication, how long obesity had been a problem, and what goals she had set in terms of weight loss. The worker was astonished to find that a pound a day was an unrealistic goal. She also expressed interest in learning more about calories. The nurse scheduled weekly visits so as to help her deal with the weight problem and to check her progress. By beginning with the experience, the nurse fostered an integrative learning experience. An alternative course of action would have been to administer a relief-giving drug and then to lecture on the dangers of not following specific instructions about dosage of prescribed drugs. Such an alternative does not constitute counseling; in fact it does not meet the standard of care of an expert occupational health nurse.

Crisis Intervention Skills

"Crisis occurs when a person faces an obstacle to important life goals that, for a time, is insurmountable through the utilization of customary methods of problem solving. A period of disorganization ensues, a period of upset, during which abortive attempts at solutions may be made."[13] A person who is in crisis feels helpless and unable to take action or to resolve the situation. Crisis intervention involves psychological resolution of the individual's immediate crisis and restoration to at least the level of functioning that existed prior to the event that caused the crisis.[14]

The purpose of intervention as provided by occupational health nurses is to help the employee identify the problem and the alternative solutions and to help the person to accept one of these solutions or to accept referral to a mental health professional. However, many emotional problems that workers bring to nurses may require only the intervention of a caring person, such as the nurse, who can help the individual to select an adaptive way of dealing with the problem.

Counseling Activities

Workers often ask questions about their health, and they expect the nurse to give honest, forthright answers. This type of interchange between nurse and worker is neither advice giving nor counseling; it is simply giving information that the worker has need of and has requested. The purpose of such interchange, like counseling, is to help workers achieve new knowledge or understanding. The fact that nurses are there, are seen as helping persons, and know the workers, who in turn know and trust them, makes nurses key persons in providing care to workers who are having interpersonal relationship problems.

It is imperative for nurses to have counseling skills; to know the mental health resources of the community; and to have time, quiet, and privacy to counsel workers. They also need skill and understanding when they have to help the disturbed deal with anxiety. Neither worker nor nurse may know the cause of the anxiety. All a nurse may have to go on is appreciation of the amount of panic a person is experiencing. The nurse's aim is to help the person reduce this feeling of panic, and to do so as quickly as possible. The nurse stays with the person and asks others to get help if needed. If the episode involves more than one person, the nurse may have to call on others to provide first aid if other workers have been involved.

At other times anxiety is less obvious. Change in one's life-style or change in one's job can cause anxiety that some people cannot understand or handle. Marriage, divorce, the birth of one's first child, debts, or the children going off to college can and do cause difficulty for some people. Anxiety may be caused by the need to move to a different town as a worker accepts a new job and the family must leave familiar surroundings and friends. The person who accepts the job may get into serious trouble because the family's coping behavior that was successful and appropriate "back home" is hopelessly ineffectual in the new environment. This worker and family need someone to help them deal with the situation; an occupational health nurse can be this person. Sometimes all that is needed is to help a worker recognize that his wife needs help learning how to get about in this new community; others may need family counseling.

Adult workers often have families and are the parents of the community. Disruptions that occur at home and in the community have the potential for being felt at work. Divorce, an alcoholic wife or husband, a very sick child, an ill parent who must be placed in a nursing home, a lost pregnancy, or a teenager picked up by the police are often precipitating factors that cause anxiety, and sometimes, grief reactions, that interfere with a person's ability to cope, that in turn causes his or her work behavior to be less than satisfactory.

When a person has lost something of importance—a job, a part of the body, or someone dear—the occupational health nurse needs to be aware of this fact and understand that the person will experience a period of grief. It is essential for the grieving to be helped to understand the dynamics of loss to be able to resolve their feelings and accept the loss. Nurses can function as helping, caring persons in such instances. They must understand how people cope and be able to help them utilize their own strengths and patterns of behavior and to adopt new ones. Nurses counsel to help the workers over the stage of just worrying about something and get them to the point of utilizing patterns of behavior that will resolve the problem. Grieving should not extend over a protracted period of time and if it does, the nurse's function is to persuade the person to accept referral to a mental health professional.

There are times when occupational health nurses must be able to communicate clearly with management personnel. For example problems peculiar to the work setting can result when a person who is a supervisor develops alcoholism or an illness that interferes with her or his judgment or when a worker's neurotic behavior causes other workers to become anxious or angry. These persons may have little or no insight into what their behavior does to others. Such behavior is frequently the cause of unproductive work groups and causes many visits to the health unit by workers who are influenced by it. The person who is responsible for evaluating the supervisor's work is the one who must deal with his work behavior, but this is not always easy to arrange. However, until action is taken by the "boss," little that is positive will happen. The "boss" must deal with the work behavior; the occupational health unit staff must deal with the illness. They may also have to help the "boss" to deal with the supervisor.

Nurses may be the first to recognize a problem in a department as they see workers who come into the health unit with ill-defined problems and headaches. Others come in saying, "I'll be O.K.; I just need to get away from the job for a minute," or "I just need a break—he is impossible; can I stay here for a minute?" By questioning, nurses gain information that they must use carefully so as not to condemn the person whose behavior is at fault. Nurses may share what they know with unit physicians to determine how to proceed. At other times they attempt to help someone in management to deal with the situation.

When a worker's disruptive behavior disturbs other workers, management must become involved. Nurses and physicians can and should be involved when the disturbing person's problem is alcoholism, illness, or inability to cope with a work situation or a family problem. Sometimes the solution may involve helping such a person to recognize that he or she needs to learn how to be a supervisor. At other times a nurse may help an employee arrange for care of his mentally ill wife and for someone to care for the children. At others, after "the boss" has had a confrontation with the person, a nurse may help her to go to talk with the alcoholism counselor.

When occupational health nurses are providing care for the disturbed, they use many of the skills and understandings basic to the determination of a person's needs for nursing care. Nurses assess as quickly as possible what happened to produce a worker's anxiety. They assess the level of the worker's anxiety. A very anxious person cannot see or hear accurately and has great difficulty making relevant connections. Nurses must recognize this difficulty and compensate for it. Nurses aim to learn what information gaps exist. They use these two pieces of information—level of anxiety and information gap—to determine a person's need for care. When the person is very upset and the level of anxiety is high, it is essential that a nurse help the worker to know, for example, the extent of the damage or trauma and the nurse's immediate plans for relieving the pain or discomfort. If there has been any loss of consciousness, a nurse needs to discover with the patient the last thing he or she is able to recall and then to fill in on what has happened.

To illustrate this last point, an occupational health nurse was at the scene of an explosion in an oil refinery. Among the injured was a secretary who had suffered only superficial scalp wounds and a slight concussion from being thrown against the wall. When she regained consciousness after being transported to the occupational health unit, the young woman began to look around and attempted to piece together what had happened. She suddenly screamed and said, "Oh no. Oh no. It couldn't be." The nurse said, "What couldn't be?" The patient began to sob violently, repeating the same phrases over and over. The nurse said, "Tell me in words." After several more minutes of crying, the patient was able to speak and said, "My skirt—it's all wet. I just never thought it would happen." "What are you referring to?" was the nurse's question. With much difficulty the woman searched for the words while the nurse waited. At last, in a whisper, the woman told her that she had finally had a seizure, that she must be an epileptic, like her uncle who was in a state hospital, and that the pain in her head and her drenched skirt were the evidence. The nurse waited long enough to estimate the extent of the information gap, then filled in the details. There had been an explosion; the patient had not had a seizure; and her skirt was wet because several bottles of solution had been broken and their contents spattered about the office. There were more tears—this time tears of relief. Consider the state this young worker would have been in if she had been taken directly to the hospital for head X rays without having had this communication. It is not unusual for such an incident, poorly managed, to result in a full-blown psychosis.[15]

References

1. Caplan, G. *Principles of Preventive Psychiatry*. New York: Basic Books, 1964, pp. 17, 18.
2. Kleinfeld, M. "The Trouble-shooting Industrial Hygiene Survey," *AMA Archives of Industrial Hygiene*, Vol. 18, No. 2, Aug. 1958, pp. 120–125.
3. Colligan, M. J., Cohen, B. G. V., Webster, W., and Smith, M. J. "An

Investigation of Job Satisfaction Factors in an Incidence of Mass Psychogenic Illness at the Work Place," *Occupational Health Nursing*, Vol. 26, No. 1, Jan. 1978, pp. 10–16.
4. Goldwater, L. J., Kleinfeld, M., and Berger, A. R. "Mercury Exposure in a University Laboratory," *New York State Department of Labor Monthly Review*, Vol. 35, No. 4, Apr. 1956, pp. 13–16.
5. NIOSH. *Occupational Diseases: A Guide to Their Recognition*, Pub. No. 79-116. Washington, D.C.: GPO, 1977, p. 214.
6. Caplan, G. *An Approach to Community Mental Health*, New York: Grune & Stratton, 1961, p. 176.
7. Acquilera, D. C., Messick, J. M., and Farrell, M. S. *Crisis Intervention in Theory and Methodology*. St. Louis: Mosby, 1970, p. 22.
8. Peplau, H. E. *Interpersonal Relations in Nursing*. New York: Putnam's, 1952.
9. Acquilera et al., op. cit.
10. Caplan, G. *Concepts of Mental Health and Consultation*. Washington, D.C.: GPO, 1959, pp. 176–177.
11. Hinsie, L., and Jacob, S. *Psychiatric Dictionary*, 3rd Ed. New York: Oxford University Press, 1960, p. 615.
12. Smoyak, S. *Psychiatric First Aid in Occupational Health Nursing*, Pub. No. 100-2-65. New York: ANA, 1964, p. 2.
13. Caplan G. *An Approach to Community Health*, op. cit., p. 18.
14. Acquilera et al., op. cit., p. 13.
15. Smoyak, op. cit., p. 6.

Selected Readings

AAOHN. *Guide to Interviewing and Counseling for the Occupational Health Nurse*. New York, 1972.
Aline, L. E., Kelsey, J., Visser, M. J., and Daly, T. "Moving as Perceived by Executives and Their Families," *Journal of Occupational Medicine*, Vol. 18, No. 8, Aug. 1976, pp. 546–550.
AMA Council on Occupational Health. *Guide for Evaluating Employability after Psychiatric Illness*. Chicago, 1962.
Anders, R. "When a Patient Becomes Violent," *AJN*, Vol. 77, No. 7, July 1977, pp. 1144–1148.
Baughn, S. L. "The Role of the Nurse in Dealing with Stress in the Industrial Setting," *Occupational Health Nursing*, Vol. 24, No. 4, 1976, pp. 15–16.
Block, G. R., and Block, H. "Traumatic and Post Traumatic Neuroses," *Industrial Medicine*, Vol. 41, No. 10, Oct. 1972, pp. 5–8.
Brown, M. L. "The Extended Role of the Nurse in Occupational Mental Health Programs," *Industrial Medicine*, Vol. 40, No. 9, Dec. 1971, pp. 17–23.
Burton, G. *Interpersonal Relations: A Guide for Nurses*. New York: Springer, 1977.
Cobb, S., Brook, G. W., Kasl, S. V., and Connelly, W. E. "The Health of People Changing Jobs—A Description of a Longitudinal Study," *American Journal of Public Health*, Vol. 56, No. 5, May 1966, pp. 1476–1481.

Cooper, C. L., and Crump, J. "Prevention and Coping with Occupational Stress," *Journal of Occupational Medicine*, Vol. 20, No. 6, June 1978, pp. 420–422.

Enelow, A. J. "Industrial Injuries: Prediction and Prevention of Psychological Complications," *Journal of Occupational Medicine*, Vol. 10, No. 12, Dec. 1968, pp. 683–687.

Jacobson, G. F., Strickler, M., and Morley, W. E. "Generic and Individual Approaches to Crisis Intervention," *American Journal of Public Health*, Vol. 58, No. 2, Feb. 1968, pp. 338–343.

Kiev, A. "Crisis Intervention," *Journal of Occupational Medicine*, Vol. 12, No. 5, May 1970, pp. 158–163.

Levinson, H. "Emotional Toxicity of the Work Environment," *Archives of Environmental Health*, Vol. 19, No. 9, Aug. 1969, pp. 234–243.

Levinson, H. "Various Approaches to Understanding Man at Work," *Archives of Environmental Health*, Vol. 22, No. 5, May 1971, pp. 612–618.

Melchiode, G., and Jacobson, M. "Psychiatric Treatment: A Barrier to Employment Progress," *Journal of Occupational Medicine*, Vol. 18, No. 2, Feb. 1976, pp. 98–101.

NIOSH. *Proceedings—Reducing Occupational Stress*, Pub. No. 78-140, GPO: 017-033-00293-Z. Washington, D.C., 1979, price $3.25.

Noland, R. L. *Industrial Mental Health and Employee Counseling*. New York: Behavioral Publications, 1973.

Ross, D. W. "How to Get a Neurotic Worker Back on the Job Successfully," *Occupational Health & Safety 77*, Vol. 46, No. 1, Jan.–Feb. 1977, pp. 20–22.

Schwartz, G. E. "Stress Management in Occupational Settings," *Public Health Reports*, Vol. 95. No. 2, March–April, 1980, pp. 99–108.

Selye, H. *Stress without Distress*. Philadelphia: Lippincott, 1974.

Sohn, D., and Simon J. "Narcotics Detection in Industry," *Journal of Occupational Medicine*, Vol. 12, No. 1, Jan. 1970, pp. 6–9.

Trickett, J. M. "A Positive Approach to Mental Health in Industry," *American Association of Industrial Nurses Journal*, Vol. 11, No. 7, July 1963, pp. 16–20.

Walke, M. A. K. "When a Patient Needs to Unburden His Feelings," *AJN*, Vol. 77, No. 7, July 1977, pp. 1164–1166.

Xintaras, C. (Ed.). *Behavioral Toxicology*, NIOSH Pub. No. 74–126 Washington, D.C.: GPO, 1974.

CHAPTER 15

Alcoholism and the Worker

One of society's oldest and most familiar toxic substances is alcohol. Research has clearly established that beverage alcohol is the most abused drug in the United States.[1] Moreover its abuse is increasing by significant proportions each year. An estimated 10 million men and women, approximately 7% of the adult population, suffer from alcohol abuse and alcoholism.[2] Among adolescents, 1975 data permits an estimate of problem drinking among 19–23% (approximately 3.3 million) of youths in the 14- to 17-year age range.[3] Only a minority, 3–5%, comprise the highly visible skid row population, as most alcoholics are hidden among the nation's working, school-going, and homemaking population.[4]

Alcoholism is a treatable illness that can be reached through a broad range of health, rehabilitative, and social services, depending upon individual treatment needs and the progression of the illness. The causal factors in alcohol abuse and alcoholism have not yet been isolated. Social, psychological, cultural, and physiological variables have all been shown to be factors in its development and progression. Besides intoxication, alcoholism has been found to be associated with emotional disorders, chronic progressive diseases of the central and peripheral nervous system, and diseases of the liver, heart, muscles, and gastrointestinal tract, as well as other organs and tissues.

Not all people who drink or get drunk on occasion are alcoholics. The true alcoholic has a chronic, progressive disease and is unable to control the amount, the time, or the place of her or his alcohol use. Initially alcoholics drink for the same reasons as nonalcoholics; however the alcoholic becomes addicted. Psychiatrists and others who have worked with alcoholics have found that many of them have personality problems. When the desire to escape a problem or frustration and worry is consistently responsible for the person's drinking, than a personality problem may be the basic cause of the person's alcoholism.

The far-reaching consequences of alcoholism affect all aspects of American life, impacting the nondrinker as well as the drinker. The total economic cost to the nation has been established at nearly $42 billion per year.[5] Of special concern is the finding that approximately $12.7 billion is expended annually on alcohol-related health and medical problems.[6] It is especially notable that the $8.4 billion expended for hospital care of alcoholics in 1975 was nearly 20% of the total hospital expenditures for adults.[7] Almost $20 billion of the estimated $47 billion bill for alcoholism in the United States is caused by lost production.[8]

Alcohol . . . has been seriously implicated in death and injury resulting from home, industrial, and recreational accidents. A national survey found that 36 percent of regular drinkers and only 9 percent of nondrinkers reported two or more accidental injuries in the previous year. Heavier drinkers appear to have more accidents than other people, and alcoholics have a considerably higher rate of accidental death than the general population.[9]

Occupational accidents affect a substantial portion of the population. One researcher estimates up to 47 percent of nonfatal industrial accidents and up to 40 percent of fatal industrial accidents are alcohol related.[10]

Experimental evidence has shown that alcohol inhibits coordination and judgment, lengthens reaction time, and decreases motor performance and sensory skill in simulated industrial work. Studies show that problem drinkers are as much as three times more likely to be involved in industrial accidents than the general population.[11]

Those workers who come to work drunk present less of a problem. They may be dealt with by being given time off without pay and some may be fired. It is important that they be made to understand that their behavior is not acceptable and when indicated they should be referred for care. Some of these people are alcoholics, others are not. The referral may be to the employee assistance program if the company has one in place. These people present less of a problem than the so-called half-man, a term coined by the staff of the Yale Plan for Business and Industry in the 1950s. This person may be a valued employee. He may report to work not feeling up to par. This may occur on a day or two after payday, or on a Monday or even Tuesday after the weekend. This worker goes about his job, and probably only another alcoholic would recognize that he is covering up a hangover. The worker may or may not make a mistake, get hurt, or hurt someone else. Few if any suspect that this person is an alcoholic. Those who are suspicious cover up for him, and the foreman knows the worker to be a good worker most of the time. Industry's problem drinker is the half-man. As the disease progresses the alcoholic becomes better recognized by coworkers, supervisors, and others.

Occupational health nurses must be alert to the possibility that a worker has a drinking problem when he or she has frequent day-after-payday absences or repeatedly reports to the health unit with a headache or gastrointestinal upset on a Monday morning. Counseling these workers involves talking with them about the nature of their problem and the sources of help available to them. Once an alcoholic has faced up to the fact that the "boss" will no longer put up with poor work performance and frequent absence, the worker will be more receptive to suggestions about services that may be helpful. These are two essential characteristics of an occupational alcoholism program: confrontation by the supervisor concerning work behavior and health counseling to help the worker recognize his need and accept help for the problem.[12]

Definitions

Alcoholism is a complex illness. Many definitions have been written for it, none of which has pleased every one. The following definition is one developed at a conference on treatment

Alcoholism is a progressive disease but one which can be arrested at any point. It is initially characterized by a psychological dependence on alcohol. At some point, the person loses control over his drinking and then is considered biologically dependent or addicted. If his drinking continues, it increasingly impinges on the alcoholic's life and health until he either receives treatment or dies.[13]

Alcoholism is also defined as alcohol dependence syndrome by WHO and in the ninth revision of the International Classification of Diseases. Alcoholism is characterized by a compulsion to take alcohol on a continuous or periodic basis to experience its psychological and physical effects, and sometimes to avoid the discomfort of its absence. Tolerance may or may not be present.[14]

Alcohol abuse is a generic term applied to the misuse of alcohol, which is manifested in one or more alcohol-related problems or disabilities.

Alcohol-related problems can be classified by three broad categories:

1. Psychological: loss of control over drinking; dependence; and depressive and suicidal states of mind.
2. Medical: acute and chronic illnesses and injuries; and
3. Social: problems of demeanor and default of major social roles.[15]

Alcohol-related disability is a broad term that includes alcoholism but does not require that alcoholism be present. An alcohol-related disability exists when there is an impairment in the physical, mental, or social functioning of an individual, so that it may be reasonably inferred that alcohol is part of the cause of that disability. Impairment includes actual health problems related to a specific drinking bout; offensive behavior caused by heavy drinking; injuries, death, and property loss caused by accidents related to drinking; failure of the chronic excessive drinker to fulfill his or her role in the family or on the job; and mental problems, such as depression and anxiety, related to drinking. People manifesting alcohol-related disabilities, although not necessarily alcoholics, have an increased risk of becoming alcoholics. The fact that a person is addicted to alcohol (an alcoholic) implies a probable impaired behavioral responsiveness to social control.[16]

A *problem drinker* is a person who drinks alcohol to an extent or in a manner such that an alcohol-related disability is manifested. Therefore the term *problem drinker* generally is applied to those who demonstrate problems in relation to drinking alcohol.[17]

Federal Alcoholism Legislation

Public concern about alcohol abuse and alcoholism reached a high point in the mid-1960s. As a result many of the social, health, and educational programs newly enacted at the federal level became vehicles in the search for more effective means of dealing with alcoholism. Particularly notable among these federal programs were the following.[18]

1966. The Office of Alcohol Countermeasures was established within the National Highway Traffic Safety Administration of the Department of Transportation. This office funded, on a demonstration basis, Alcohol Safety Action Programs (ASAP). Many of these programs proved highly successful in the reduction of alcohol-related traffic accidents. A number of these programs received continued funding by state and local governments following the demonstration.

1966. The Law Enforcement Assistance Act made funding available for detoxification centers.

1966. The National Center for the Prevention and Control of Alcoholism, the forerunner to the National Institute on Alcohol Abuse and Alcoholism (NIAAA), was established by presidential mandate. The act followed two federal court decisions that chronic alcoholics could not be held criminally liable for public inebriety.

1968. Title III of the Public Health Service Act Amendments, PL 90-574, added to the Community Mental Health Centers Act an authorization of federal grants for constructing and staffing alcoholism prevention and treatment facilities.

1970. The amendments to the Community Mental Health Centers Act, PL 91-211, extended and expanded the provisions of PL 90-574 by authorizing funds for training, program evaluation, treatment and prevention, and demonstration of new or relatively effective or efficient methods of delivering services.

1970. The passing of the Comprehensive Alcohol Abuse and Alcoholism Prevention, Treatment, and Rehabilitation Act, PL 91-616, made alcohol abuse and alcoholism a national priority. This law established NIAAA as the primary vehicle for federal activities in the area of alcoholism and alcohol-related problems.

PL 91-616 created the National Advisory Council on Alcohol Abuse and Alcoholism, whose responsibility it is to advise, consult with, and make recommendations to the Secretary of the DHHS on all matters relating to alcohol abuse and alcoholism. This council must approve treatment, prevention, and training projects as well as review research projects and grant applications received by the various divisions of NIAAA.

Title II of PL 91-616 charges the United States Civil Service Commission with the responsibility for developing and maintaining prevention, treatment, and rehabilitation programs for alcohol abuse and alcoholism among federal employees. NIAAA is likewise responsible for fostering similar programs for employees of DHHS, state and local governments, and private industry. This federal commitment to a partnership with state and local communities is clearly enunciated in the formula grant program and in NIAAA grants and contracts for prevention and treatment.

Of particular note to health planners is the PL 91-616 mandate (Sec. 321) that all private and public hospitals receiving federal alcoholism funds must not discriminate against alcohol abusers and alcoholics suffering from medical conditions solely because of their alcoholism. PL 93-282 tightens this provision by adding, "any private or public hospital or outpatient facility which receives support in any form from any program supported in whole or in part by funds appropriated to any federal department or agency shall not discriminate in its admission policies against alcohol abusers and alcoholics solely because of their alcohol abuse and alcoholism. Discrimination can result in suspension or revocation of all federal support received by the hospital or outpatient facility."

1974. One amendment to the Comprehensive Alcohol Abuse and Alcohol Prevention, Treatment, and Rehabilitation Act of 1970 that was made in 1974 (PL 93-282) made NIAAA a part of the Alcohol, Drug Abuse, and Mental Health Administration (ADAMHA), one of six agencies that report directly to the Assistant Secretary for Health of the DHHS. The significant concern of Congress was displayed when NIAAA was charged with responsibility for formulating and recommending national policies and goals regarding the prevention, control, and treatment of alcoholism, and for developing and conducting "comprehensive health education, training, research, and planning programs for the prevention and treatment of alcoholic abuse and alcoholism for the rehabilitation of alcohol users and abusers."[20] Further amendments in May 1974 (PL 94-371) continued and expanded NIAAA's spending authority and required that specific action be taken by the states and NIAAA to improve the nation's alcohol abuse programs.

Occupational Alcoholism Programs

Management personnel are becoming increasingly aware of the incidence of alcoholism in workers. Among the many companies that have introduced alcoholism programs for their employees are the Kemper Insurance Companies, Allis-Chalmers Manufacturing Company, and the Consolidated Edison Company of New York, to name only a few. Probably none of these companies have more alcoholics among their work force than others, but the difference is that they have recognized the existence of alcoholism among their workers and others have not. A clipping from the (McKeesport) *Daily News* summarizes industries' concern and sets forth what Westinghouse Electric Corporation plans to do:

Yesterday, some 300 Westinghouse managers, medical personnel and training supervisors attended the first in a series of workshops at the Green Tree Marriott that will provide them training and information on alcoholism and how to deal with it. "We are not certain of the full impact of alcoholism on Westinghouse employees and on the company, but we are sure it is a serious one," said Harry B. Burr, medical services administrator.

U.S. industry estimates state that nearly 6 percent of the nation's workforce have job-related problems stemming from alcoholism. This means, according to Burr, that upwards of 7,000 Westinghouse workers "could be alcoholics."'

"We estimate that alcoholism costs Westinghouse more than $24 million a year in those kinds of productivity losses which can be identified," he added.

Westinghouse in the past has had programs for dealing with alcoholism, but they were planned and administered at the local level. This is the first time a corporate policy has been developed to attack the problem.[21]

Essential Components

One of the projects funded by NIAAA was the New York–based Corporate Headquarters Alcoholism Project operational from 1974 to 1977. The experience of the staff of this project was that there is no one model for an industrial alcoholism project that is universally applicable. They were of the opinion that there are identifiable components which must be adapted to each company's program for it to succeed:

1. Commitment of the persons responsible for the program to give sufficient time and effort toward educating employees about alcoholism and to training appropriate staff. Ideally, program direction is provided by a member of top management.
2. A written policy statement about the company's attitude toward alcohol abuse and its efforts towards arresting it.
3. Frequent, regular reinforcement of the policy statement in a variety of ways to insure that all employees are familiar with it.
4. Dissemination of information about the program so that employees are aware of the specific services offered and the extent of the insurance coverage and benefits.

5. Assurances to the employee that the program is confidential and that its purpose is to help him maintain his job and health, so that self-referrals would be encouraged.
6. A flexible approach with respect to the employee's treatment needs.
7. Training of supervisors in maximally effective confrontation and referral techniques when an employee's job performance and/or on-the-job behavior show a pattern of deterioration.
8. Collection, analysis, and interpretation of data regarding the costs and success rates of the program.
9. Establishing techniques for collecting data that maintain confidentiality so that the issue of confidentiality cannot be used as a rationalization for avoiding data collection and analysis.[22]

A Plan

Any plan for helping alcoholic workers includes measures to identify those who need help and those who can help. In the industrial setting those in the best position to determine who needs help are likely to be foremen or supervisors. They must be aided in learning to recognize such persons and to realize that covering up for them does not help problem drinkers. They must confront alcoholics with their poor work attendance and deteriorating work practices and insist that they seek professional help in identifying and treating the cause. They then send these persons to the occupational health unit or to the employee assistance program counselor for consultation about how, where, and who can help with the health aspects of their drinking problems.

The following outline suggests a framework for an industrial alcoholism program:

1. Purpose
    a. Early detection of alcohol abusers
    b. Restoration of the employees' health to enable them to meet satisfactory attendance and job-performance standards
2. Process
    a. Supervisory identification and referrals based on work-performance standards and attendance or other criteria established by the company, or on self-referrals to a skilled and trained counselor and/or health professional
    b. Determination by the counselor or physician of the underlying cause of poor work performance and referral of troubled employees to an appropriate resource for treatment, counseling, and/or rehabilitation
    c. Health personnel follow-up of those referred, in terms of their cooperation with treatment and improvement in work performance, including a conference among the employee, the treatment

　　　　facility, and the supervisor, and with the primary focus always on
　　　　employee productivity
3. Components
　　a. A policy statement by both management and labor indicating their
　　　　attitude toward alcoholism as a treatable disease
　　b. A statement describing how the program works, how employees
　　　　will be treated, and how their jobs will be protected
　　c. Health insurance coverage for detoxification and for psychiatric or
　　　　other consultations
　　d. Training and education for managers, occupational health staff, supervisors, shop stewards, and employees with respect to alcoholism, its recognition, and how they are individually involved in the
　　　　program process
　　e. Identification of diagnostic, treatment, and counseling services
　　f. The maintenance of records in order to be able to evaluate the cost
　　　　and success of the program and its effect on both the individuals
　　　　treated and the corporation.

Worker Compliance

Some companies identify and designate specific services that they provide for employees. Some workers decide to go to their family doctor for treatment. Some seek psychiatric help, on either a private, clinic, or outpatient basis, and very frequently in group therapy. However it is necessary to ensure that any psychiatric service to which an alcoholic is referred has the understanding needed for working with alcoholics. Many go to what seems to be one of the best sources of help for the alcoholic, Alcoholics Anonymous (AA).

Alcoholics Anonymous

Alcoholics Anonymous is an informal society of over a million men and women throughout the world who once drank irresponsibly but now stay sober by sharing their experiences and knowledge and by helping others to achieve and maintain sobriety. There may be an AA unit in the industry, and there are many in the community; and someone from such a group will be glad to try to help a person. The answer to how AA works apparently lies in the fact that only an alcoholic can make sense to another alcoholic who is still drinking. The alcoholic who has stopped drinking brings twofold understanding to the man or woman who needs help. The nondrinking alcoholic can approach the drinker with sympathy born of having shared the same compulsions, broken promises, and remorse in the past. His or her own drinking experience makes the person familiar with the shame, subterfuges, and alibis with which the chronic alcohlic attempts to deceive family, friends, employer, and self. Upon turning to AA for help, the newcomer soon learns that the only thing hoped for is a sincere and earnest desire to stop drinking. The alcoholic who is honest in his desire to stop and keeps an open mind will very likely succeed in becoming and remaining sober. The AA philosophy is based on 12 steps which are suggested to its participants as a guide to recovery. The first and most significant step is the person's admission of his powerlessness over alcohol. Others include deciding to turn one's will and one's life over to God as one understands God; the searching out of wrongs done to others and making amends to these people: and willingness to work with other alcoholics who need help.[23]

The Nurse in an Alcoholism Program

In an occupational health setting a considerable number of employees who come to the occupational health unit and are first seen by the nurse may be alcohol abusers although the presenting symptoms may not appear to be alcohol related. These workers may complain of a variety of physical ailments and describe a wide range of difficulties including marital, familial, financial, social, and legal problems. Therefore the nurse must know the signs and symptoms of alcoholism and appreciate the fact that alcohol may act synergically with various toxic substances to which industrial workers are exposed. The nurse must be aware that the ingestion of certain neurotoxins, such as trichloroethylene, may result in clinical syndromes that simulate alcoholism and may be incorrectly diagnosed as such.[24]

Frequently alcoholic employees are aware that their drinking pattern is unlike that of their friends; and yet many factors, particularly the social and moral stigma associated with alcoholism, make them reluctant to admit their problem. The alert nurse will identify the need for intervention. Taking the initiative and saying to such a person, "Do you think, as I do, that your drinking too much is the problem?" is a risk the nurse may have to take. She should not ask this question unless she is willing to help the person understand why she asked it and to stay involved until he is able to accept referral to an alcoholism counselor.

In the May 1976 issue of the *American Journal of Nursing*, E. Heinemann and N. Estes present a "Nursing History Tool for Use With Patients with Alcohol Problems." It contains 91 questions arranged in seven sections:

1. Drinking history
2. Symptoms related to gastrointestinal systems
3. Symptoms related to neurological systems

4. Symptoms relating to cardiovascular and pulmonary systems
5. Psychosocial status
6. Drug taking, other than alcohol
7. Final questions.[25]

Occupational health nurses will find this tool helpful as they interview workers to determine to what extent their health problems are related to misuse of alcohol. The information can be gathered in one sitting or over a period of time. Depending on a person's difficulties and whether or not the person accepts the idea that alcohol contributes to the health problem, a nurse may start with the questions related to the drinking history.

If nurses have the stereotyped image of the alcoholic as a trembling, skid-row bum with bloodshot eyes, they must seek educational opportunities that will help them to reverse this attitude. Failure to recognize the early manifestations of alcoholism still continues even among today's health professionals. Nurses should select training programs that include information about the sociological, psychological, physiological, and spiritual implications of alcoholism, since within the nursing role they may be called upon to deal with aspects of any or all of these areas in work with alcoholic employees.

Nurses need to know what resources are available for treatment and rehabilitation of the alcoholic and what facilities are available for inpatient detoxification. They must also be aware of the various outpatient resources for alcoholics as well as services for their family members: AA, Al-Anon, and Al-Teens, for example. In addition they need to know what voluntary agencies, such as the National Council on Alcoholism (NCA) and its local affiliates, are available as resources for information in matters relating to alcoholism and what governmental agencies at the state and federal levels are doing.

With appropriate training and understanding, occupational health nurses can function as an integral part of an occupational alcoholism program. Their involvement can be coordinated with their already-established duties and may be expressed in several types of activity:

1. As health professionals they can advise management personnel of the need for a definitive policy for the handling of alcoholic employees.
2. As educators in matters relating to physical and mental health they are in a position to help educate employees, including first-line supervisors, in the various implications of alcohol abuse.
3. As interventionists when crises arise they are often the ones called upon to assist in the emergency care of an employee who is exhibiting acute symptoms resulting from alcohol abuse.
4. As counselors they often have access to information about an em-

ployee's drinking problem (or that of an employee's spouse) before it comes to the attention of the supervisor in the form of deteriorating work performance; they can use this information to help the person realize and admit the need to do something about the problem.
5. As health care providers they may assume responsibility for identification of the extent of the alcohol-related health problem, for referral to care, and for follow-up after treatment has been started; they may act as liaison between the treatment facilities, the employee, and the employer.

Occupational health nurses can function in all of these areas because they are already recognized by employees as professionals knowledgeable in health matters and who will not betray confidentiality. Their activities will be determined by any existing programs as well as by corporate and health department policies. Whatever their role an understanding of alcoholism and its treatment, and of the person who is an alcoholic, will assist nurses to provide needed care for workers and to work cooperatively with those who have other responsibilities for the success of a company's alcoholism program.

References

1. Human Services Horizons. *Alcohol Abuse and Alcohol Programs: A Technical Assistance Manual for Health Service Agencies*. Washington, D. C.: U.S. Department of Commerce, National Technical Information Service, 1978, p. 1.
2. Ibid.
3. Ibid.
4. Ibid.
5. Ibid.
6. Ibid.
7. Ibid.
8. Ibid., p. 2.
9. Noble, E. P. (Ed.). *Third Special Report to the Congress on Alcohol and Health*. DHEW, Alcohol, Drug Abuse, and Mental Health Department. Rockville, Md., GPO, 1978, p. 87.
10. Ibid.
11. Ibid.
12. Guida, M. A. "Occupational Health Nurses are in the Best Position to Help Workers Fight Alcoholism," *Occupational Health & Safety 78*, Sept.–Oct. 1978, pp. 48–52.
13. Capital Blue Cross, Provider Affairs Division. *Alcoholism Treatment: Considerations for Third Party Payers*. Harrisburg, Pa., 1974.
14. Noble, op. cit., p. 9.

15. Ibid.
16. Ibid.
17. Ibid.
18. Human Services Horizons, op. cit., pp. 4–6.
19. Ibid., p. 6.
20. Ibid.
21. *Daily News*, McKeesport, Pa., 1978.
22. NIAAA. *Corporate Headquarters Alcoholism Project*, Grant No. AN01755-02.
23. "Alcoholics Anonymous' Twelve Steps and Twelve Traditions," AA World Services, New York, 1939.
24. NIOSH. *Occupational Diseases: A Guide to Their Recognition*, Pub. No. 79-116. Washington, D.C.: GPO, 1977, p. 218.
25. Heinemann, E., and Estes, N. "Assessing Alcoholic Patients," *AJN*, Vol. 76, No. 5, May 1976, pp. 786–789.

Selected Reading

AMA. *Manual on Alcoholism*. Chicago, 1973.
Block, M. V. *Alcohol and Alcoholism*. Belmont, Calif.: Wadsworth, 1970.
Bourne, G., and Fox, R. (Eds.). *Alcoholism: Progress in Research and Treatment*. New York and London: Academic, 1973.
Cline, S. *Alcohol and Drugs at Work*. Washington, D.C.: Drug Abuse Council, 1975.
Daghestani, A. N., Barglow, P., Hilker, R., and Asma, F. E. "The Supervisor's Role with the Problem Drinker Employee," *Journal of Occupational Medicine*, Vol. 18, No. 2, Feb. 1976, pp. 85–90.
Dupont, R. L., and Basen, M. M. "Control of Alcohol and Drug Abuse in Industry—A Literature Review," *Public Health Reports*, Vol. 95, No. 2, March–April, 1980, pp. 137–148.
Estes, N. J. and Heinemann, E. *Alcoholism: Development, Consequences, and Interventions*. St. Louis: Mosby, 1977.
Fox, R. "Disulfiram (Antabuse) as an Adjunct in the Treatment of Alcoholism," in *Alcoholism: Behavioral Research, Therapeutic Approaches*. New York: Springer, 1967.
Health Communications. Focus on Alcohol and Drug Issues Series: 1. *Alcohol in the Workplace;* 2. *The Supervisor's Handbook on Substance Abuse;* 3. *Manager and Supervisor Sensitivity Training Program*. Hollywood, Fl., 1973.
Helms, D. J. "A Guide to the New Federal Rules Governing the Confidentiality of Alcohol and Drug Abuse Patient Records," *Medical Records News*, Aug. 1976, pp. 7–19.
Jellinek, E. M. *The Disease Concept of Alcoholism*. New Haven, Conn.: Hillhouse, 1960.
Kemper Insurance Companies. *Management Guide on Alcoholism*. Long Grove, Ill., 1977.
Kemper Insurance Companies. *What to Do about the Employee with a Drinking Problem*. Long Grove, Ill., 1975.

Marlatt, G. A., and Nathan, P. E. *Behavioral Approaches to Alcoholism*. New Brunswick, N.J.: Rutgers Center for Alcohol Studies, 1978.

McCabe, T. R. *Victims No More*. Center City, Minn.: Hazelden Books, 1978.

National Clearinghouse for Alcohol Information. *Selected Publications on Occupational Alcoholism Programs*. Rockville, Md.: Acquisition and Reference Service, 1979.

National Industrial Conference Board. *Company Controls for Drinking Problems*. New York, 1970.

New York City Central Labor Council of the AFL-CIO. *Union Peer Counseling in Substance Abuse*. New York: Central Labor Rehabilitation Council of New York, 1979.

Schramm, C. J. (Ed.). *Alcoholism*. Baltimore: Johns Hopkins University Press, 1977.

Trice, H. M. *Alcoholism in Industry*. New York: Christopher D. Smithers Foundation, 1972.

Trice, H. M., and Roman, P. M. *Spirits and Demons at Work*. Ithaca, N.Y.: Cornell University Press, 1972.

Warshaw, L. J. *Managing Stress*. Reading, Mass.: Addison-Wesley, 1979.

Wrich, J. L. *The Employee Assistance Program*. Center City, Minn.: Hazelden Press, 1974.

CHAPTER 16

Health Insurance

An important part of occupational health nurses' work is to help workers with a serious nonoccupational illness get adequate medical care and hospital services when required. Nurses need to know how these services are provided and financed. They must be aware of the extent of the several insurances that workers may select and know the major features of each.

The traditional purpose of insurance other than health insurance is to protect the insured against catastrophic events that would be too costly for the individual to bear. The husband who dies in his early 50s and whose wife and child are protected through the life insurance he bought has prepared for just such an eventuality. Health insurance plans, on the other hand, emphasize low-risk coverage; most people covered by health insurance incur small losses at a fairly constant rate.

Gallup estimated in 1970 that 157.6 million, or 78%, of the resident civilian population of the United States were enrolled in public and private insurance plans that included hospital coverage.[1] Current public plans include Medicare, Medicaid, Crippled Children's Services, and Civilian Health and Medical Programs for the uniformed services, referred to as "Champus." Although it does not have a definite health insurance program, the Veterans' Administration procures medical care for veterans in VA hospitals, clinics, and long-term care facilities, as do the USPHS's hospitals and clinics for selected beneficiaries. Private health insurance plans are written by the stock and mutual insurance associations. Blue Cross and Blue Shield are nonprofit programs. Kaiser Permanente is an example of the prepaid group plan.

It is estimated that 34 million Americans under 65 years of age have no health insurance. Only two in every five have insurance that pays the doctor's bills outside the hospital. Only 4 people in 100 have insurance for dental care. These estimates are derived from *Q and A on Health Security,* a pamphlet published by the AFL-CIO Department of Social Security, that spells out one possible approach to national health insurance. It is pointed out that many families having a health insurance plan started the plan because it was a fringe benefit in the union contract. Both in and out of Congress debate about national health insurance continues, with many

191

views being expressed as to what should be mandatory and whether policies should have coinsurance and deductible features.

In 1966 the Medicare and Medicaid provisions were added (as Title XVIII) to the Social Security Act of 1935. In 1973 the Health Maintenance Organization Act (PL 93-222) was passed.

Health Maintenance Organizations

A health maintenance organization (HMO) is based on four principles: (a) It is an organized system of health care which accepts responsibility to provide or otherwise assure the delivery of (b) an agreed upon set of comprehensive health maintenance and treatment services for (c) a voluntary enrolled group of persons in a geographic area and (d) is reimbursed through a prenegotiated and fixed periodic payment made by or on behalf of each person or family unit enrolled in the plan. The enrolled group includes those individuals or groups of people who voluntarily join the HMO through a contractual arrangement in which the enrollee (or head of household) agrees to pay a fixed monthly or other periodic payment (or have it paid on his or her behalf) to the HMO. The enrollee agrees to use the HMO as his or her principal source of health care if he or she becomes ill or needs care. The contract is for a specified period of time, a year for example.

The HMO concept grew from the success of a variety of medical foundations and prepaid group-practice organizations in various parts of the United States that are now providing health care services for more than 7 million persons. The Kaiser Foundation Health Plan, for example, now cares for almost 2 million persons, mainly in California. The Health Insurance Plan of Greater New York cares for three-quarters of a million people. The Group Health Cooperative of Puget Sound in Seattle, Washington, the Group Health Association of Washington, D.C., and the San Joaquin Medical Care Foundation of California are other examples of plans which have proven themselves during the past decade.

These organizations were started and now operate under a variety of sponsors and financing mechanisms. Their continued effectiveness has led to the conviction that a much greater number of HMO organizations could be created if additional financial and technical assistance were made available and that thereby the health services delivery system in our country would be markedly improved.

An HMO can be organized and sponsored either by a medical foundation (usually organized by physicians), by community groups, by labor unions, by a governmental unit, by a profit or nonprofit group allied with an insurance company or some other financing institution, or by some other arrangement. The HMO may be based in a hospital or a medical school, or it may be a free-standing outpatient facility or group of such facilities.

The HMO Act identified two types of HMOs—the group-practice type and the individual-practice type—and established criteria under which each type must function in order to qualify for the benefits of the act. These benefits are financial assistance, the overriding of restrictive state laws, and mandatory dual choice. One item in this legislation is of special importance to the occupational health nurse. This is the requirement that employers who employ an average of 25 or more people during any calendar quarter and who are required to pay their employees the minimum wage must include in their health benefits plan qualified HMOs that provide services in the area in which their employees reside. This requirement applies only to employers who offer some sort of health benefit insurance package to their employees. A health benefit program is any arrangement for the provision of or payment for any of the basic supplemental health benefits described in the HMO Act to eligible employees by or on behalf of the employer.

In an article in the October 1975 issue of the *Journal of Occupational Medicine,* Leon Warshaw suggested that *HMO* be used "to denote not any particular organizational structure, form or sponsorship, but rather the general concept of an organized arrangement for providing a comprehensive range of health services to a defined, voluntarily enrolled population of subscribers in exchange for a predetermined premium calculated on a per capita basis,"[2] a definition that includes all the major points about an HMO.

Basic Hospital Insurance

Basic hospital insurance is what most persons have. It provides protection against such hospital charges as room, food, X rays, laboratory tests, drugs, use of operating room, and other normal hospital services. Some plans—Blue Cross for example—cover the full cost of these expenses up to a specified number of days. Others pay a stated amount per day toward room and board, plus additional sums for the various services.

Basic Medical-Surgical Insurance

Basic medical-surgical protection can be bought separately or in combination with a hospital expense policy. Its primary purpose is to cover those doctor bills which occur while a person is hospitalized. Surgery is the biggest single benefit, and a policy generally includes a list of cash allowances provided for each surgical procedure. These may or may not be as much as the surgeon's fee, depending on the policy and the premium. Some of the higher cost plans also include reimbursement for a doctor's services at the office or at the individual's home.

Major Medical Insurance

Designed to protect against the catastrophic cost of prolonged illness or serious injury, major medical insurance takes over where basic coverage stops. Total benefits may be as much as $25,000–50,000 or higher and include expenses both in and out of the hospital. While such policies differ from company to company, they seldom cover the full cost of any sickness or injury. To keep the policy premium within reach of most persons, there is usually a deductible of several hundred dollars. This means that a person must pay the first, say $500, of the bills before the benefits begin. For individual policies the higher the deductible, the lower the premium.

Comprehensive Major Medical Insurance

Comprehensive major medical insurance is actually a combination of hospital, surgical, and major medical protection in a single policy. The difference is that, unlike most hospital and surgical plans, there is a deductible and a person is required to pay a small percentage of all bills. For this reason it usually costs less than separate policies with similar benefits.

Disability Income Insurance

Sometimes called loss-of-income insurance, disability income policies vary widely by company, and so do the benefits. There are policies that pay a specified income from the first day of hospitalization, while others require a waiting period of 2–3 months before benefits begin. The amount a person receives also ranges from a modest sum during each month of disability to about two-thirds of the regular earnings. Likewise the maximum limits on these payments vary. Obviously, higher and longer payments generally demand larger premiums, although the amount is also determined by age.

Prepaid Group-practice Programs

Prepaid group-practice programs are local programs which enable participants to pay in advance for health services performed by an approved group of physicians and hospitals. In some instances they are sponsored and paid for by employers exclusively for the protection of their employees. The benefits offered differ from program to program. Some provide only basic coverage; some cover almost all expenses when the patient uses the program's own group of doctors and health-care facilities.

Medicare includes two different plans. Part A for hospital expenses is for those aged 65 and on Social Security or Railroad Retirement Program, and others who do not have enough work credits may obtain Medicare by paying monthly premiums. The local Social Security office can supply full details and current information on costs and coverage. Part B of Medicare is not free; there is a monthly fee. This part of Medicare is similar to major medical coverage. There is a deductible after which Medicare pays the percentage of what is considered to be a "reasonable fee" for medical and surgical care.

The Nurse's Responsibility

To help workers use their health insurance plan wisely, nurses as well as workers must have answers to the following questions:

1. What services are covered and to what extent?
2. How many days of coverage does the policy provide for?
3. What are the deductibles and how much are they?
4. What are the exclusions?
5. How long are the waiting periods?
6. Are preexisting conditions covered?
7. Is the policy noncancelable by the company?
8. Are maternity benefits included?

In fact occupational health nurses must know as much as possible about the health insurance plans employees have access to. If it is an HMO or other form of health insurance, nurses should have copies of the promotional brochures that describe the benefits and know someone in the insurance company or HMO who can answer questions regarding what is and what is not covered. Occupational health nurses must be careful not to give misinformation. They cannot speak for the insurance company or the HMO. They can assist both by helping workers who have such protection to use the HMO's services and/or their health insurance coverage wisely.

References

1. Krizay, J. (Ed.). *The Patient as a Consumer*. Lexington, Mass.: Lexington Books, 1974, p. 190.

2. Warshaw, L. J. "The HMO Concept and Its Current Status," *Journal of Occupational Medicine*, Vol. 17, No. 10, Oct. 1975, p. 629.

Selected Readings

Banta, H. D., and Bosch, S. J. "Organized Labor and the Pre-paid Group Practice Movement," *Archives of Environmental Health*, Vol. 29, No. 7, July 1974, pp. 43–49.

Bowman, R. A., and Culpepper, R. C. "National Health Insurance: Some of the Issues," *AJN*, Vol. 75, No. 11, Nov. 1975, pp. 2017–2021.

DHEW, Health Resources Adminstration. *How to Shop for Health Insurance*. Washington, D.C.: GPO, 1978.

Kisch, A. I. "Planning for a Sensible Health Care System," *Nursing Outlook*, Vol. 20, No. 10, Oct. 1972, p. 640.

Leininger, M. "An Open Health Care System Model," *Nursing Outlook*, Vol. 21, No. 3, Mar. 1973, p. 171.

McClure, W. "National Health Insurance and HMOs," *Nursing Outlook*, Vol. 21, No. 1, Jan. 1973, p. 44.

Myers, B. *Health Maintenance Organizations: Objectives and Issues*. DHEW, Health Services and Mental Health Administration. Washington, D.C.: GPO, 1972.

Quinn, N. K., and Somers, A. R. "The Patient's Bill of Rights: A Significant Aspect of the Consumer Revolution," *Nursing Outlook*, Vol. 22, No. 4, Apr. 1974, p. 240.

Roemer, M. I. "Health Care-Financing and Delivery around the World," *AJN*, Vol. 71, No. 6, June 1971, p. 1158.

Silver, G. A. "National Health Insurance, National Health Policy and the National Health," *AJN*, Vol. 71, No. 9, Sept. 1971, p. 1730.

PART V

Health and Safety Education

The worker's right to know and the worker's right to be involved in the conservation of his or her own health requires that the occupational safety and health professional be able to help the worker to have sufficient and meaningful information so as to be able to make informed decisions, develop work-related behavior that is safe, and practice health habits that contribute to the maintenance of health and well-being. Part V of this book deals with how health and safety education is practiced in an occupational setting and how the nurse can and does help workers understand, develop, and use safe work and good health practices. The fourth set of correlative activities that are the parameters of a comprehensive occupational safety and health program is:

WORKER EDUCATION

Continuing awareness of employee needs and environmental conditions to determine what are safe work practices and good health procedures

Instruction to increase the worker's understanding of the exposure and its effects and of preventive health measures and to develop the worker's ability to follow safe work practices and good health procedures; supervision of work practices and follow-up of health-related behavior to ensure each worker's continued well-being

The nurse, as a member of the occupational safety and health team:

- Teaches workers how they can protect their own health, use health resources, and follow good health and safety practices

- Fulfills an ombudsman's role for those workers who require help in understanding their rights and how they may benefit from the legal, social, and health resources that are available to them; assists workers to enter and utilize the health care system.

CHAPTER 17

Education for Health and Safety

Education for health and safety is a process with intellectual, psychological, and social dimensions relating to activities that influence the abilities of people to make informed decisions affecting their personal, family, and community well-being. The process is based on scientific principles. It aims to facilitate learning and behavioral change in both health professionals and consumers.

In his foreword to the book *Healthy People: The Surgeon General's Report on Health Promotion and Disease Prevention*, President Carter said in part:

We Americans are healthier today than we have ever been. Our understanding of the causes of health problems has grown enormously, and with it our ability to prevent and treat illness and injury. . . .

I have long advocated a greater emphasis on preventing illness and injury by reducing environmental and occupational hazards and by urging people to choose to lead healthier lives. So I welcome this Surgeon General's Report on Health Promotion and Disease Prevention. It sets out a national program for improving the health of our people—a program that relies on prevention along with cure. This program is ambitious but achievable. It can substantially reduce the suffering of our people and the burden on our expensive system of medical care.

Government, business, labor, schools, and health professions must all contribute to the prevention of injury and disease. And all of these efforts must ultimately rely on the individual decisions of millions of Americans—decisions to protect and promote their own good health. Together, we can make the goals expressed in this report a reality.

This book was published in 1979 by the GPO (order number 017-001-00416-Z). It should be in every occupational health unit library. The price is $5.00. *Healthy People* is the first Surgeon General's report on health promotion and disease prevention. Its purpose is to encourage the second public health revolution in the history of the United States. The first was the struggles against infectious disease which spanned the late 19th century and the first half of the 20th century. In 1900 the leading causes of death were influenza, pneumonia, diphtheria, tuberculosis, and gastrointestinal infections. Today, as we move into the second health revolution, cardiovascular disease, including both heart disease and strokes, accounts for about half of all deaths in the United States, and cancer accounts for another 20%. In 1900 the death rate was 17 per 1,000 persons per year; in 1979 it was 9 per 1,000. The cost of health care is great. From 1960 to 1978 this grew from $27 billion to $192 billion dollars. The Surgeon General said, "Clearly, the American people are deeply interested in improving their health. The increased attention now being paid to exercise, nutrition, environmental health, and occupational safety testify to their interest and concern with health promotion and disease prevention." Occupational health nurses, as they help workers learn, are helping make the second public health revolution succeed.

Programs designed to improve the health of workers and to stimulate the use of both occupational and community health care systems encompass the activities associated with the initiative *education for health*. This term is being used by health systems agencies, especially the North East New York Health Systems Agency, to describe educational activities designed to improve health status and health care delivery. The agency believes that education on health topics can occur successfully in a wide variety of settings, involving persons from all walks of life as teachers and students, and using many different approaches. The activities associated with the education for health initiative reinforce those that make up environmental monitoring, health surveillance, and primary care. Workers need to know what hazards exist in their work environment and what the consequences can be of not wearing personal protective equipment or of not controlling their weight or of not giving up smoking.

The purpose of health and safety education in an industrial setting is to bring about changes in the knowledge, feelings, and behavior of workers as these relate to safe work and health practices. For such an educational program to be effective, the planning and the teaching methods must be in accord with current understanding of how adults learn. Those who teach must utilize techniques that influence feelings and behavior. Those who plan and conduct worker training programs must accept the fact that people learn more readily when they view what they have to learn as being knowledge they want or need. Equally important, workers must believe that what they are being asked to learn is acceptable and important to their family and their work group. The nurse who plans health and safety educational programs needs to remember that discussions of real-life experiences are usually more effective than formal lectures or the presentation of physiological arguments about why an action should be taken.

Like it or not, health educators must accept that people will change behavior only when they understand what they must do and when they see the recommended action as a means to an end they themselves value. Frequently nurses and the safety professionals have to determine what is important to workers and be certain the information is being presented in a form that they can readily understand.

The worker's right to know what the hazards of the job are and the employer's responsibility to provide a safe and healthful work environment are basic to an understanding of the intent of the Occupational Safety and Health Act. Hence the teaching done by the health professional has as its purpose helping the worker to recognize and, when indicated, to report hazards to OSHA and/or to request NIOSH to do a health hazard evaluation (see App. B for additional information).

Education-for-health programs for workers include teaching employees what they must do to prevent harm to themselves, to fellow workers, and to their families. Health education for workers must be adapted to fit into the overall health program of the industry. Since workers cannot be taken away from their work for long periods of time, nurses must make maximum use of their contacts with employees to teach and to demonstrate good health practices as they provide care or do health assessments.

Occupational health and safety education programs should be attuned to the needs of worker and industry. The aim should be to help employees learn how to take responsibility for the promotion, maintenance, and protection of their own and their families' health. The Chinese saying, "If I hear it, I forget it; if I see it, I remember; if I do it, I know," points out how people learn. All people, no matter how old or how young, can learn. What they learn is influenced by many factors. The speed at which they learn depends on how deeply they are involved in the process and how much they are interested in learning.

The following factors influence how people learn and should be given maximum consideration:

- The way members of a work group feel about and act toward each other, the way workers are supervised, including the recognition by supervisors of the special individual needs of each person and respect for each individual as a person
- The orientation program provided for new employees that aims to help them know how to work in a safe and healthful manner
- The policy of the company about safety and health and the way this is made known to the workers
- The policies concerning housekeeping and sanitation that are developed and implemented by management
- The activities associated with membership on safety and health committees
- The learning that comes with an experience and is reinforced when the foreman or the nurse uses the moment of the unsafe act or the safe act to help the worker understand and to benefit from the experience

- The attitude and the example set by management, including top, middle, and first-line, regarding health and safety, for example wearing protective gear when indicated
- The prompt and appropropriate care that is provided for occupational injuries and illnesses and which demonstrates the value of secondary prevention.
- The provision by management and the supervised use of personal protective equipment
- OSHA inspections; posting of OSHA reports
- The type and variety of food available to workers
- The health assessment program provided by management, The Wise Owl Club, and other safety promotion activities to reward workers for safe work behavior
- Modification of processes and the substitution of less toxic substances that enhance the safety and healthfulness of the work environment
- Environmental monitoring
- Health surveillance activities.

Education-for-health-and-safety initiatives planned for workers and carried out as part of a comprehensive occupational and safety health program have the potential for closing the gap between what the professionals know about prevention and how the workers utilize this knowledge and the positive health services that are available to them. Because nurses have frequent contact with workers and because workers learn to trust nurses, they are in an ideal position to engage in health and safety education. Nurses need the skills, understanding, and willingness to do so.

Health Education Programs in Industry

Education for health programs has proved successful in reducing cardiovascular risk factors among people at high risk, in shortening hospital stays, in increasing use of breast cancer screening services, in reducing hospital readmissions among congestive heart disease patients, in reducing blood pressure, and in providing low-income families with skills to improve their overall life styles.

Two Approaches

The concepts of prevention and wellness provide two frameworks about which to build education for health programs. Prevention-oriented education for health programs centers on preventing the onset of disease, promoting recuperation and rehabilitation of persons who are ill, and promoting community activities that combat illness and its onset. Medical surveillance activities incorporated into the health guidelines of the SCP of OSHA/NIOSH have similar objectives.

Wellness-oriented education for health programs focuses on advances beyond the normal state of nonillness toward higher levels of well-being. They concentrate on four major topics: nutrition, physical awareness, stress reduction, and self-responsibility. The wellness concept promotes the understanding of individuals' needs and how to meet them, activities of self-care, the development of humanistic skills on the part of health providers, and the consideration of alternate approaches to healing. By fostering individual activity, the likelihood of citizen participation in promoting "health" in the community is increased.

Both the wellness approach and the preventive approach to health focus on the maintenance of good health. The preventive approach is more medically oriented, focusing as it does on the prevention, treatment, and amelioration of illness, particularly among high-risk groups. The wellness approach, on the other hand, focuses on improving the existing levels of health of all persons, sick and well.

The environmental monitoring required by OSHA and by good occupational health practices focuses on the wellness approach. If the quantities of a toxic substance in the work environment are under control, workers will not be harmed; and if the mechanical hazards are guarded, workers will not be injured. Medical surveillance activities that provide for adequate assessment of worker health often find deviations early when they are reversible; they focus on the preventive approach. The workers' right to know as stated in the Occupational Safety and Health Act of 1970 is another way of saying "education-for-health."

In recent years the leading causes of death and disability have been those diseases and conditions which are either chronic in nature or are related to risk-taking behavior: cardiovascular diseases, cerebrovascular and neoplastic diseases, and accidents. In contrast to acute diseases, which have a fairly abrupt onset and a finite duration, chronic illnesses have a gradual onset and an indefinite duration. Health resources that are needed for the treatment and rehabilitation of persons with these conditions contribute heavily to the increasing costs of health care.

Educational programs designed to teach the use of health resources include instruction in the selection and use of health services, increasing awareness of health care options, how to choose from among these options, and how to deal assertively with health professionals. Each of these aspects of education in the use of health care resources provides people with the skills to make decisions regarding the types of health care they will choose to accept. An example of such an option is self-care programs that encourage people to take the responsibility for maintaining their health; these programs have proved effective in containing costs and in reducing inappropriate demand on the health care system.

Education for health is a less costly method of dealing with life-style–related diseases and conditions like cardiovascular disease. As life-styles contribute significantly to health status, and as education is a powerful method of promoting healthful behavior, a prime target in education to promote wellness is change in life-style. In occupational health there is an additional emphasis, that of safe work practices as well as good health practices. The experience of effective occupational safety and health training programs reinforces the value of education for health and for safety.

The Health Education Committee

Many occupational health nurses have found it is a good idea for management to establish a health education committee to assist the nurse in formulating and implementing a master plan for the health education program. This committee has representatives of the personnel department, one or more of the operating units, the labor union, the front office, the safety department, and the occupational health department. Its activities are coordinated with those of the safety committee as these relate to worker education and learning.

When an occupational health education committee takes the initiative in setting up a health education program which deals with the identification and control of non-work-related chronic illness, this program can and should be arranged so as to be correlative with the health education plan in the community. Many community health agencies, both official and voluntary, have programs for industrial workers. Health educators serving in the local health department or voluntary health agencies can be asked to be consultants to the committee and/or to the nurse.

The committee will need to meet at regular intervals, more frequently while formulating the program and less frequently after the plan has been made and is being implemented. When formulating the master plan for a health education program, it is helpful for the committee members to study absenteeism in the plant as well as the monthly reports of the health department in order to identify problem areas. The special hazards of the industry must also be identified, and plans must be made to incorporate learning about toxic substances along with planning how to teach workers to acquire protective work practices and health habits. For example workers who are exposed to one or more of the federally regulated carcinogens need to understand what is meant by "cancer-causing substances." They need to learn about the special control measures that must be carried out, for example that they may not eat or smoke in the work area. They also need to learn what signs and symptoms to watch for and to whom these are to be reported. Table 2 (pp. 210–211) shows how an overall health education plan can be drawn up; it is included here as a guide for nurses in compiling a program for the workers in their industries.

Intrastaff Communication

The various educational backgrounds and work experiences among the members of the safety and health occupational team may result in poor communication. Efforts should be made to assure that the health personnel and the safety and supervisory staff understand each other, because effective communication between them governs the overall effectiveness of the team. Communication may be defined as the interchange of ideas, thoughts, or opinions. The nature of thought requires that it be couched in words in order for it to be transmitted from the mind of the sender to the mind of the receiver. Too often the sender (in this case, the nurse) and the receiver (the worker or the safety professional) give the same words different meanings when they engage in conversation. Frequently the specialized jargon that exists within the various disciplines complicates communication to such an extent that either decoding messages is impossible, or worse, their meanings become garbled.

Occasionally the nurse hears from a worker that his protective equipment hurts or is uncomfortable and hence he is not wearing it. Sharing this information with the foreman or the safety professional can result in the worker being assigned a different piece of equipment that fits better. In addition the worker also needs to have added instruction as to why it is needed and how to use it. Wearing it is the behavioral change the worker must develop, but getting him to wear it is the challenge for the nurse and the safety professional. The nurse must work and communicate with others in an intrastaff relationship to try to identify what needs to be done and by whom, and the nurse should be involved in helping to get it done.

Program Planning

Program planning is an exercise that requires certain steps:

1. Identifying the problem or condition involving people and/or their environment which has a current or potential harmful effect on the achievement of the aims of the occupational safety and health program.
2. Stating the condition of the people and/or the environment that is considered by experts to be desirable to attain and to maintain. The objective should be specific as to condition to be attained, degree of intended achievement, and time interval.
3. Listing the work that must be accomplished to achieve the objective. These are the program activities and should be stated as actions.

4. Evaluating to determine the extent to which the predetermined objectives have been attained; determining what effort was put into the doing of the project, what were the end results, and what level of attainment was achieved.

Sample Programs

The value of measurable outcomes that indicate behavioral change is easier to expound than is stating the objective. The following health and safety education program modules provide examples of the points made in this chapter concerning formulation and implementation of health and safety education and training activities.

Glaucoma Screening

The purpose of a glaucoma screening program as defined by the occupational health committee is to test the intraocular tension of all workers 35 years of age or older on whom this test has not been performed within the previous 12 months.

The aims of the program are to provide the workers with educational material about glaucoma so they can understand the disease and the value of screening as a means of identifying persons at risk and can make informed decisions to participate in the glaucoma screening program. This is a measurable behavioral objective. If there are 150 workers 35 years of age or older who have not been seen by an ophthalmologist and/or who have not had a health assessment that included measuring intraocular tension with a tonometer, this is the population at risk. The proportion of this population that participates is a measure of the effectiveness of the program and the degree of importance that the people in this industry give to the identification of glaucoma at an early stage.

The procedure for a glaucoma screening program might be to:

1. Develop the list of workers eligible to take part.
2. Develop the plan for scheduling performance of the test.
3. Discuss the plan with the physician on the health team. Establish the level of elevation above normal at which the test is to be repeated and/or the employee referred to an ophthalmologist.
4. Plan with the ophthalmologist to evaluate your technique. Perform several measurements under supervision.
5. Select informational material for distribution.
6. Develop a bulletin board display.
7. Announce the program and the place and procedure for making an appointment to have the test done.
8. Check the participant's name against the list of those eligible to take part.

Education for Health and Safety

9. Conduct the test.
10. Refer patients with intraocular tension greater than the predetermined acceptable level to an ophthalmologist.
11. Determine if the referral has been completed and if the referral was appropriate. If not completed, find out why and attempt to help the worker understand why the referral was made and what must be done.
12. Write a report. Identify the purpose of the program and indicate the percentage of the population at risk that participated. Note the number of persons with elevated tension readings and the number of persons referred. Note also the number of persons already under treatment.
13. Determine the next step. For example if participation was less than 1 in 10 of those who were eligible, reevaluate the informational program. Ask a few key people who did not take part to tell you why and then modify the educational part of the program accordingly.
14. Evaluate results in regard to: (a) benefits achieved (number of cases disclosed and referrals completed), (b) need to repeat program, and (c) timetable for giving repeat programs.

OSHA Required Worker Training for Those Working with Benzene

The purposes of the program as defined by the occupational health committee are:

1. To explain the OSHA medical surveillance requirements to workers whose jobs involve possible contact with benzene
2. To explain the terms *cancer, leukemia,* and *aplastic anemia*
3. To discuss the plan and what tests will be conducted
4. To answer workers' questions about the hazards of exposure to benzene

The aim of the program is to inform the workers of the hazards of working with benzene so they can decide to participate in the medical surveillance program.

The procedure for a required training program for workers exposed to benzene in the work place might be to:

1. Study the OSHA Standards
2. Confer with the physician, union representative, and management representative on the occupational health committee to get their input and support
3. Make a plan to meet the requirements of the OSHA Standards

4. Develop a timetable for the program activities
5. Arrange with the first-line supervisors and the union representative for a meeting of all the workers who are at risk; in planning for this meeting:
    a. Study the blood diseases associated with benzene (leukemia, aplastic anemia) and benzene as a chemical that is an occupational carcinogen
    b. Read "Conceptual Model for Preventive Health Behavior" by Nola J. Pender in the June 1975 *Nursing Outlook*, pp. 385–395 (or a similar article) to increase knowledge of personal, interpersonal, and situational factors that are motivating or inhibiting determinants of preventive health actions
6. Meet with the workers
    a. Explain the medical surveillance plan that will be followed
    b. Explain the OSHA requirements
    c. Define *cancer, leukemia,* and *aplastic* anemia
    d. Review each worker's health history to determine whether it is accurate and complete
    e. Describe the tests that will be done and what the test results mean
    f. Schedule workers for their appointments
7. Arrange with the laboratory to do the required tests and blood studies
8. Call each worker back for a final conference, and share with him or her the results of the tests and the overall results of the medical surveillance program
9. Complete all necessary records
10. Evaluate the results of the program and make suggestions for modification of the plan.

Safety Education

Safety education is provided primarily by safety professionals and the first-line supervisors responsible for establishing safe work practices. They train the workers to carry out these practices and supervise their work behavior to assure that these practices are in fact followed. The aim of safety training should be to develop safety consciousness on the part of the worker. Correlatively, the essential aim of safety education in relation to OSHA is to teach workers to recognize and to avoid work hazards and to make suggestions when they feel that safer equipment or operation can be achieved.

Safety training in the industrial setting has traditionally been carried on separately from health education. To meet the intent of the OSHA Standards these two services must cooperate in planning and executing their activities. Otherwise workers will be confused, and little or nothing will be accomplished. The subject matter will vary of course, and whenever possible it should be determined by the workers themselves. All information should be presented in a simple and practical manner, since effective safety education not only shows why workers should be careful but also teaches them how to work safely. Much of this teaching is done by the safety professionals and first-line supervisors, but it is important that the nurse and the doctor on the team know in general what is being taught and by whom so that they may reinforce this teaching whenever possible.

Program Evaluation

Periodic evaluation of the progress of a worker education program is necessary to find out whether the program is accomplishing its aims. There is no single way to measure the effectiveness of a health education program. Each worker responds differently to the many and varied activities of a well-planned program. How each person promotes, maintains, and protects his own and his family's health is an individual matter. Some need to develop different attitudes and learn new health habits, while others need only to modify their present attitudes and habits. The importance that members of the occupational health team attach to health education and the amount of attention they give to it are overriding factors in determining the success of the program.

Although it is hard to measure such long-term results as changed attitudes about health, certain other results can be measured. Insofar as possible, specific objectives for the program should be included in the master plan, so that progress can be checked against them. For example one objective may be to cut down on the number of eye accidents in a particular department. Progress toward meeting this objective is fairly easy to evaluate in that the number of injuries before the program of eye safety was started can be compared with the number after it was put into operation. Lost time and medical costs are measurable.

When the objective is to help workers know the danger signals of cancer, the results are less easy to evaluate. One measure could be the number of pamphlets taken from the health literature rack over a certain period of time. A more revealing indication of success might be an increase in the rate of completed referrals, that is, the number of people who sought care from their physician or community clinic for one of the danger signals. The number of men who took advantage of a chest X-ray survey can be counted, as can the number of women who saw the film "Breast Self-Examination." In the latter case a better check would be to ask the women who did see the film if they are following the suggestion and are performing breast self-examinations once a month.

Table 2
Sample Health Education Program Plan

Aim	Time Table	Coordinate with
To inform workers about high blood pressure; to promote weight control	Feburary is heart month; plan for full impact at that time; order material and new scale in November and arrange with editor for space in February issue of company paper.	Local heart association and editor of company paper; set up policy or renew policy concerning blood pressure with the physician that requires referral.
To help the worker learn the seven danger signals of cancer; to promote stopping smoking	Over 7-month period, feature one of the seven danger signals on the bulletin board and in the information rack in the OHS unit.	Local American Cancer Society; order *Cancer and the Worker* from N.Y. Academy of Sciences meet with management and the union and the physician concerning medical surveillance for workers in department.
To inform the worker about eye health; to promote participation in glaucoma screening program	Conduct glaucoma screening program in March and April; order materials in February; bulletin board and company paper focus in March.	NSPB; set up policy and/or review policy with the physician on level of elevation of tension requiring referral.
To inform the worker about skin care and to promote personal hygiene	Develop slide film show on hand washing; show at intervals in the waiting room throughout the year; use in January safety meeting with men working outdoors.	Safety department physician; Workmen's compensation representative to discuss the plan and script for the slide film show; order material; work with company photographer or create a slide show on how to care for hands; tape message.

Bulletin Board	Literature Rack	Company Paper	Other Activities
Plan 3 displays: What is high blood pressure? Why control weight? Why stay on medication?	Copies of OSHA governmental publications in English and Spanish.	What you need to know about blood pressure. Alert workers to the 1980 DHHS & Agriculture's publication "Nutrition and Your Health."	Hold blood pressure clinics 1 hour per week; put scale in waiting room; set up chart so people can record weight loss.
Plan seven displays, one each for seven danger signals; Plan one for stopping smoking.	Copies of American Chemical Society publication for distribution; have copies of *Cancer and the Worker* on hand for loan.	Explain the company's medical surveillance program.	Meet with union representatives and safety department; plan special health education session for workers at risk.
Plan two displays: The eye and What is glaucoma?	Copies of booklet from NSPB.		Conduct glaucoma screening program.
Plan one display on care of skin; focus on harm to skin from the cold and from chemicals.		Show at safety meeting. Develop a 50-film slide projector program with taped message on how to wash and dry hands and on special attention needed during cold weather for those working outdoors;	

Health Education Aids

Literature

Much worker education can be accomplished through the use of a well-planned literature display and exhibit. Bulletin boards and health literature racks in the cafeteria, rest rooms, and throughout the plant can be used to make health information freely available to workers. Such display material should be chosen carefully and changed frequently. There should be a bulletin board in the occupational health unit for posters and for a display of health and safety information. Carefully chosen pamphlets on health topics should be available at the nurse's station for workers to read if they have to wait a few minutes for the nurse or physician.

Some of the almost endless supply of information pamphlets are excellent; others are worthless. All literature used in an employee health and safety education program needs to be critically chosen and evaluated. Expert members of the occupational health team should be responsible for checking the accuracy of specific information offered. The physician and the nurse should read all health information pamphlets before they are given to workers and ask the safety engineer to review those dealing with safety subjects. In addition to printed matter, many posters, exhibits, and films are available. These too should be reviewed critically to assure that they are correct and that the message is pertinent to the program and written with clarity for the worker. When English is not the first language of the employee, foreign-language publications are of special importance and value.

When a nurse needs pamphlets, posters, films, or displays to use for a health education program, it is important to decide what idea is to be put across. It is helpful to review the resources in the community to see which agencies might be able to help. Contact one or more of the local or state offices of these agencies and tell the representative about your plan, approximately how many there are in the group, their sex, their average age, and what you can of their interests and educational backgrounds, and ask for suggestions.

The department's policy and procedural manual should include the agencies' addresses and, if possible, the names of the persons to be contacted and the type of service offered by local official and voluntary agencies. Many state health and labor departments have bureaus or divisions for public health information. The nurse will find it helpful to become familiar with the resources of these official agencies and learn how to use them. Many insurance companies also supply a wide variety of health and safety education materials that can be used to good advantage. The nurse should be familiar particularly with the materials available from the insur-

Education for Health and Safety

ance carrier that provides the workmen's compensation, health, hospital, and life insurance for the company's employees. The cost of publications has so increased that most health care agencies and insurance companies no longer make these available in quantity for mass distribution.

Single copies or limited quantities of publications are made available free and additional quantities are for sale. Many health and safety publications, especially those developed by the government, can be reprinted. Permission to reprint can be granted if the request to do so is made officially to the author and the publisher. When the occupational health budget is developed each year, a line item for health publications should be included so that the necessary films can be rented or purchased and pamphlets and posters purchased to support the health education program.

Nurses will find it most helpful to have their names on the list of those to whom announcements of new publications and/or sample copies are mailed by commerical, voluntary, and official agencies. In this way they can keep up to date on what is available and can share this with the members of the health and safety committee.

Health and Safety Guides

Soon after NIOSH was created by the Occupational Safety and Health Act, a decision was made to commit funds and professional staff time to the development of health and safety guides. The purpose of the guides is to provide management with information they require to determine whether their establishment is or is not in compliance with the OSHA Standards. The guides have been developed for industry groups like hospitals, laundries, dry cleaners, plastic fabricators, and so on and are available for sale from the GPO (see page 312 for additional information).

NIOSH's staff also developed a series of guides to good work practices that are very useful as training aids. Single copies are available free from NIOSH and they are also for sale by the GPO. Examples are *A Guide to Good Work Practices for Operators of Cranes; Welding Safety;* and *Working with Cutting Oils*.

NIOSH also publishes an annual *Publication Catalog,* and it is recommended that a copy be on file in the health unit so that the availability of specialized publications will be known by the staff. A catalog of OSHA publications is also available; it provides information about this agency's publications.

OSHA Standards

The OSHA Standards require that workers be offered a medical surveillance program they can participate in or reject. The health teaching program offered in support of the prevention of illness from exposure to toxic substances must be so planned and conducted as to give the workers the amount and kind of information that will allow them to make informed decisions and encourage them to participate in the medical surveillance program. The number of workers who participate in the medical surveillance program and who respond to the recommendations of the nurse and the safety professionals can be used as one measure of the effectiveness of the teaching program.

The OSHA Standard on vinyl chloride in Appendix D is an example of information that nurses can use as the basis for their health teaching. Similar information is included in the OSHA health standards and in the publications that have been generated as a result of the SCP, a joint undertaking of NIOSH and OSHA (see page 306 for added information as to availability).

The objective of the SCP, which was begun in 1973, was to develop more comprehensive standards for the 390 substances whose environmental limit standards were promulgated by the DOL in 1971. For each of the substances, the Draft Technical Standards developed by SCP include provisions pertinent to the potential hazards; engineering monitoring and control mechanisms; sampling techniques and sampling intervals; medical surveillance and physiological testing procedures; the fire, explosion, and safety hazards; record keeping; and retention and accessibility to records for each substance. NIOSH has published some of this material as the *Pocket Guide to Chemical Hazards*. It is based on the standard completion information for some 385 chemicals and is available from the GPO (order number 017-033-00342-4); the price, as of 1979, was $5.00.

Incidental Teaching Aids

Pamphlets and other printed matter alone do not constitute a health education program. Planned training sessions to discuss some aspect of health, individual conferences, the distribution of selected printed materials, and well-planned displays all play a part. Audiovisual presentations, some of which are designed especially for a work group, can be and often are used to great advantage. Television sets in waiting rooms that show specially designed tape recordings are an effective teaching device. The use of movie films and slides adds a further dimension to a health and safety training session if the material presented is carefully selected and used to reinforce what the worker is being told.

Cartoons and pictures depicting actual events can be most effective. There are many examples of programs in industry where the safety professional uses pictures taken at the work sites to show both good and poor work practices. At other times and places the safety professional or the nurse routinely have pictures taken to illustrate an accident. These are displayed on a bulletin board or used to illustrate a report to management or an article in the company's magazine. Workers with talent in taking pictures or drawing cartoons can be most helpful members of a health and safety committee. Such people like to be asked to participate in activities to inform other workers.

The provision of adequate sanitary facilities, food service, and occupational health and safety services are important components of a health education program. None of these services is intended exclusively to influence the worker's knowledge, feelings, and actions about health, but they do nevertheless. Just the fact that they are available indicates that someone thinks that health and safety are important. Also the nutritionist or the food service manager can be enlisted to help develop an effective health education program. The program planners should capitalize on the many teaching opportunities available in the cafeteria. Here the workers are free from their job responsibilities and interested in food. Here teaching by example is carried out when adequate and nourishing meals are served.

Various teaching aids can be used to help workers to understand the food value of fruit juice compared to a soft drink or of milk compared to coffee. Also the cafeteria is the ideal place to stress the importance of weight control. An example is the nurse who, once a week, had her lunch with a group of workers who wanted to learn more about food values and calories and talked with them about nutrition. Other nurses occasionally show a film during the lunch hour and have interested workers join them in viewing it and discussing it afterward.

Occupational health team members should remember that they teach health and safety by their attitude and example as well as by participating as teachers in the planned program. Every action of every occupational health team member is noticed by the workers, and everything they do or do not say has an influence on attitudes and behavior. People also accept new ideas and practices only after they have become familiar with them, have used them, and are convinced that they are important. The following example shows how health teaching may be carried on as an adjunct to other occupational health services or to other activities in which workers take part.

An overweight nurse suddenly realized that she was setting a bad example. Her credibility was challenged when she counseled workers on diet. She organized a seven-session diet therapy group. The purpose was to deepen her understanding and that of the eight other overweight workers of their self-image and of the causes of their overweight condition. They explored nonphysiological blocks to weight loss. The result was a consciousness-raising experience, with members of the group being extremely supportive of each other, and they all lost weight.

The Nurse as Occupational Health Educator

The role of the occupational health nurse in a health education program includes being a facilitator of learning with the goal of arousing the workers' interest and developing their understanding. To do so the nurse provides meaningful information that workers can accept and use as the basis for altering their health habits and work practices.

Health and safety education activities are an integral part of every occupational health program. If nurses are to help workers learn how to protect their health and how to make use of health care resources and safe work practices, the nurses must understand the concept of self-responsibility, that is, each person responsible for determining and enhancing his or her own health potential. Health is much more than the absence of illness; it is a dynamic state in which people do their best with the capacities they have and act the best they know how to maximize their strengths. Helping workers understand this concept is a challenge occupational health nurses must deal with as they assess the health status of employees in relation to their work. Helping workers to recognize hazards and to know when and how to see that the employer carries out his responsibility under OSHA is an integral part of an occupational health nurse's responsibilities.

One of the staff work responsibilities of nurses is to provide management with information about the health and safety of the work environment that permits their making decisions as to what must be done to assure that the establishment is in compliance. When a nurse has found a useful publication or hears of a conference that will provide current and necessary information, she forwards the information, over her signature, to management. Occupational health nurses provide information about health, not only for workers, but for management, who must make decisions, often about subjects they do not truly understand or when they do not appreciate the significance of their decisions.

An excellent way for nurses to contribute to the effectiveness of occupational health education programs is to contribute articles on health and/or safety to the company's and other publications. Most nurses do not like to write, and many say that they can't write. Writing is a skill that requires practice and one which occupational health nurses would do well to develop. Editors of company publications are usually more than willing to help a nurse who feels insecure about her writing skill. The health information units of state health departments and many of the voluntary health agencies will supply information and facts for articles. Many also provide appropriate articles that may be adapted to serve the needs of the industry's health education program.

Selected Readings

AMA. "Guide to Health Education and Counseling of Employees," *Occupational Health Nursing*, Vol. 19, No. 8, Aug. 1971, pp. 17–19.
ANA, Division of Community Health Nursing Practice. *The Professional Nurse and Health Education*, ANA Pub. Code VP 483000. Kansas City, Mo., 1975.
Cantor, N. *The Teaching-Learning Process*. New York: Holt, Rinehart & Winston, 1953.
DOL. *Teaching Safety and Health in the Workplace, An Instructor Guide*, OSHA 2255. Washington, D.C.: GPO, 1976.
Engel, P. G. "The Re-emerging Priority Safety Education and Training," *Occupational Hazards*, Nov. 1977, p. 31.
Hollister, W. G., and Edgerton, J. W. "Teaching Relationship-Building Skills," *American Journal of Public Health*, Vol. 64, No. 1, Jan. 1974, pp. 41–46.
Leventhal, H. "Changing Attitudes and Habits to Reduce Risk Factors in Chronic Disease," *American Journal of Cardiology*, Vol. 31, No. 5, May 1973, pp. 571–580.
Mager, R. F. *Preparing Instructional Objectives*. Belmont, Calif.: Fearon, 1962.
Milio, N. "A Broad Perspective on Health: A Teaching-Learning Tool," *Nursing Outlook*, Vol. 24, No. 3, Mar. 1976, pp. 160–163.
Pender, N. J. "A Conceptual Model for Preventive Health Behavior," *Nursing Outlook*, Vol. 23, No. 6, June 1975, pp. 385–388.
Redman, B. (Ed.). "Patient Teaching," *Nursing Digest*, Vol. 6, No. 1, Special Issue, Spring 1978.
ReVelle, J. B. "Safety Education: Which Way to Go," *Professional Safety*, Vol. 24, No. 6, June 1979, pp. 18–22.
Simmons, J. (Chairperson-Ed.). "Making Health Education Work," *American Journal of Public Health*, Vol. 65, No. 10, Supple., Oct. 1975, p. 1.
WHO. *Expert Committee on Health Education of the Public*, Technical Rep. No. 89. Geneva, 1954.
Wilson, H. *Employee Training and Development*. Deerfield, Ill.: Administrative Research Association, 1960.

PART **VI**

Management of the Occupational Health Unit and Program

Basic principles of administration apply to an occupational health service as they do for the conduct of any other unit of the company. Someone provides administrative direction and in doing so delegates to others responsibility for program planning, implementation, and evaluation. Because the occupational health unit staff provides therapeutic care for workers who are injured or become ill at work, provision must be made for a physician to provide medical direction. Part VI of this book deals with the role of the nurse in the management of the occupational health unit: the staff, the program, the budget, and the usefulness of the service to the industry and the employees. The nurse as a member of the occupational health service staff:

- Participates in planning and evaluating the occupational health program, which aims to meet the needs of the workers and the industry
- Participates in the establishment of and, when required, the use of a disaster plan and in teaching and coordinating the activities of the first-aid personnel
- Develops and maintains a health record for each worker
- Prepares reports that reflect the range of activities of the occupational health service and permit drawing conclusions about cause, frequency, and severity of illnesses and injuries; identifies needs; and proposes program plans that permit an evaluation of the effectiveness of the occupational health service
- Establishes and maintains liaison with community health and social agencies.

CHAPTER 18

Administration of Occupational Health Services and Units

The word *administration* is derived from the Latin verb meaning *to serve*. Today, however, the word means *to manage*. Management is the process of making decisions, the coordinating of activities, the handling of people, and the evaluation of performance directed toward group objectives.

This chapter deals with the application of basic principles of administration to the management of an occupational health service. These principles are well known, enjoy wide acceptance, and are as applicable to the effective management of an occupational health service as they are to that of any health service or, for that matter, to any department of the company. Of concern are two levels of administration: industry level and health unit level. It is at industry level that policy is established, budgets are approved, and areas of responsibility are delegated. At the health unit level the person to whom the responsibility for the day-to-day operation of the health service has been delegated is accountable.

Administration is an enabling process. It requires that someone provide leadership who has the ability to make policy and to plan. This person must also be able to execute the plan by providing the services or by delegating this responsibility to others. The person who administers a health unit has six key functions, three that constitute process and three that constitute effect:

PROCESS	EFFECT
To forecast	Development of plan and policy
To organize	Coordination of the efforts of workers, materials, and equipment
To command	Control of the budget, hence of the actions of the staff and the scope of the service

These six functions follow each other in logical sequence. They are as essential for the effective management of an occupational health service organized to serve the employees of an establishment that employs less than 500 people as they are for a health unit organized to provide services for many thousands of employees. In the large establishment the full-time medical director is a member of the top management of the company and as such formulates the company's occupational health care plan and is responsible for its execution. The medical director may set administrative and medical policies and exercise control over these activities at both the industry and the health unit levels.[1] (Occupational Medicine Practice Committee, 1979). In the smaller establishment, when the physician is a part-time employee or consultant, all too often someone in management who has administrative responsibility retains control of the budget in such a way as to limit the authority of the nurse to manage the health unit's day-to-day operation.

The occupational health staff should be administratively responsible to someone at the policy-making level. A nurse who is the only full-time health unit employee should have clearly defined areas of responsibility and lines of communication that permit direct access to the decision-making member of management. The practice of having a nurse report through a part-time physician or to the person responsible for safety is to be discouraged. These employees and the nurse are co-workers and, if they do not all work in one department, they should report individually to someone in management for administrative direction. A nurse who is to be the establishment's only full-time health unit employee needs to be aware of the problems that can arise if she has the opportunity to manage the health unit but has not been delegated the responsibility to do so. This needs to be clarified at time of employment and shown in the nurse's job description. Because many health units do not have full-time medical directors, company management must see that there be a physician appointed to provide medical direction for the program that the nurse is to carry out. The physician may be employed part time or serve as a health consultant, but a physician must be involved if the industry is to meet the health assessment requirements of the OSHA Standards for medical surveillance. Medical direction is different from administrative direction; both are required. The person who provides medical direction for the program can also provide administrative direction if he has the authority to control the expenditure of funds. The person who is not a physician but who has administrative responsibility cannot provide medical direction for the program.

Managing the Occupational Health Unit

Except in the very large establishment the occupational health unit will be a relatively small department. In all establishments, large or small, the health department will be a nonmonetary profit-producing unit of the company. It will require a specialized staff of health professionals. It tends not to fit the mold and method of functioning of other units of the company that are organized to produce the company product or to provide services. Often the need for and nature of an occupational health unit is not well understood or appreciated by those responsible for company management; hence there is need for special input from an expert consultant as to the purpose of the health unit and how the health professional functions.

Several health-related activities require input from a health professional, and if the person who must make the decision is not knowledgeable about occupational health, then some provision must be made for meaningful input in all three of the processes of administration: forecasting, organizing, and commanding. This is easier said than done. Physicians are often so busy that they tend not to take on consultation commitments. Many do not want to be responsible for determining the extent of a medical surveillance program or to provide medical orders for use by a nurse they do not know. Problems sometimes arise because the management person responsible for the administration of the occupational health unit and program is not sufficiently informed and hence unable to make administrative decisions. Our society continues to think of the physician as leader of the occupational health unit; but when the physician is only a part-time employee or consultant, the nurse should be selected for leadership ability and given administrative responsibility for the unit and for providing guidance to the management person who provides the administrative direction. When indicated, this nurse should have access to a physician willing to discuss the recommendations the nurse will make to management.

In any work situation someone must decide what should be done. Too often someone decides to employ a nurse, but no one has done any forecasting of needs and no program has been formulated. Forecasting requires facts, classified and analysed. The plan that evolves must correspond to the realities of the situation. The person who makes the plan needs to consider the limitations of the situation. For example the industry is in business to make a product or to provide a service that can be sold; hence the occupational health program plan needs to be so designed that it can be implemented at and through the place of employment. To be workable, a health plan for an industry should (a) be simple, (b) be flexible, (c) fit the needs of the people it aims to serve and the industry that employs them, (d) utilize existing resources, and (e) have clearly defined objectives.

The process of organization involves finding the means, both human and material, to meet the forecasted needs and the program plan. It also requires that someone determine what jobs are to be done; what workers are to do them; and what materials, tools, and equipment are needed to accomplish the work required for the plan to be carried out. Someone must be responsible for the overall direction of the service to ensure that things are being done in accordance with the plan. A health care program needs to be under the direction of someone who has health care knowledge and expertise. The nurse can direct the program if the responsibility is so delegated, if opportunities for input into the planning process are provided, and if there is recognition by top management that the nurse is in this role to facilitate the administration of the establishment's occupational health service.

Staffing Patterns

Occupational health services exist because individuals have occupations and work together in groups. The size of the group, the nature of the organization (service or manufacuring, commercial or governmental), and the willingness of the management to provide the occupational health service determines whether there will be a health service at the place of employment. It is a truism that workers' need of a health and safety program at their place of employment is the same whether they work for a company that employs 20,000 or 20 persons. Quantitatively the need is less in the small establishment and less likely to be met. The concept of what an occupational health service is has developed from the experience of the large manufacturing establishments and service industries that have employed occupational safety and health professionals to develop and to conduct such services.

The number and variety of personnel who staff an occupational health service depends upon the size of the industry. The health departments of very large industries employ a full complement of staff with a full-time medical director as the administrator. The director has on the staff full- and part-time physicians and medical consultants. The nursing personnel include a nursing supervisor, head nurses, staff nurses, and occasionally, nurses who visit workers at home. In addition there are technicians, clerks, and maintenance workers. Sometimes assigned to the health department but more frequently to separate departments are the engineer members of the occupational health team—the safety and industrial hygiene specialists and their staffs. A special staff concerned with medical insurance programs is also a part of some medical departments.

The complete occupational health team is seldom found in companies that employ less than 5,000 workers, and only in the health services of large industries are all the members of the occupational health team full-time employees of the company. As the size of the industry increases so does the number of full-time professional members of the team. In the small companies, those that employ less than 500 workers, the nurse usually works alone and receives medical direction from a part-time doctor who may or may not be a salaried member of the industry's health service staff. Other programs may be staffed by two or more nurses. Occasionally a small company with special needs may employ a full-time physician, but more often the doctor is part time. The clerical and maintenance personnel in such health services are usually part time or are sent into the health unit from other departments of the establishment. Such establishments may have one or more persons responsible for safety. Seldom is a person with industrial hygiene expertise employed full time.

Increasingly in the larger occupational health units nonmedical administrators are responsible for the management of the units or unit. There may be a staff of full-time and/or part-time physicians including a selected list of consultants. The largest proportion of the positions are for nurses. The members of the nursing service staff report to the occupational health nursing service director, who is a member of the occupational health unit's decision-making management team. There are head nurse positions in the various units and for the several work shifts if the occupational health service is operational for more than 8 hours. In many chemical and heavy-manufacturing establishments, the occupational health units are staffed 24 hours a day throughout the year. There may be positions for licensed practical nurses, although most of the nurses working in occupational health are registered professional nurses. On the staffs of the large industrial occupational health units, there may be technicians who staff the X-ray units and the clinical laboratory. There may be specially prepared personnel to do audiometric and pulmonary-function testing, especially if the work load for these procedures is great. There is a clerical staff, and in the very large units there may be a record librarian or supervisor of health records. Sometimes as an integral part of the occupational health department, but usually in a separate department, are the environmental and safety professionals, who are also members of the occupational health team. This unit may have its own industrial hygiene laboratory staffed by specialized chemists. The number of persons on the staff of the environmental facet of the occupational health team frequently exceeds that of the health unit. Here the majority work in safety and accident prevention. In addition, there usually is a special staff concerned with the worker's compensation and health insurance programs.

No realistic formula has yet been developed for estimating the number of nurses, doctors, and allied personnel needed to staff an occupational health unit. Where employees live and work influences the size of the staff. In a metropolitan area, an occupational health service usually provides care for workers with occupational diseases or injuries and gives emergency care and counseling for nonoccupational conditions. In underdeveloped areas the service may provide complete care for workers as well as their families, so the variety and number of unit personnel would be much greater.

One standard for estimating the minimum number of nurses needed to staff a health service of an industry employing between 500 and 2,000 employees is 8 hours of nursing coverage per week for each 100 workers. Using this formula an industry employing 500 workers would need 40 hours of nursing time for the first 8 hours of operation. If it is a continuous-operation establishment then some decision must be made for what coverage is to be provided for workers on the other work shifts. One employing 2,000 workers would by this standard require 160 hours per week and four nurses. If this is an around-the-clock operation, two nurses may work 8–4 when the large majority of the workers are on duty, and one nurse may work 4–12. The fourth nurse will fill in for the days off of the 8–4 and 4–12 nurses.

Another rule of thumb is 1 hour of doctor time for each 6 hours of nursing time. This would provide 7 doctor-hours per week for the industry with 500 workers and 30 doctor-hours for the larger ones. The addition of one nurse for each additional 1,000 workers has been found to be satisfactory in all but very hazardous continous-process industries. These figures are suggested as minimums, although it is recognized that they are much higher than is the practice in many occupational health services now in operation.

The need for clerical help is also hard to estimate. In larger occupational health services, the need for clerical staff and laboratory technicians is obvious. This is not true in a smaller service, and the only solution seems to be that clerical help should be assigned to the department on a part-time basis. Someone who can do both clerical work and simple laboratory and screening procedures is a welcome addition to the occupational health department staff.

Wise use of professional time is an important part of good management of the occupational health department. The activities of the nurse and the physician should be studied regularly, and as the service grows, it may be necessary to make staff changes. This may involve the use of a clerk or a technician for those nonnursing and nonmedical activities that are an important part of the program. In small services or in new ones, it is sometimes the pattern for the nurse and the doctor to carry on all the activities until the weight of the work load is established and then to add personnel as needed. Neither the nurse nor the physician should be so burdened with clerical, routine health assessment activities, and health unit maintenance responsibilities that they cannot carry out their professional responsibilities of providing a positive health program.

Nursing Service Personnel

Several levels of nursing positions are recognized in occupational health services. Some of the more commonly used terms are occupational health nurse, occupational health nurse practitioner, director of nursing services, nursing supervisor, head nurse, and nurse coordinator. The larger the staff the more need for several levels of positions that involve directing the activities of the staff nurse. The AAOHN defines the *occupational health nurse coordinator* as "a registered professional nurse who is proficient as an occupational health nurse clinician, and who is able to develop, implement, evaluate, supervise, and coordinate the delivery of health care services to employees."[2] What is important is the delegation to a nurse of the responsibility for setting the standards for nursing service and for the direction of the work of the nurses. The title of this position is of less importance than is the assignment of both the responsibility and the opportunity to determine the extent of the nurse's involvement in the program. The person who has these responsibilities is more able to function effectively if she or he has had experience at several levels of occupational health nursing practice and has had academic preparation for this leadership position.

Some corporations have established a consultant position instead of a director position because of the autonomy of its separate units in the corporation. The nurse selected to fill this position is on the staff of the corporate medical director, a consultant to the director in nursing matters, and the nurse member of the corporation's health department management team. Each of the several occupational health units have a head nurse, and the corporate-level occupational health nurse consultant provides assistance to these head nurses as well as to the physicians and managment of the company, not only on questions of nursing practice, but on questions relating to the occupational program. This nurse consultant frequently represents the corporate medical director on committees within the corporation and in the community.

The director of nursing service or the consultant nurse forecasts the number and type of nursing positions and sets the standards for nursing practice. The nurse in the leadership job is responsible for evaluating the performance of the nurses and speaks for the nurses in the overall planning and organizing of the occupational health service. She consults with the medical director and a representative of top management on budgetary matters.

When several levels of positions exist, the staff nurses report to the nurse who is their supervisor. A good working relationship between the nurse supervisor and the staff is important for the efficiency of the health unit and the job satisfaction of supervisor and staff. The supervisor and the nurse director or nurse consultant must have a similar good working relationship. Both turn to their supervisor or consultant for orientation to the job and for direction in nursing matters and interpretation of health unit policy.

The employer's concept of the job that the nurse is to perform will be influenced by what the personnel director or the manager thinks to be the role of the nurse. This all too often is to give care to people who are sick or hurt. Time not used to give such care is then expected to be used to do "something else." This may be to do the insurance forms, to be an assistant in the personnel office, and/or to be involved in health promotion and health conservation activities. These latter functions are not understood by many people in industry, who also do not see the nurse as the person who can do the planning of the program and the required activities. The job description provided by a company may be as simple as "Nurse—nonexempt salary level; reports to the director of personnel."

In such cases nurses have to spell out what a nurse can do and what constitutes the required support system: medical direction for the program the nurse is to carry on and access to the skills and understandings of the industrial hygienist and the safety professional. The job description of the position filled by the nurse should provide the basis for evaluation of the nurse's performance and spell out the channels of communication between the nurse and management, the nurse and the safety professional, and the nurse and the physician. The job description should specify the several areas of responsibility and the particular functions of the nurse. It is suggested that these be stated as actions, for example making recommendations to management regarding the extent of the hearing conservation program. The statement of functions should show the amount of independent decision making to be undertaken by the nurse as well as the nurse's degree of involvement in the planning for accomplishment of the specific activities. The following list of functions includes examples of statements that may be incorporated into a job description for an occupational health nurse:

- Plan and conduct screening programs for the workers.
- Provide nursing care for workers who become sick or are injured while at work.
- Prepare an annual plan of work and the first draft of the budget.
- Prepare monthly reports for management, including all heads of departments, to show use of occupational health unit and for what reasons.
- Represent the company and occupational health nursing on the local heart association's health education committee.
- Serve as a member of the establishment's safety committee.

Supervision

Supervision is the process of setting standards of nursing practice and helping the staff to accept and be able to meet them. It is a creative process that results in growth for both the supervisor and the staff nurses. The results are seen in the development of leadership skills on the part of the supervisor and a strengthening of skills and abilities of the staff nurses.

The major responsibilities of the supervisor are to:

Administration of Occupational Health Services and Units

1. Serve as a member of the occupational health unit's management staff
2. Participate in the planning of the occupational health unit's program
3. Determine what contributions the nurse can make to the achievement of the occupational health unit's program goals
4. Set standards of nursing practice
5. Select staff for employment
6. Evaluate staff performance
7. Conduct staff education
8. Involve the staff in the development of work practices as well as policies and procedures for the unit.

Supervision is not administration; it is an adjunct to administration. Supervisors support the administration and the manager; they enlist the manager's help and endorsement for the staff's needs and concerns. When more than one nurse is employed, one should be designated the nurse supervisor and be assigned the responsibility and given the opportunity to fulfill the duties of the supervisor. When only one nurse is employed, she must be able to participate in the six functions of administration of the occupational health unit. This nurse must be self-directive as to nursing functions and professional growth.

Communication

An important aspect of supervision is good communication. Those who give direction to staff must remember that it is the recipient of their communications who determines whether they have made themselves understood. The recipient's behavior is the indicator of whether communication has been anything other than interpersonal static. Effective communication on the part of the supervisor involves both receiving and providing information and ideas.

Standards

Standards of performance should be spelled out so that quality as well as quantity of performance can be measured. Standards should be broad in scope, clearly stated, relevant to the plan, reasonable, and possible to achieve. They ought to be definite enough that the professional can know whether he or she has met the standards but at the same time be flexible enough to allow for creativity and be adaptive to changing conditions.

Evaluation

Evaluation is the process of considering evidence or facts measured against a value or set of standards. When doing a nursing audit, a nurse supervisor looks for evidence that:

1. The care provided by the nurse was in line with the physician's orders
2. The nurse made observations
3. The nurse directed the nursing care provided
4. The nurse coordinated the care given by others
5. The nurse recorded the care given
6. The nursing care provided met the standards established for the occupational health unit
7. The nursing care included teaching the worker-patient
8. The nursing care included recognition of the environmental hazards of the worker's job
9. The nursing care took into consideration the worker's basic human needs and was planned to meet them
10. The nursing care included the five levels of prevention and had as its purpose the worker-patient's earliest possible return to work and to independent functioning.

Delegation

Delegation is the act of empowering someone to act for another. In all too many situations delegation just sort of happens when someone starts to do what needs to be done but hasn't been. Delegation is most effective when someone higher up in the organization plan asks a staff member who has special expertise to carry out an activity. This person willingly accepts and supports the taking of an action or the making of a decision by an employee at one or more levels below his or her own. The key words are *accept*, *support*, and *taking* or *making*. The end results are usually more efficient delivery of services and the acquisition by the staff person of new skills and more confidence. Delegation of responsibility from the management representative to the nurse permits the nurse to purchase certain items or to order a taxi to transport a sick worker home.

The day-to-day administration of the health unit is often delegated to a health unit manager or the nurse. In such instances clarification of what is delegated is required, and it would be well for the nurse to explain to management how she makes decisions. Trust needs to be developed. Therefore when the nurse becomes aware of questions or problems that have not been dealt with, she will find it useful to make the decision and then check it with the person who has delegated the responsibility. For example, "I'll have to deal with this situation and for these reasons. . . . I plan to do the following things . . . . Do you have any suggestions or reasons to think I should not proceed in this fashion?" Working together in this way helps to develop trust.

Consultation

The consultation process involves advising and the use of educational techniques whereby one with more knowledge and experience shares this expertise with another to help that person identify and solve a problem and thereby acquire new professional work-related behavior. The occupational health consultant will:

- Define a problem and suggest means whereby it can be solved
- Offer advice on a given subject in such a way that the consultee can use all, part, or none of it
- Serve as an arbitrator in organizational conflicts
- Serve as a role model for an occupational health nurse and demonstrate how to perform certain specialized activities.

Consultation involves the identification of a problem. The major service of the consultant is to help the consultee to formulate a clear definition of the problem. This delineation of the problem often leads to its solution.

Consultants are change agents. They bring their expertise in occupational health nursing to an interchange between themselves and the occupational health nurse, management, and the physician. They are specialists with particular knowledge, although they have no authority in the occupational health unit. They come into a situation upon request. Often a consultant's employer is an insurance company or a state agency. Increasingly the consultant will be a member of the headquarter's staff or of a consulting firm that sells service to industry.

Mental health nurse consultants are experts in human relations and interpersonal problems who aim to teach new ways of relating and serve as role models for the occupational health nurses. They do this by creating an environment in which previous behavior patterns can be examined without censure and in which nurses can learn new behaviors to use when a situation arises involving the patterns that are the subject of the consultation.

Maintenance of the Health Unit

Provision should also be made for adequate maintenance of the department. This is a company management responsibility which includes the formulation of administrative policies and the provision of a sufficient operating budget to provide for adequate personnel, equipment, and facilities and for keeping them at optimum efficiency.

The occupational health unit must be clean. The nurse's responsibility in this is to supervise the activities of the people who do the cleaning. Good housekeeping pays off, and a well-planned program of maintenance that includes routine wall and window washing, floor scrubbing, and cleaning of equipment and storage cupboards is recommended. A systematic plan should be developed for painting and other major maintenance activities. The equipment should be serviced by a trained technician; dates when equipment has been purchased, serviced, and calibrated should be recorded and an administrative report should be maintained. There should be a systematic checking (daily, weekly) made of all equipment to assure that it is in working order. There should be a plan for the rotation of supplies; those set aside for the disaster plan should be utilized and replaced as indicated by the lifetime usefulness of the drugs, equipment, and other supplies.

Maintenance of an adequate supply of materials and equipment is also necessary. This requires wise planning and study, so that sufficient quantities of the most useful types of equipment and medical supplies are always on hand. These supplies include drugs, dressings, records, linens, and many other things, depending on the extent of the service. Some keep only a 2 months' supply on hand. It is poor economy indeed to buy a quantity that cannot be stored safely or that will not be used before it is out of date. The physician should be consulted about medications and medical supplies; and new medications, dressings, and equipment should not be ordered unless the physician has approved their use. The nurse should keep up to date and be on the lookout for dressings and other supplies that are particularly adaptable to the care the unit provides.

Budget Process

Budgeting is a process that requires a statement of aims and goals. The first step consists of delineating what must be done, by whom, and in what time frame. The second step is to price these activities, including staff salaries, fringe benefits, and relief staff. The costs of supplies, equipment, space, and utilities must be determined. The associated costs of using consultants and medical specialists need to be shown as well as the overhead charge for the specific services from other departments. If cars and/or ambulances are assigned to the occupational health unit, then the cost of gasoline and maintenance as well as the monthly garage rent must be shown in the budget. The purchase and rent of audio visual equipment and supplies should be estimated, as should the purchase of health and safety pamphlets, books, and posters. These and money to cover the cost of the staff's participation in professional meetings, continuing educational programs, and for the purchase of professional journals and professional books should be routine in the budget. The third step in the budgeting process is getting the budget approved and funded. The fourth step is using the funds as allocated, and when major shifts must be made, justifying these and seeking administrative approval.

Physical Facilities

The space requirements of an occupational health department are governed by many of the same factors that influence the planning of the health program: the number of employees, the inherent hazards of production, and the availability of community health facilities. The principles of wise planning apply whether the health department is to serve the workers of a small or a very large industry. These include meeting the present needs, providing for growth, and affording adequate space so that the staff may function at optimum efficiency and so that employees may be served in privacy.

The appearance of the health unit is also important. It should be bright, cheerful, and easy to keep clean and orderly. The space allocated should provide for at least two rooms: a waiting room and a treatment room. When possible, the treatment room should be divided into two separate units so that two persons can be cared for at the same time. This will also permit a consultation or health examination to be carried on while a worker is receiving treatment.

Equipment

The equipment needed will vary with the industry, and the overall cost of setting up the unit will be determined by the amount and kind of equipment purchased. It is wise to start with essentials and to add to these as the need arises. It is also wise to buy good-quality equipment; this does not necessarily mean that it must be the most expensive.

The publication *Organization and Operation of an Occupational Health Program*, distributed by the Occupational Health Institute (OHI), includes floor plans of large, medium, and small occupational health units, one of which shows a mobile multiphasic screening setup in three mobile trailers or as a floor plan for a health facility. For this reason, no discussion of this topic is included here. The publication is available from the OHI office (see App. C for information on how to order). Appendix D of the NIOSH publication *The New Nurse in Industry* also includes samples of floor plans in addition to a list of equipment and supplies.

Policy and Procedure Manual

One of the activities essential to the smooth administration of an occupational health unit is the development of a policy and procedure manual. The nurse supervisor is primarily responsible for preparing the manual. Both the staff nurse and the nurse who works alone will find that they too need such a manual and should be involved in its preparation.

The occupational health procedure manual should contain, in usable form, the information the nurse needs for effective management of the health unit. It is a reservoir of medical and administrative policies, nursing protocols, and information concerning the health service, the industry, and the community. Specifically, it should include:

1. A list of services provided by the health program and the policies that regulate these services
2. Written medical policies and medical standing orders
3. A list of nurses' responsibilities in the occupational health program
4. A list of potential occupational hazards of the industry, including signs and symptoms of acute and chronic poisoning, and required personal protective equipment
5. Copies of the state workmen's compensation law, state health and labor laws, and OSHA Standards that relate to work or health
6. An inventory of controlled drugs and solutions
7. Samples of all records and reports and directions for their use
8. A chart showing administrative organization of the company, the names of the officers and department heads, and lines of communication between the health service and other departments in the industry
9. An organizational chart showing staff and administrative lines of the occupational health unit
10. A list of nurses' responsibilities in the occupational health program or a copy of the job description if it has been prepared in sufficient detail.

The procedure manual grows with the department. It should be revised and reviewed periodically; hence it is wise to use a loose-leaf notebook and standard-sized paper so that additions can be made when necessary. AAHON has published *Guide for the Preparation of a Manual of Policies and Procedures for the Occupational Health Nurse*, available from them (see App. C for address). The Wisconsin State Health Department, in cooperation with the State Nurses' Association and the State Medical Society, have published a manual that can be personalized for the establishment by the addition of appropriate policies and other materials as indicated. Both of these are for sale and provide a framework for the person who has the responsibility for developing and keeping the manual current. As new problems arise and as decisions for handling them are made by either the management, the occupational health physician, or the nurse, this information should be added to the manual.

Compiling the manual, like running the occupational health service, requires teamwork. The nurse needs the assistance of someone who represents management and of the physician to assure that the administrative policies and medical orders and policies included are as these individuals would have them. The nurse should try to be original and to include any

Administration of Occupational Health Services and Units

pertinent or helpful information so that the manual will serve both her needs and those of the health service's relief nurses.

As a reservoir of policy statements and protocols that are the basis of nursing care and medical surveillance, the manual can be used for the orientation of new staff and can help to assure continuity and uniformity of services. Samples of record and report forms and an explanation of their use, distribution, and storage will be of great assistance to the person who substitutes when the nurse is off duty or to a new nurse learning to work in the health unit.

A profile of the industry should be included in the manual. Answers to the following questions will help the nurse to draw such a profile:

1. Is the establishment the only one in the corporation or is it one of several?
2. What is the type of industry according to SIC?
3. What products or services does the establishment produce?
4. Does administrative direction for the health unit originate at the corporate level or at the occupational health unit level?
5. Does the establishment employ a medical director? If so, what is the extent of his or her influence on the direction of the unit?
6. Is there an industrial hygienist on the occupational health and safety team?
7. Is there a director of nursing service on the staff? Or a nurse consultant? In either case, what is the extent of his or her influence?
8. Does the establishment employ a director of safety and loss control?
9. What is the size (number of employees) of the work force for whom the nurse will provide care?
10. What is the average age, sex, salary, and hourly distribution of the work force?
11. Do employees work on morning, afternoon, and evening shifts?
12. What hazardous operations or toxic substances are involved?
13. What community resources (hospitals, clinics, rehabilitation centers, medical specialists) are available?
14. What health insurance coverage or HMOs are available to the employees?
15. What insurance company is responsible for the workmen's compensation? Does it provide for nursing consultation?

Toxic Substances Reference File

Every establishment in which toxic substances are used should have a ready reference file on these substances. The occupational health nurse frequently is responsible for developing this file and keeping it current. The criteria documents prepared by NIOSH as a basis for standards development by OSHA are available from the Superintendent of Documents,

GPO. These publications contain pertinent data on overexposure, the suggested medical surveillance procedures, how to handle an emergency spill, environmental monitoring activities, the recommended personal protective equipment, and an extensive bibliography.

The criteria documents, the technical guidelines, and the safety data sheet are sources of information for the nurse and others on the occupational health and safety team. Because of the extensive data available on toxic and hazardous substances, carefully documented files on the particular hazards of an establishment should be developed and kept current for ready reference.

The following list includes data that should be on file and available to employees who work with any toxic substance:

1. The name and nature (liquid, powder, etc.) of the substance. In the case of a trade name, list the ingredients of the preparation. (Keep a copy of the manufacturer's safety data sheet in the file.)
2. The areas in the establishment where the substance is used.
3. The body system at greatest risk and routes of entry into the body.
4. Signs and symptoms of acute exposure.
5. Signs and symptoms of chronic exposure.
6. The current OSHA standard.
7. Environmental monitoring procedures in force.
8. Worker training programs.
9. Personal protective equipment required.
10. Emergency procedures to be followed (reference to protocol for care of acute illness).

Protocol Development

The following examples of how protocols can be written are shown here to indicate the kind of information that should be included. There is no one way to develop such forms. It is suggested that, once a format has been decided upon, all protocols be prepared accordingly.

Example 1

CONDITION: DERMATITIS—
INFLAMMATION OF THE SKIN

Signs and Symptoms
erythema, edema, papules, itching
History
It is essential that a careful and detailed history be taken and recorded, including information as to when this episode began. Take history of past similar episodes if any, including childhood, the characteristics of the skin at time the condition was first noticed, any home therapy if attempted.

What does the employee think to be the cause? What substances—at work, at home, or at play—has the worker used that are different from those used normally? Record information about food-intake.

Examination of the Skin

Observe and record the condition of the skin; determine the extent of involvement. Is secondary infection present? Describe and locate the lesions.

The nurse is reminded that the definitive medical diagnosis can be made only by the physician. This is contingent upon certain criteria, and it is essential that nurse's observations and the history as provided by the worker be recorded carefully and completely. This is to include what the lesions look like, the location of the lesions, the time of appearance and periods of remission if these occur.

Primary Care:
  I. Take careful history.
  II. Observe the condition of the skin; determine extent of involvement.
  III. Make a determination.
     A. When the above information is reviewed and the condition is determined to exceed that which meets the criteria for the nurse to handle, arrange for the worker to be seen by the dermatologist.
     B. When the above information is reviewed and the condition is determined not to be extensive, the nurse will:
        1. Cleanse the area.
        2. Apply wet compresses of 2% Burrow's solution for 15 minutes.
        3. Apply appropriate dressing.
        4. Teach the worker to apply solution and dressing.
        5. Teach worker handwashing techniques, if indicated; and discuss personal hygiene.
        6. Make appointment for worker to be seen again within 24 hours at which time, plan of care is reevaluated and/or worker is seen by physician.
        7. Cover with sterile dressing those areas of the skin that are not intact, so as to minimize secondary infection.
        8. Discuss problem with safety engineer and foreman in order to limit worker's exposure and to determine the need for protective equipment, apron, gloves, and the possibility or advisability of reassignment to a different job.

Developed by _____ RN
             _____ MD

Date:
  Original _____
  Revised _____

Example 2

CONDITION: LACERATION—
A WOUND MADE BY CUTTING OR TEARING

1. Major lacerations.
   a. Lacerations involving deeper structures (nerves, tendons, and muscles) or those about the face.
   b. Lacerations involving embedded bodies, often accompanied by hemorrhage.
   c. Lacerations that have become infected.
2. Primary care for major lacerations (those that require care by the physician).
   a. Make patient comfortable on chair or table.
   b. Wash hands before giving care.
   c. Make careful examination to determine extent of injury (take into consideration cause of injury as well as objective signs).
   d. Control bleeding by direct pressure (tourniquet is seldom needed).
   e. Cover injured area with sterile gauze; cleanse surrounding area with soap and water.
   f. Again check for bleeding.
   g. Apply dry sterile dressing; immobilize as indicated; prepare patient for transfer to the doctor's office or to the hospital.
   h. Prepare all required records and reports.
   i. Arrange for transport of injured worker in taxi or ambulance, arrange for someone to accompany worker.
   j. Call doctor and brief him on condition of worker.
3. Minor lacerations.
   a. Superficial lacerations.
   b. Simple lacerations whose edges approximate easily and evenly.
   c. Those in which tests of sensation and function show that nerves and tendons are intact.
   d. Noncontaminated wounds.
4. Primary care for minor lacerations.
   a. Make patient comfortable on chair or table.
   b. Wash hands before giving care.
   c. Make careful examination to determine extent of injury (take into consideration cause of injury as well as objective signs).
   d. Control bleeding by direct pressure.
   e. Cover injured area; cleanse surrounding area with soap and water.
   f. Irrigate wound with sterile normal saline solution.
   g. Again check for bleeding; recheck extent of injury.
   h. Approximate edges of laceration, using tape strips.
   i. Apply dry sterile dressing.

j. Record all pertinent information.
k. Make appointment for follow-up care.
5. Follow-up care for lacerations. Lacerations are to be dressed daily. Instruct worker to return for redressing whenever dressings become wet or dirty from work.
   a. Check carefully; evaluate healing process and the worker's attitude about the injury and care being given.
   b. Apply dry sterile dressing.*
   c. Counsel worker concerning the need for adequate care.
   d. Record all pertinent information.
   e. Make appointment for follow-up care.

N.B. The nurse will continue to redress as necessary all minor lacerations. If the wound does not heal in 3 days the advisability of having it and the plan of care evaluated by the physician should be considered. Major lacerations are to be redressed by the nurse as per doctor's orders. If sutures were used, these are to be removed on the 5th day unless ordered to the contrary or removed by the physician.

Example 3

CONDITION: HEADACHE—PAIN
IN THE HEAD DUE TO ANY ONE OF MANY
PHYSICAL OR EMOTIONAL CONDITIONS

1. Headache associated with a toxicologic or pathological condition.
   a. Headache associated with industrial intoxication caused by exposure to chlorinated hydrocarbons or carbon monoxide.
   b. Headache associated with vertigo.
   c. Headache associated with elevated TPR or blood pressure.
2. Simple headache—no toxicologic or pathological condition apparent.
3. Primary care for workers with headache.
   a. Take careful history. Determine what medications, if any, the person takes routinely. Determine whether worker has been exposed to any hazardous substance.
   b. Take TPR. When temperature is 100° F. or more, worker should be urged to go home and to consult his family physician and must not be allowed to return to work.
   c. Take blood pressure. If this deviates from "normal" and from that recorded on worker's health examination, counsel worker to check with his family physician.

*Doctor's standing order. These should be as sophisticated as the physician and the nurse believe to be indicated for the condition to be treated.

     d. When history and symptoms indicate that headache, as far as the nurse can determine, is uncomplicated, give aspirin, grains X. If allergic to aspirin, give Tylenol, grains X. This may be repeated once after a time lapse of 4 hours.
     e. Record all pertinent information on worker's record.
4. Follow-up care.
     a. Check to determine how the person is feeling and whether headache has subsided. Recheck blood pressure if indicated; if elevated, counsel worker and urge him to see family doctor.
     b. Check worker's health record; if he has reported to the health unit frequently for headache, make an appointment for worker to be seen by the physician.
     c. Repeat medication (aspirin, grains X or Tylenol, grains X) if indicated to help worker be more comfortable and thus be able to continue work.
     d. Record all pertinent information.

Example 4

CONDITION: CARBON MONOXIDE POISONING— TWA = 50 PARTS PER MILLION PARTS OF AIR

I. Incidence—occurs most frequently in garage workers.
II. Systemic effect—combines with hemoglobin to form carboxyhemoglobin, thus depriving the body cells of oxygen.
III. Symptoms and signs of poisoning.
    A. Mild.
       1. Frontal headache.
       2. Feeling of tightness across forehead.
    B. Moderate.
       1. Weakness and dizziness.
       2. Increased respiration and fast pulse.
       3. Pale skin tone in later stage; the mucous membranes are cherry red.
    C. Severe.
       1. Collapse—patient no longer breathing.
       2. Bright discoloration of skin, or dusky cyanosis.
       3. Tongue is cherry red.
       4. Death.
IV. Primary care.
    A. Remove both the affected worker and all other workers from the contaminated area *immediately*.
    B. If the affected worker is not breathing, start artificial respiration *immediately*.

- C. Administer oxygen.
- D. Keep person at rest.
- E. Always take a careful history of each garage worker who reports complaining of headache.
- F. Check with worker's foreman if in doubt concerning the work environment.
- V. Engineering controls.
  - A. Adequate general ventilation.
  - B. Special ventilation through flexible hose attachments for engine exhaust pipes.
  - C. Maintenance of ventilation equipment.
- VI. Medical controls.
  - A. Education of workers concerning danger and how to protect themselves.
  - B. Preplacement and periodic medical examination should give special attention to cardiovascular and smoking history.

Example 5

PROGRAM TO CONTROL TETANUS INFECTION

Uses and Indications for Tetanus Toxoid*

For active immunization against tetanus: Clients with known sensitivity to horse serum and those with asthma or other allergies should be urged to maintain immunity with tetanus toxoid in order to avoid the hazards of antitoxin (horse serum) therapy.

Dosage and Frequency

1. Primary course of immunization (without wounds or with clean minor wounds)
   a. First dose: 0.5 milliliters
   b. Second dose: 0.5 milliliters 4–6 weeks later
   c. Third dose: 0.5 milliliters 1 year after the second dose
2. Booster doses: 0.5 milliliters every 10 years thereafter to maintain adequate protection

Route of Administration
   Intramuscular

Contraindications
1. Known hypersensitivity   2. Acute illness

*Ingredients: Tetanus toxoid, sodium chloride solution, mercury preservative, aluminum potassium sulfate.

3. Current allergen therapy
4. Current immunosuppressive therapy
5. Severe or grossly contaminated wounds by *unimmunized* clients

Possible Adverse Reactions

Note: Manufacturers recommend a test dose for previously immunized persons over 25 years of age who are more likely to develop the following reactions:

1. Anaphylactic shock
2. Local redness
3. Induration
4. Tenderness
5. Malaise
6. Low-grade transient fever

Prophylaxis after Injury

I. Clean minor wounds (work and nonwork related). No prophylaxis needed except when:
   A. A primary course of immunization was not completed; then give the second and/or third dose of 0.5 milliliters to complete the course.
   B. The most recent toxoid injection was administered more than 10 years before the injury; then give one dose of 0.5 milliliters.
II. All other wounds (work and nonwork related).
   A. Give 9.5 milliliters stat if the client has had a primary course of immunization but has not had a booster dose in the preceding 5 years, except in instances where:
      1. Any *contraindications* listed in this protocol are present.
      2. The history of the client's immunization is uncertain.

Refer to Physician or Medical Facility for Tetanus Immunization Those Workers with a:

1. History of adverse reaction to tetanus immunization
2. Wound that obviously requires medical attention
3. Contaminated wound more than 24 hours old
4. Fresh contaminated wound and immunization lacking or history of immunization uncertain

Remarks

1. Store tetanus toxoid at 2–8° C. (35–46° F.). *Do not freeze.*
2. It is mandatory that appropriate consent form be signed by the client before administering toxoid.

3. It is mandatory to observe the client in nursing station for 20 minutes after administration of toxoid.
4. Enter date and dose in the record; complete worker's personal immunization record card.
5. Do not give booster injections to active reservists in any service; refer them to their reserve centers.

N.B. This example is based on format used in the manual of the New York State Department of Civil Service Employee Health Service.

References

1. Occupational Medicine Practice Committee. "Scope of Occupational Health Programs and Occupational Medical Practice," *Journal of Occupational Medicine*, Vol. 21, No. 7, July 1979, pp. 497–499.
2. AAOHN. *Guide for On-the-Job Orientation of the Occupational Health Nurse*. The Association, New York. 1976, p. 4.

Selected Readings

AAOHN. "Standard for Evaluating an Occupational Health Nursing Service," *Occupational Health Nursing*, Vol. 23, No. 11, Nov. 1975, pp 25–24.
AIHA. *Standards, Interpretation, and Audit Criteria for Performance of Occupational Health Programs*. Akron, Ohio, 1977.
AMA. *Company Medical Policies*. Chicago, 1973.
ANA, Commission on Nursing Services. *Standards for Nursing Services in Hospitals, Community Health Agencies, Nursing Homes, Industry, Schools, Ambulatory Services, and Related Health Care Organizations*. Kansas City, Mo. 1973.
Boccuzzi, N. "Head Nurse Growth: A Priority for the Supervisor," *AJN*, Vol. 79, No. 8, Aug. 1979, pp. 1389–1392.
Boydstein, S. M. "Design of an Occupational Health Unit." *Occupational Health Nursing*, Vol. 27, No. 1, Jan. 1979, pp. 7–11.
Carter, J. H., Hilliard, M., Castles, M. R., Stoll, L. D., and Cowan, A. *Standards of Nursing Care: A Guide for Evaluation*, 2nd Ed. New York: Springer, 1976.
Goldbeck, W. B. *A Business Perspective on Industry and Health Care*. New York: Springer-Verlag, 1978.
Hughes, J. P. (Ed.). "Cost Effectiveness of Occupational Health Programs," *Journal of Occupational Medicine*, Vol. 16, No. 3, Mar. 1974, pp 153–186.
Klutas, E. "Nursing Administration," *Occupational Health and Safety 78*, Vol. 47, No. 3, May–June 1978, pp. 44–47.
Mager, R. F., and Pipe, P. *Analyzing Performance Problems*. Belmont, Calif. Fearon, 1973.
Miner, J. B., and Miner, M. G. *Personnel and Industrial Relations*, 2nd Ed. New York: Macmillan, 1973.

Mintzberg, H. *The Nature of Managerial Work*. New York: Harper & Row, 1973.
Phaneuf, M. C. *The Nursing Audit Profile for Excellence in Nursing*. New York: Appleton-Century-Crofts, 1972.
Webb, S. B., Jr. "Objective Criteria for Evaluating Occupational Health Programs," *American Journal of Public Health*, Vol. 65, No. 1, Jan. 1975.

CHAPTER **19**

Administrative Reports

As a verb, the word *record* means to set down in writing, as for the purpose of preserving evidence; as a noun, the word defines the form on which the information is written. A *report* is an account or statement that describes in detail an event or situation, as in a medical report on the condition of a patient. To be meaningful, a report requires the use of an adjective to delineate what the report is about.

Administrative reports are useful in explaining the activities of the occupational health unit staff. They provide an effective means of communication with other departments and with management, and they establish a record of what was considered important data when making decisions concerning the operation of the occupational health unit. A copy of each report should be maintained on file in the unit.

This chapter deals with the several administrative reports that are prepared by occupational health unit personnel to:

1. Reflect the extent of the programs and activities carried on by the occupational health unit staff
2. Permit the drawing of conclusions as to the effectiveness of the various programs and activities
3. Put on record the utilization of the staff's time and their professional competencies
4. Provide information that will facilitate the making of recommendations as to the need for change in the conduct of the unit and in any or all of its programs and activities.

Three types of administrative reports are used:

1. Official reports are prepared by management for the DOL and the administrator of the workmen's compensation insurance program of the state. The one that goes to the DOL is the annual report to OSHA of reportable injuries and illnesses. The workmen's compensation report may be sent to the insurance carrier, who in turn reports to the state. Both reports require data generated by reports for which the nurse has some responsibility.

2. Managerial reports are from the occupational health unit staff to the member of top management who provides administrative direction for the unit. Copies of these reports are also often sent to the supervisors of the several operating units and to the safety director. They are made monthly and include data on the work load of the occupational health unit staff and on the number and type of occupational injuries and illnesses covered by workmen's compensation and reportable to OSHA.

3. Occupational health unit reports are specific reports sent by a member of the occupational health unit staff to another employee, for example, RN to MD, RN or MD to management, RN to safety and industrial hygiene personnel, RN to supervisors, or RN to a department of the company. These reports usually take the form of a memo which explains a modification of a program, requests a change in a program, explains a happening, or deals with such topics as staff changes, sick leaves, special leaves, or special problems.

The first two types of reports require some procedure for keeping track of the items to be reported. The occupational health unit has traditionally kept a daily log for the purpose of recording the number and types of injuries and illnesses treated. Now, however, the OSHA Log (Form 200), which is required by law, is kept to accumulate data as to the number and severity of industrial injuries and illnesses. Because the OSHA Log is used only for reporting certain specific conditions, a second log or other means of accumulating information is kept for all other illnesses and injuries. It is recommended that information about first-time care, about subsequent treatment, and about the cause of the injury or illness be made directly onto the individual's health record. In fact all information about a person's illness and injury experience—both occupational and nonoccupational—should be incorporated into the individual's personal health record, as discussed in Chapter 2.

Preparation of Monthly and Annual Reports

A checklist can be utilized to assure the inclusion of all required data in the monthly and annual reports. This list should include the following several categories of occupational injuries and illnesses that have been identified as important:

1. Those that require
    a. First-aid care only
    b. Care by the occupational health unit staff
    c. Care by a physician in his or her office

Administrative Reports 247

    d. Care at a hospital emergency room
    e. Care requiring hospitalization
2. All OSHA-reportable illnesses and injuries.

These illnesses and injuries are usually reported by diagnosis; for example, second-degree burn, foreign object in eye, fracture of right leg, and personal problems. Causes of these conditions are usually reported as occupational or nonoccupational. Since the number and kind of retreatments provided for persons who have occupational illness or injury are also reported, the checklist should include (a) redressings done, (b) physiotherapy treatments performed, and (c) other treatments as ordered.

Because people often come to work with such health problems as an acute illness or an injury sustained on the way to work, the occupational health unit staff provides primary care for workers with conditions that would be reported as nonoccupational in origin. The amount of primary care given for such conditions may be anywhere from 1 to 100 times as great as that given for occupational illnesses and injuries. Therefore the statistics should reflect the nature of the nonoccupational health problems treated and what care was provided by the health staff.

Data about medical surveillance programs that should be included in reports are: (a) the percentage of eligible employees who took part in the program; (b) the number of positive and negative biological test results; (c) the number of workers transferred to different positions, if this was the case; and (d) the number of hours of instruction given to workers who, in accordance with OSHA Standards, must be informed concerning the hazards of their work environment.

The number of referrals by the occupational health unit staff to the safety and industrial hygiene staffs should be reported. It is also important to show the referrals to first-line supervisors by the nurse. For example, if the nurse finds a worker who should be wearing safety shoes but is not doing so, the nurse calls this to the attention of the supervisor or the safety engineer, or both. Information that the nurse picks up from workers who tell her about a malfunctioning safety device that has been reported but still has not been corrected should also be reported; this will help to show the interrelationship between the health care and safety aspects of the occupational health program.

Data about screening programs that should be included in monthly and annual reports include the number of workers who (a) take part, for example come to a hypertension screening clinic or have their blood pressure taken; (b) take advantage of the influenza immunization program; and (c) have completed their tetanus innoculation series.

It is also useful to report the amount of time the nurse spends in such activities as:

1. Conferring with first-line supervisors about environmental conditions, workers' problems, and problem workers
2. Making inspection tours, either as a nursing function or in collaboration with safety personnel
3. Checking on the sanitation in all areas including food service and wash-up areas
4. Meeting with members of the health education and the safety committees
5. Counseling workers who have health problems.

Characteristics of a Good Report

The statistical report will be more interesting and helpful to management personnel, to the medical director, to the administrator of the health unit, and to the safety engineer if the main items are reported by department, date, and time when care was provided. In addition, if the statistics for the current month can be shown next to those of the preceding month and in relation to those of the same period 1 year previously, helpful comparisons can be made.

When appropriate, reports should contain conclusions as drawn by the occupational health unit staff. If for example there is a sudden peak in the number of workers reporting with minor lacerations from a work area where few if any have occurred in the past, this fact needs to be highlighted, as should the fact that an increasing number of workers are reporting to the health unit with such ill-defined symptoms as slight headache, fatigue, and stress. One such episode is of little concern, but if a pattern is discernable it would be wise to suggest an investigation of the cause. That is to say that administrative reports from the occupational health unit to management and to safety personnel should not only outline what the staff has done but indicate areas that require attention in order to meet the aim of protecting the workers' health. Data presented in such a way as to permit the drawing of conclusions and making comparisons is much more useful than isolated numbers. The reporting should also give evidence that the occupational health unit staff recognizes the possible relationship between workers' health and the environment of their work areas.

Increasingly in the future it will be important to be able to show the incidence, by department, of such symptoms as headache, muscle and joint pain, and neurological problems, whether these be work connected or not. Often an important but missed relationship between workers' health and their jobs can be picked up when minor illness problems are recorded so as to be retrievable for the monthly summary report. Such information may help to pinpoint areas where environmental hazards exist that had not been previously suspected.

Memoranda

The administrative direction of an occupational health unit is provided by a member of management who may or may not be knowledgeable about health program planning, medical care, and treatment facilities, but this person must often make decisions about activities that will extend or eliminate a program or require additional space, equipment, and personnel. The occupational health nurse who suggests that something new be added or that something old be dropped can expect any one of three answers: yes, no, and maybe.

The memorandum is an effective means of providing information that the decision maker can study as a basis for making a decision, but it must be as specific as possible. For example, if the current health assessment protocols do not include a hearing test for workers assigned or about to be assigned to an area where a noise hazard exists and if OSHA then promulgates a new standard that requires audiograms for those workers, a request or recommendation must be made to add this procedure to the program.

Often the entire occupational health staff will need to collaborate in formulating the memorandum. The first question to be answered is whether there is any alternative and if so, what are the advantages, disadvantages, and relative cost of the alternative? Having decided that there is no feasible alternative, the next thing to be decided is what additional space will be required and what the cost of building a hearing booth will be. Other questions that arise and must be answered before the request can be sent to management are: What is the cost of an audiometer and what are the features of the various models? Can anyone on the staff be taught to give the tests or must a specialist be engaged? What would be the comparative cost of utilizing a local hospital's hearing clinic instead of inaugurating a hearing conservation program? Should a policy be established that all workers be given a screening audiogram so as to have the pertinent data against which to compare changes as each person ages and as they work in a noisy department?

When the answers to these questions are in hand, the memorandum can be written. It should contain all the information the decision maker will need. In this particular situation the request should obviously receive a yes answer, and the writer might conclude the memo by stating, "Unless I hear from you to the contrary by [a specific date], I will proceed to prepare the purchase order for your signature so that the program can be started without further delay."

Another type of memorandum often sent by the occupational health staff to management contains information about something that has already happened. Using the example cited above, such a memo might simply state: "In view of the new OSHA Standard, we will proceed in the following manner," and then give an outline of the plan to start the new program. Whenever a new program has been initiated it is wise to send a report to the member of management responsible for the direction of the occupational health unit. Such a report should include the highlights of the program, the participation, whether the objectives of the program were achieved, what problems arose, and recommendations as to when and how this program should be carried out if it is to be repeated.

The occupational health nurse should report periodically to management on how the essential services for the workers are being carried out and whether any problems have arisen in connection with these services. Nurses involved in programs they are proud of should make a point of telling others about what they are doing and the results of their activities.

CHAPTER 20

Records

Occupational health records are written accounts of facts concerning the health of workers. Health facts to be recorded are primarily those generated by the procedures performed by health professionals: (a) assessment of each individual's state of health at the time of job placement and at periodic intervals throughout the person's employment, (b) assessment of the extent of an injury or illness of the employee who reports for care to the occupational health unit, (c) the care provided, and (d) conclusions and recommendations. Every effort should be made to assure that the information recorded is correct and complete, recorded on the correct form, and filed in the person's individual health record folder. (Increasingly, occupational health records are being computerized, and the impact of this is dealt with later in this chapter.)

The individual record folder permits the accumulation in one place of all pertinent health information for each individual worker with the least time, effort, and space. This requires the use of a folder sufficiently large to hold all of the required information including:

1. The forms on which medical and nursing notes have been entered by the physician and the nurse who have provided care for the injured or ill worker
2. Completed workers' compensation forms and/or copies of the OSHA forms for illness or injury the worker sustains
3. Completed health examination forms for every examination and screening
4. All pertinent and related forms and letters and medical surveillance, reports, and all laboratory and X-ray reports.

Many different types of folders are used; what is important is that the type selected be sturdy and expandable. The folder and the place where it is filed must provide safe, fireproof storage and be readily accessible to the health professionals on the staff but inaccessible to others who have no right to use the records.

It is essential that occupational health nurses understand the purpose of the health unit's record system and be able to communicate this effectively to management. The main purpose of records is to have available data that can be used to protect the worker; the employer; and the health professional who made the decision, provided the care, and recorded the information. The occupational health records system should provide:

1. Specific and continuous information concerning each worker's state of health
2. Specific information concerning injuries and disease conditions (both occupational and nonoccupational), the care provided, and by whom
3. The basis for an evaluation of the health service
4. The basis for planning and evaluating the occupational health program activities
5. Data for research studies.

Three words are suggested as guidelines for all who are responsible for developing, using, and evaluating an occupational health service record system. The first two are *simplicity* and *convenience*, particularly in referring to the use of the system and the purposes the forms are designed to serve. Equally important is the third word, *why?* Why this record form? Why this report? No form should be initiated or continued past the time that it has a direct bearing on the fulfillment of the purposes of the occupational health program, namely:

- To identify the health hazards in the work environment or to control them
- To assure optimum compatibility between the individual's capabilities and limitations and the physical, mental, and emotional demands of the job
- To provide optimum care and rehabilitation for workers whose illnesses or injuries are due to work-related causes.

Legal Implications of Records

Workmen's Compensation

The health records containing information, as they do, about the worker's occupational injury and disease experiences that are covered by Workers' Compensation legislation are particularly liable to summons by courts of law. To be of value, the record should contain all pertinent facts about the injury or illness, the cause, and the care provided. Failure to present a legible, factual record can embarrass the nurse, the physician, and the employer as well as the injured worker. An inadequate record will make it difficult or even impossible for the compensation commissioner to reach a fair decision in a disputed case. Records should not be kept just to be taken into court, but on the other hand, complete, detailed factual records will be of value in court.

Malpractice Defense

The increasing number of malpractice suits makes it essential that all health professionals record complete data about the health problems they deal with, the causes of the problems, and what was done for the injured or ill person, so as to have a record to use in their own defense if it is ever needed. A complete record should provide the needed information if a question ever arises as to the correctness of the professional person's judgment and actions. When called upon to testify in court, the occupational health nurse will find that complete, well-written records are very helpful.

The Employer's Right to Know

The employer is entitled to a report on the health status of an employee as it relates to his ability to perform job tasks, but the employer need not know the specific details of the individual's physical and mental condition. When, however, the data in a health record is related to an occupational or potentially compensable condition, this information becomes legally available to the employer and to the insurance company. Compensation is a form of third-party payment, and the person paying the bills is entitled to certain information. The employer is considered to have a valid interest if, by law, necessity, or agreement, he is responsible for part or all of the cost of care or indemnity. Having a valid interest as the third party, the employer is entitled to know the facts about the specific condition, the prognosis, and the treatment. Otherwise employers should not have access to health information without the consent of the individual.

Forms and How to Use Them

Medical and Nursing Notes

The form for recording medical and nursing notes should provide space for a running account of all data pertaining to the injury or illness of the worker. It is the source of the basic information needed for all reports, legal and statistical, which refer to the worker's health status. Each entry should include the date and time of the visit to the health service, the reason for the visit, a detailed description of the worker's condition (signs, symptoms, and part of the body involved), a description of the care or services rendered, the disposition of the case, and all other pertinent information. Entries need not be long to include all necessary information.

Somewhere on the page, preferably at the top, the worker's name, department, and social security number and/or payroll number should be recorded as a way of identifying the individual so that one John Brown can be differentiated from another John Brown should need arise 1 week or 20 years after the information was recorded. When an OSHA file number is assigned to the injury or illness, this too must be recorded so that the notes can be identified with the injury data.

EXAMPLE A

Mary L. Brown	182-12-1670	79-611
Name	SS#	OSHA File #

4/6/79 1:00 P.M. While removing gear from packing box, worker caught left hand on bent nail in lid. Abrasion of dorsal surface, left hand. Area cleaned, and dry sterile dressing applied. To return 4/7/79 for redressing.

EXAMPLE B

James Andersen	172-12-1400	N/A
Name	SS#	OSHA File #

4/19/79 2:30 A.M. Complains of not feeling well—thinks he is getting flu. TPR 100^2-120-24. Face flushed. Coryza. No history of allergy. 10 grains of aspirin administered; suggested the dose be repeated in 4 hours. Suggested he see family physician if symptoms continue. Suggested bed rest, forced fluids. Sent home in taxi, 3:10 A.M.

M. Doe, RN

The information in Example A concerns an occupational injury. The worker's foreman will need to know about this accident and, under the workmen's compensation law, other company representatives may also have reason to see the record. This injury will also be recorded on the OSHA Log and have an OSHA number. The information in Example B concerns a nonoccupational condition, and the worker's supervisor will be told only that the man is ill and not able to work.

Problem-oriented Medical Records

Lawrence Weed developed a medical record system designed to assist the various members of a team to give effective care to persons with many problems. With the help of the patient, the team lists the problems and identifies which are the most pressing and what means are proposed to solve them. The so-called Weed system can be used effectively in occupational health.[1] This record format permits listing of health, work, and family problems that have the potential for interfering with the person's ability to reach his or her potential on the job. Special environmental hazards can and should be incorporated into the list along with the plans that have been made to deal with and to help the person deal with the problems. For example if the worker refused to take part in the medical surveillance program when it was first made available, this fact is recorded, as are the efforts made to find a way to help the person understand the program and take part in it. Weed says of the record system: "The first page should consist of a numbered problem list. It is a table of contents and an index combined, and the care with which it is constructed determines the quality of the whole record."[2]

Health Examination Form

The health examination form should provide space for recording data obtained at the preplacement health examination and at all subsequent health examinations. The following data are usually called for:

1. Complete identification of the individual. Name, date of birth, sex, social security number, and payroll number if one is assigned.
2. The individual's position, title, job description number, and the division or place in the establishment where the individual will work.
3. A complete health history. The health history form should provide space for updating health and illness data on subsequent examinations.
4. A reproductive history. The form should also provide space for updating the data on subsequent examinations.
5. A work history. It is essential that changes in the person's work assignment be noted in the appropriate space on the health record along with the appropriate dates. The work history form should provide space for recording all past work experiences, including summer employment and the type of job, length of time on the job, and any hazards the person can identify associated with past employment, including history of the use of personal protective equipment.
6. Data generated by laboratory tests (blood and urine tests, for example).
7. Data generated by screening procedures. The format for recording information from screening procedures should be such as to enable the health professional to identify change. Space should be provided for recording audiometric, electrocardiographic, visual, and pulmonary functions; test results; reports of X rays with identification of X-ray film and where it is stored.
8. Data generated by physical examination including the dates of the examination and the signature of the person who performed the examination.
9. Conclusions and recommendations.

The requirements of medical surveillance, environmental monitoring, and record keeping in the OSHA Standards give proof of the importance placed on occupational health records. Records of persons working with certain toxic substances (see App. D) must be maintained for the duration of employment plus 20 years or 30 years, whichever is longer. The exact number of years is stated in each standard (See App. D, p. 328). If the establishment goes out of business, then OSHA requires that the records be sent to the director of NIOSH for safekeeping.

Increasingly in the future, data that are recorded when a person is working may be called for after the person has retired or goes to work for another employer. For example data in an individual's occupational health record may be used to establish whether the cancer the person has developed was or was not caused by exposure during previous employment.

Use of Classification Systems

There are several approaches to the classification of disease. The anatomist, for example, may desire a classification based on the part of the body affected. The pathologist is primarily interested in the nature of the disease process. The clinician will consider disease from these two angles but needs further knowledge of etiology. In other words there are many areas of classification, and the particular axis selected will be determined by the interests of the investigator. A statistical classification of disease and injury will depend therefore upon the use to be made of the statistics to be compiled. In occupational health this classification will need to permit the identification of work-connected disease and non-work-caused illness or injury. It is also important to be able to identify the non-work-connected illness and disease information that has been gathered from the family and the worker's past health history at the time of employment.

When one speaks of statistics it is at once inferred that the interest is in a group of cases and not in individual occurrences. The purpose of a statistical compilation of disease data is primarily to furnish quantitative data that will answer questions about groups of cases. Two classification manuals are recommended for use in the record-keeping system of an occupational health unit: the *Standard Industrial Classification* and the *International Classification of Disease, Ammended*, (ICDA). The SIC is used to identify various industrial institutions, and the IDIC provides for uniform coding of diseases. The occupational nurse needs to be familiar with both of these classification manuals and know how to use them. The person in industry responsible for reporting the employment data will know the SIC number or numbers to be used in reports to the DOL. The record librarian of the local hospital will know how to use the IDIC manual.

Many occupational health unit record systems use the IDIC three- or four-digit numbers so data on these classifications can be retrieved. This system makes it possible to select from all the records those workers who, for example, have had an injury that resulted from being struck by something or those who had a blood pressure of at least 150/100 on their last physical examination.

Record-keeping Requirements, State and Federal

In order to carry out the purposes of OSHA, employers are required to keep and make available to the Secretary of Labor (and also to the Secretary of DHHS) records on certain employer activities covered by the act. Employers are also required to maintain accurate records (and to make periodic reports) of work-related deaths, injuries, and illnesses. Minor injuries which require only first-aid treatment need not be recorded, but a record must be made of any injury that involves medical treatment, loss of consciousness, restriction of work or motion, or transfer to another job.

Log of Occupational Injuries and Illnesses

Each recordable occupational injury and occupational illness must be entered on a log of cases (OSHA Form No. 200) within 2 working days of receiving information that a recordable case has occurred. Logs must be kept current and retained for 5 years following the end of the calendar year to which they relate. Logs are to be maintained for three reasons:

1. Logs for the prior 5-year period must be available in the establishment without delay and at reasonable times for examination by representatives of the DOL or the DHHS or by representatives of states accorded jurisdiction under the act.
2. The log will be used in preparing the annual summary of Occupational Injuries and Illnesses (OSHA Form No. 202), which must be posted in every establishment.
3. The log will be needed for preparation of reports by those establishments selected to participate in a statistical program.

In addition, the log will aid in reviewing the occupational injury and illness experience of the establishment and in the calculation of incidence rates and lost-day rates.

The Occupational Health and Safety Act places the responsibility for keeping the OSHA records and for being in compliance with the OSHA record-keeping requirements on personnel at the top management level. Granted, the "boss" may delegate this responsibility, and it is well for the nurse to remember this fact. Keeping the OSHA Log, Form 200, is not necessarily the responsibility of the nurse, although many, perhaps most, do.

The nurse's responsibility is to record the care provided and sufficient information about the worker's injury or illness and its cause (as told to the nurse by the employee) to assure that whoever uses the record will know why the nurse proceeded as he or she did and will be able to complete the required OSHA forms. The director of the establishment's safety department may be assigned by management the responsibility for keeping the OSHA Log, and other record-keeping requirements may be assigned to a secretary or to the director of the personnel department or to the nurse. What is essential is that the OSHA Log be maintained according to the current OSHA requirements and that it be available for reviewing by the compliance officer.

Workmen's Compensation Records

The forms on which the information required by the workers' compensation insurance company is written are usually supplied by that company or by the state agency. These are usually identified as the first notice of injury and the supplemental report of the injury. Another form that must be completed for occupational injuries and illnesses is the OSHA Form 201, Supplementary Record of Occupational Injuries and Illnesses. If the compensation form for the first notice of injury provides a space for recording the information required by OSHA, then one form can be used for both purposes.

The Essentials of Good Record Keeping

Completeness

Records kept by members of the occupational health team should be detailed enough to permit evaluation of the cause-and-effect relationship of any toxic substance found in the environment by the person doing the environmental monitoring and any signs and symptoms of illness found by the person performing the health surveillance examination. The long delay that may occur between exposure and the development of signs of illness makes it necessary that both sets of data be easily retrievable, not only currently but at any time in the future, perhaps as many as 20–40 years after the data were collected.

Data generated through environmental monitoring must be so recorded that it can be related to specific workers doing specific jobs for a specific period of time. It should also include what techniques were utilized to collect the exposure data and the length of time over which the data were collected. It is essential that it be possible to relate the TWA or TLV currently "the standard" to the levels recorded, and the date when collected is most important.

Confidentiality and Protecting Records from Misuse

The confidential nature of the physician-worker and nurse-worker relationship should never be jeopardized, so the health history and health examination records of an individual must be considered confidential. A good rule to follow is that only health personnel should have access to health records, and no information about a worker's state of health should be released without the worker's written permission.

The nurse's attention is directed to the "Rule" that relates to the protection of information in records concerning the person's problems with alcoholism. The *Federal Register* of July 1, 1975, 42 CFR, Part 2, 40, is the reference for the "Rules" that relate to the protection of information in records concerning alcoholism and drug abuse. When the establishment has an alcoholism program, there must be recognition of the federal rules governing the confidentiality of alcohol and drug-abuse patient records. What can be released by whom to whom is controlled, as explained by D. J. Helms:

> In these times of freedom of information when laws and regulations enforcing the public's right to know are in the ascendancy, it might appear that federal rules governing the confidentiality of alcohol and drug abuse patient records (42 CFR Part 2, The Rules) based on the need-to-know principle are something of an anomaly. Further consideration of the matter, however, reveals that the Rules are really a means of accomplishing a parallel objective; namely, to enforce an individual's right to privacy. That is, the right to know enables an individual citizen to obtain more information about himself from government, while the Rules prevent government and others from obtaining more information about the individual than they are deemed to need to know. Thus, understanding of the need-to-know concept is essential to grasping the theoretical framework within which the Rules are constructed. This is plainly stated in Section 2.18:
> > Any disclosure made under this part whether with or without the patient's consent shall be limited to information necessary in the light of the need or purpose for the disclosure.
> To highlight this principle in another way, it could be said that an individual desiring to assert his "right to know" information about himself should be permitted to do so even if his only motivation is curiosity. Such is emphatically not the case under the Rules. To obtain information protected by the Rules, one must establish his need-to-know along explicity approved lines, and any custodian of such information would be well served to remember this precept and adhere to it strictly.[3]

All occupational health records should either be filed in locked cabinets kept in the health department or be stored in a computer program with controlled access. Only authorized members of the staff should have access to the health records. When nonprofessional people—secretaries or clerks—have reason to work on these records, they should be instructed as to their responsibility and helped to understand the importance of keeping information in medical records confidential. The professional members of the occupational health department often find that they have to explain the concept of confidentiality to others in the industry.

Under certain circumstances OSHA and NIOSH personnel have the right of access to health records. Nurses should not release any record to anyone, either a lawyer or an OSHA or NIOSH representative, without the full knowledge of the management. The signed release of the worker may, in certain situations, also be required. When a request for a record is made, the nurse asks what information is desired, then alerts both the responsible person in management and the physician of the request. The nurse must be prepared to discuss with management, the lawyer, and the governmental agency representative how the record system is set up and what is recorded on each form, so that the person requesting information will have a realistic expection of what information is contained in the records and whether it will be useful for the purpose for which it is sought.

Two influences have complicated the maintenance of confidentiality in regard to occupational health information: (a) third-party payment for medical care in health and accident insurance programs and (b) the needs of the occupational safety and health personnel for information from which to develop standards. Occupational health and workmen's compensation are a part of the so-called third-party payment system, as are the hospital and health insurance programs provided by management. What is needed most is judgment on the part of all people who handle records and reports and, equally important, the good sense to "keep quiet." Perhaps the following example will help to explain these influences.

Mr. S. applies for a job as truck driver at the XYZ Company. One of the provisions for employment is that a health examination and certain standard laboratory tests, to be paid for by the company, be done. If Mr. S. wants the job, he must have the examination. As a child he lost the sight of his left eye when he was hit by a snowball containing a stone. The information about the blindness of the left eye is recorded on the examination form, and the examiner sends the employment officer sufficient information to enable that officer to match the man's capabilities to the demands of the jobs available. Hence a job that requires extremes of depth perception is beyond Mr. S.'s capabilities. However he does meet the requirements for a job that is open in the chemistry laboratory, and a safe match is achieved.

In the AMA's *Guide to the Development of an Industrial Medical Records System*, three health-appraisal forms are described: a medical history form, a medical examination form, and a rating form. The purpose of this last form is to convey information about a job applicant's health to the management person who makes the decision whether to hire the person. This information is usually stated in code in order to protect the applicant from disclosure of personal health and illness status to nonhealth personnel (see page 82 for an example of such a system). Staffs of both the occupational health unit and the department responsible for selecting new employees must know the code.

Having the information on file about the blindness of the man's left eye is protection for the worker if, for example, he should be unfortunate enough to have an accident which causes him to lose the sight of his right eye and is now completely blind. The second-injury fund (see page 149) protects the the employer, whose insurance company pays the costs incurred by the loss of the one eye, while the worker and his family are protected since the remainder of the permanent total disability compensation is paid by the second-injury fund.

Breaks in confidentiality of occupational health records are most likely to occur in connection with non-work-related problems. For example Mrs. B., secretary to the personnel director, has been absent from work because she has been hospitalized for surgery. Information required by the insurance company for payment of her hospital and doctor bills includes a statement from the surgeon indicating the nature of the health problem and the procedures performed. This too is third-party payment. The insurance clerk who handles the forms must not reveal to anyone that Mrs. B. has had her gallbladder removed.

Increasingly the worker will need to be involved in the decision to release information, especially when the information requested is related to job placement or rehabilitation. This privilege belongs to the worker, not the physician or the nurse. Only the employee can give the consent that permits the physician to tell what he knows about a person's health problem when it is not work connected. The occupational health physician and nurse have the obligation to interpret to workers who have chronic disease problems the reasons why it is important that they share certain information about their health with the employer. For example diabetics are in a much safer environment if someone knows about their disease and is prepared to give them care if the need arises. "Privileged communication, in the legal sense, refers to the right of protection from disclosure of confidential information to a person acting in a professional capacity in a court of law."[4]

The concept of confidentiality as it applies to how the occupational health nurse functions is somewhat less structured. The information the nurse has about an employee's health or illness status does not fit the legal description of privileged communication. For example a worker may say to the nurse who has just provided care for his knee that had been injured when he tripped and fell going up the steps into the work area, "I'd been drinking before I came to work. I can tell you because you won't tell anyone." The nurse must tell this employee the truth: that her report must include all the information she had and used to make the nursing diagnosis before providing his care. Such information is not and cannot be privileged. The worker may be angry or disappointed because he thinks the nurse is being unkind. Her job then is to help this worker to deal with his work-related behavior and the impact that his drinking is having on it.

There are times when other employees ask nurses about information they have regarding another employee's illness or injury. The foreman may ask, "What's wrong with Joe?" It is commonly known that Joe has had "a stroke" and is in the intensive care unit at the hospital. The wise nurse will deal with the supervisor's need to know without going into details. What the foreman needs to know is whether Joe's illness is major or minor, whether he is receiving good care, and when he can be expected to return to work. The foreman must decide whether or not to replace Joe. Had Joe been hospitalized for an emergency appendectomy, the nurse could and should inform the foreman that Joe has had surgery and indicate the length of time that Joe's surgeon usually keeps patients in the hospital and off work, so that together the nurse and the foreman can make an educated guess as to when he can be expected to return to work. Again it is essential that the nurse use wisely the information she has. If Joe is overweight and in his 60s or if his job requires handling heavy boxes, the nurse's guess as to when he can return to work must be guided by these facts. She provides appropriate information for decision-making persons.

A nurse may have to help a worker who has epilepsy to tell his "boss" about it. Then, together with the worker and the supervisor who assigns the worker his tasks, she can make a plan. Understanding and communicative skills are important in such instances. The nurse does not tell Mike's boss that he has epilepsy. Mike does so because he has been helped to recognize that he can have a support system necessary to enable him to work in a safe environment.

Record Storage

Storing of records can become a problem, especially if there are a great many that must be maintained for long periods of time. The use of microfilm or other means of reducing the volume while retaining the potential for using the data should be considered. Microfilm and microfiche readers are available, as are ones that not only display the information but can also print off a copy. A study of the volume of records to be maintained and a careful estimate of the use that will be made of those in storage would be helpful. Consultation with a record-system expert can provide information on possible ways of reducing the quantity of paper to be stored along with the factors that make each of the procedures more or less useful. Such information can be very helpful when a decision must be made whether to put records into dead storage. This can be expensive in the long run because of the cost of storage and the great difficulty in retrieving those that may be needed. Increasingly in occupational health the need to study the interaction of the worker and the work environment is being recognized. Record systems set up to keep track of day-to-day operations in an occupational health unit are no longer adequate for the collection of data for such studies. Consequently the use of the computer for storing health information is increasing.

In some systems the information is first recorded by hand on the various forms and then put into the system by key punch operators. In the more sophisticated systems the information is put directly into the memory by means of a keyboard. It is imperative that all who put in information know the "language" of the system, be careful and accurate, and double-check their recording. Occupational health nurses who have learned to keep records with handwritten or typed notes will need to take a training course if they are to be responsible for maintaining a computerized record system. Both the handwritten system and the computer system should be maintained until the new system is functioning effectively.

When the occupational health unit's record system is computerized, the program usually includes input from all divisions of the industry. Data in the personnel department records include the basic demographic data including age, sex, marital status, race, work location, and job assignments; data from the safety and industrial hygiene department including the causes of accidents; environmental data including the levels of toxic substances in the work room; the dates and areas when and where samples were taken; the methods used both for sampling and in the laboratory; the measurements of noise levels; and such other environmental conditions as vibrations. The health unit input includes data about the injury and illness, the health assessment records made at the time of job placement, and the data generated by the medical surveillance activities. All such information is put into the system so as to be retrievable in tandem along with the information about where and when the worker was assigned. Information recorded in 1978 may need to be meaningful in 1998 if, for example, several people who worked together in the later 1970s are found to have an uncommon chronic illness the cause of which may be work connected.

No record or record system should be in use that does not have a purpose, nor should a new record form be developed unless the following questions can be answered:

1. What information is to be recorded?
2. Why is the information to be recorded?
3. When will this information be used?
4. How will this information be used?
5. Who will use this information?
6. Do we have a form on which this information can be or is already being recorded?

The Nurse's Responsibility for Records

Occupational health nurses never give nursing care without recording it. They should make every effort to assure that the information they record is correct and complete. Scrupulousness and accuracy must characterize the observations they make, the information they gather, and the record they make of these. Their reports provide the basis for determining what needs to be done as well as what has been done both by themselves and by others on the team.

Nurses must understand the purpose of the occupational health unit's record system. Records must be so set up and kept as to provide data that will protect workers, employer, and health professionals involved. Nurses must be familiar with and use the current OSHA forms and all other forms required for recording the essential information. They must gather this data by questioning and observation that permit them to determine the probable cause and the extent of workers' problems and to so record the data that it will result in a record that:

1. The health professionals involved can and will use throughout the treatment phase of the episode
2. Assures that the employee's rights are protected
3. Provides sufficient information to meet the needs of management and/or any other third-party (insurance company) so they can satisfy their responsibility, that is, be able to provide the information required by OSHA and to determine whether an employee's illness or injury is compensable
4. Permits the establishment of cause and effect of the exposure of an employee to a health hazard
5. Permits peer review and auditing of the standards of care provided.

References

1. Hurst, J. W. "How to Implement the Weed System," *Archives of Internal Medicine*, Vol. 128, No. 9, Sept. 1971, pp. 456–462.

2. Weed, L. F. *Medical Records, Medical Education, and Patient Care*. Cleveland: Case Western Reserve Press, 1969.
3. Helms, D. J. "A Guide to the New Federal Rules Governing the Confidentiality of Alcohol and Drug Abuse Patient Records," *Medical Records News*, August 1976, pp. 7–19.
4. Lesnik, M. J., and Anderson, B. E. *Nursing Practice and the Law*, 2nd Ed. Philadelphia: Lippincott, 1962.

Selected Readings

AAOHN. *Guide for Setting Up a Record System*. New York, 1977.
AMA, Department of Environmental, Public, and Occupational Health. *Guide to Development of an Industrial Medical Records System*. Chicago, 1972.
Annas, G. "Legal Aspects of Medical Confidentiality in the Occupational Setting," *Journal of Occupational Medicine*, Vol. 18, No. 8, Aug. 1976, pp. 537–540.
ANSI, Z 16.4. *American National Standard for Uniform Recordkeeping for Occupational Injuries and Illnesses*. New York, 1977.
Att, M. G. "Linking Industrial Hygiene and Health Records," *Journal of Occupational Medicine*, Vol. 19, No. 6, June 1977, pp. 388–390.
Corn, M., and Esmen, N. A. "Workplace Exposure Zones for Classification of Employee's Exposed to Physical and Chemical Agents," *AIHA Journal*, Vol. 40, No. 1, pp. 47–57.
DOL. *Recordkeeping Requirements under the Occupational Safety and Health Act*. Washington, D.C.: GPO, 1978.
DOL, Bureau of Labor Statistics. "First Work Injury Data Available from New BLS Study," *Monthly Labor Review*, January 1979, pp. 3–7.
DOL, Bureau of Labor Statistics. *What Every Employer Needs to Know about OSHA Recordkeeping*, Rep. No. 412-3. Washington, D.C.: GPO, 1979.
Fulton, W. J. "Industrial Medical Potentials—A Time and Job Analysis of Medicine in Industry," *Industrial Medicine*, Vol. 18, No. 7, July 1949, pp. 270–282.
Hagey, A. "Charting Simplified," *Occupational Health Nursing*, Vol. 26, No. 4, Apr. 1978, pp. 16–19.
Kerr, P. S. "Recording Occupational Health Data for Future Analysis," *Journal of Occupational Medicine*, Vol. 29, No. 3, Mar. 1978, pp. 197–203.
McLean, A. "Management of Occupational Health Records," *Journal of Occupational Medicine*, Vol. 8, No. 8, Aug. 1976, pp. 530–533.
Meldman, J. A. "Centralized Information Systems and the Legal Right to Privacy," *Marquette Law Review*, Vol. 52, No. 3, Fall 1969, pp. 335–354.
OSHA 29 CFR Pt. 1910. "Access to Employee Exposure and Medical Records," *Federal Register*, July 21, 1978.
Snyder, P. J. "The Computerization of Industrial Hygiene Records," *AIHA Journal*, Vol. 40, No. 8, Aug. 1979, pp. 709–720.
Warshaw, L. J. "Confidentiality versus the Need to Know," *Journal of Occupational Medicine*, Vol. 18, No. 8, Aug. 1976, pp. 534–536.
Warshaw, L. "The Malpractice Problem and the Occupational Physician," *Journal of Occupational Medicine*, Vol. 19, No. 9., Sept. 1977, pp. 593–597.

PART VII

The Occupational Health Nurse

The occupational health nurse is a worker, and the environment in which she works influences not only what needs to be done but how the nurse functions. The final part of this book deals with the nurse as a person and as a change agent who uses her professional preparation and professional competencies to assist the management of the company and the workers to have a safe and healthful work environment and to be involved in activities that contribute to their own health and safety while performing work activities associated with the production of the company's product or the service. To do so the nurse must strive to maintain and improve her own professional competence.

CHAPTER 21

The Nurse as Person and Professional

Many factors influence occupational health nursing practice, none more so than nurses' own attitudes about their role as workers in an industrial establishment. Equally important is how they feel about their role as providers of care for people who are not patients but fellow employees. Those they care for may or may not have opinions about the health-illness continuum, the hazards of their work environment, and the options they think are important.

The intangible but all-important ingredient of successful occupational health nursing is the way nurses feel about the people they work with—the respect they have for the workers' dignity and worth and the value they place on the importance of gainful employment to good mental health. Nurses must work with all kinds of people, rich and poor, knowledgeable and ignorant, those who drink too much, those who belong to and support their unions, those who have family responsibilities which they handle easily and effectively, and those who cannot cope. The second ingredient of successful occupational health nursing is the way nurses feel about themselves and the importance they place on the nurse's contribution to the fulfillment of the health expectations of the workers and of the industry.

Occupational health nurses would do well to remember the statement by a nurse: "Occupational health nursing is the easiest job in the world to do badly and the most demanding to do well." The fact that many people in the industry do not believe they "need a nurse" means that a nurse must work hard at doing what she or he knows must be done.

Approximately two-thirds of the occupational health nurse positions in this country are on staffs of less than three nurses. Many work on different shifts to provide coverage during the several work shifts of continuous-process work, hence work alone.[1] They do not have the opportunity to work with a nurse supervisor who orients them to their role and to the health unit, nor is there a nurse supervisor to provide the stimulation that results when the nurse can interact with someone who has the ability to help with questions about nursing practice. Occupational health nurses who work alone or as the establishment's only nurse must be self-directed. At times such nurses must be able to function as manager of the occupational health unit, at other times as occupational health practitioners. They must be able to perform all those nursing functions which on a larger staff would be assigned to staff nurses and many of those that would be assigned to the supervisor of nursing.

Legal Issues

"The legal rules and principles governing the activities and performance of an occupational health nurse are those governing other nurses in different contexts."[2] In an article published in the December 1969 issue of *Occupational Health Nursing,* Louise Ede, a lawyer, reminded nurses that their legal relations are formed "not only in accordance with abstract general rules, but with a view to the particular circumstances of the case."[3]

"A nurse's diagnosis of a condition must meet the standards of learning skill and care to which nurses practicing that profession in the community are held. A nurse, in order to administer first aid properly and effectively, must make a sufficient diagnosis to enable her to apply the appropriate remedy."[4] This first legal decision on the responsibility of the nurse to make a "sufficient diagnosis" was handed down by the California District Court of Appeals in 1952, when an occupational health nurse was found guilty of malpractice on the basis that a metal splinter left in a wound by her negligence was the cause of the subsequent development of a skin cancer. By the nurse's own testimony she did not examine the wound for the presence of an embedded foreign body.

Certification and Professional Associations

The American Board of Occupational Health Nurses, Inc. (ABOHN) was established in 1972. The first examination for certification was given in 1974. The process of certification focuses on excellence in practice, and the nurses who qualify are recognized as certified occupational health nurses (COHN). The long-term impact of certification will be a higher standard of practice to which all occupational health nurses will be expected to conform.

ABOHN requires that certified nurses show evidence of continuing education if they are to keep their status as a COHN, and many states require this evidence for retention of licensure to practice as a registered nurse. This makes nurses themselves responsible for keeping up to date through continuing education programs. It also means that occupational health nurses must be able to represent to their employers the importance of time off to attend training sessions and to participate in the activities of the professional nursing organizations.

The Nurse as Person and Professional

The American Association of Occupational Health Nurses was founded in 1942 as the American Association of Industrial Nurses. The present name was adopted in 1974. This specialty organization, which has state and local chapters, holds an annual conference jointly with the American Occupational Medical Association (AOMA), the specialty organization for physicians who specialize in occupational medicine.

Active participation in the AAOHN provides nurses with professional stimulation and the opportunity to learn from other nurses who also work in occupational health. Membership in the American Nurses' Association (ANA) keeps them in touch with nursing as a profession, provides opportunities to help other nurses better understand the field of occupational health nursing, and permits them to make the voice of occupational health nurses heard.

Accountability

Accountability is defined simply as being responsible for the outcome of one's acts. Both the physician who provides medical direction for the occupational health program and the nurse who provides much of the care that the workers receive must recognize that the legal doctrine of *respondeat superior*, which once protected nurses as "agents" of the physician, no longer applies to acts performed by nurses for which they have specific training and education. The nurse alone is held accountable for these acts.

In 1972 the Congress passed the Professional Standards Review Organizations Act (PSRO) (PL 92-603). This established a system of review by physicians of their peers in federally supported health care services. It can be anticipated that similar outcome criteria will be established for the field of occupational health. The ANA was awarded a contract by the Bureau of Quality Assurance of the DHEW for the development of a model set of criteria for screening the appropriateness, necessity, and quality of nursing care in settings for which professional standards review organizations would have responsibility.

Code of Conduct

In the introduction to this book the idea that occupational health nursing is a synthesis of nursing practice and occupational health practices was proposed. It seems appropriate that this chapter, "The Occupational Health Nurse," include the Code for Nurses adopted by the ANA in 1950 and revised in 1960 and 1968. It is intended to serve the individual practitioner as a guide to the ethical principles that should govern nursing practice, conduct, and relationships.

The Code for Nurses

1. The nurse provides services with respect for the dignity of man, unrestricted by considerations of nationality, race, creed, color, or status.
2. The nurse safeguards the individual's right to privacy by judiciously protecting information of a confidential nature, sharing only that information relevant to his care.
3. The nurse maintains individual competence in nursing practice, recognizing and accepting responsibility for individual actions and judgments.
4. The nurse acts to safeguard the patient when his care and safety are affected by incompetent, unethical, or illegal conduct of any person.
5. The nurse uses individual competence as a criterion in accepting delegated responsibilities and assigning nursing activities to others.
6. The nurse participates in research activities when assured that the rights of individual subjects are protected.
7. The nurse participates in the efforts of the profession to define and upgrade standards of nursing practice and education.
8. The nurse, acting through the professional organization, participates in establishing and maintaining conditions of employment conducive to high-quality nursing care.
9. The nurse works with members of health professions and other citizens in promoting efforts to meet health needs of the public.
10. The nurse refuses to give or imply endorsement to advertising, promotion, or sales for commercial products, services, or enterprises.[5]

In the field of occupational health nursing, although it has been long recognized as a specialty area of practice, there have been few educational opportunities for preservice learning and little research into the essence of practice. The establishment of the Educational Resource Center (ERC) by NIOSH and the process of certification as established by ABOHN will influence practice, research, and the prestige of nurses who accept the challenge of working as expert occupational health nurse practitioners.

Need for a Research Orientation

The word *research* means careful and diligent search. Research methodology encompasses those activities basic to both investigation and experimentation for the discovery of facts leading to the institution of theories or laws, or to revisions, in light of the facts. Basic research has as its purpose discovering new information. Applied research is less esoteric. Its purpose is to produce a better understanding of the dynamics of the process being studied and the application of such knowledge to the solution of the problem.

The health and safety of workers is directly responsive to the extent and depth of our knowledge of the cause-and-effect relationships in the interaction of human and environmental factors. Equally important is an understanding of the dynamics of human motivation and human behavior, and nurses need to be aware of all this in order to provide the best nursing care.

There are few who will disagree with the statement that there are implications for occupational health nursing practice in the surge of research now being undertaken, even though not all of the data generated from this research, whether basic or applied, are presently used effectively by occupational health nurse practitioners. The results of much of the research are published in journals or reports that nurse practitioners do not see routinely. Consequently practitioners may not know what research is going on or what data are available. Another problem is that researchers and the nurse practitioners don't work at working together. Practitioners' motivations and methods of working are different from those of researchers, and all too often there is little respect for each other's ability or for the end result of each other's efforts—a situation that need not and should not continue.

It is imperative that occupational health nurses have a research orientation. It makes them ask why; it makes them look for relationships; and it makes them use the problem-solving method. Equally important it helps them recognize the need for data generated by research as the basis for program planning. When occupational health nurses understand research methods they recognize the part their records can contribute to retrospective studies. When this fact is recognized nurses realize that what they record as current events and put into employee health records may many years later be used as data in a retrospective study. Such studies are set up to determine a cause-and-effect relationship between present ill health and the work environment perhaps 10–20 years before. The information nurses record can constitute a significant resource for a study team.

Research projects to determine the toxicity of chemicals and field studies to determine the attack rate of illness of a worker population so exposed are of great importance to the total occupational health community. It is noted with alarm that in some reports members of field study teams determined that occupational health nurses, when interviewed, contributed meaningful information, but that the data about illness they had recorded did not prove to be useful. All too frequently the record contains only a notation, for example, "headache." Such a notation does not permit drawing inference about work environmental influences nor permit use by a study team of the objective evidence that the nurse had solicited and used to make the "nursing diagnosis" of headache.

Although some of the cause-and-effect relationships are well known, such as those in lead poisoning, silicosis, or radiation sickness, others are just now becoming manifest. Examples of new occupational diseases are the angiosarcomas of the liver caused by exposure to vinyl chloride[6] and peripheral neuropathy caused by exposure to methyl butyl ketone.[7] It is for these reasons that occupational health nurses must be acutely aware of man-environment health problems. They must seek information about the environment of workers and must look for relationships between the signs and symptoms that are presented and the toxic substances and other hazards associated with the occupation. What they have learned from workers must be recorded so that others can use the data.

One need only to reflect on the 20-year exposure-disease relationship of vinyl chloride and angiosarcoma to understand the occupational disease problems of tomorrow and the importance of record keeping of current health events. Every notation about a health problem should be recorded by nurses as if they were a part of a study team that had as its purpose the identification of the health effects of the work environment. Equally important is the ability to match environmental monitoring data by date, time, and place with individual employee health record data.

Practically all occupational diseases mimic diseases found in the general population. The occupational disease process may have a long latency period, often 20 or more years from onset of exposure. Data which clearly distinguish the effects of massive doses intermittently received from the effects of small insults over a longer period of time are not available. The same chemical may, with long-term chronic exposure, affect one organ of the body and, with high-dose short-term acute exposure, affect a completely different body organ. Only a diagnosis that considers the possible effect of the environment, and a complete recording of all the data upon which it was based, will contribute to a better understanding of disease etiology and to the correction of work place conditions. Knowing this, occupational health nurses can play a part in research that identifies the problem.

The practical implication of this kind of research wherein data can serve as a basis for program planning can be illustrated. A review of the research literature dealing with physical fitness, for example, concluded that "a relationship existed between low back pain, physical fitness and other individual physiological and psychological factors."[8] This was based in part on an NSC survey conducted in 1967 of over 400,000 back injuries and reported by Snook and Cirriello. This shows that "those workers in the middle age group the 30's and 40's appear to be the most susceptible to back injuries."[9] J. R. Brown of Canada, in *Manual Lifting and Related Fields*, commented on the problems of this age group. He stated, "Our observations would indicate that most of the problems arise during the period of years 31–40 and it is, of course, during this period that the intervertebral disc is undergoing a considerable change in structure and in consistency and mechanical strength. Under those conditions it is not surprising, therefore, that most back injuries occur in this age group."[10] This knowledge has meaning and can be used in plans involving job placement, health and safety education, and developing work practices. In addition incorporation of such knowledge into a health education program for workers could result in a behavior change to a more active life-style. The conclusion of an investigation of low back pain and occupations seems to back up this suggestion in that A. Magora found the lowest incidence of low back pain in a highly physical-fitness-oriented occupational group.[11]

A summary of data concerning the health effects of obesity provides reasons for occupational health nurses to intervene to protect the overweight worker's health. Evidence supports the illness-accident–obesity relationship. This is, people who are overweight have an increased chance of heat stroke and heat exhaustion, especially if they do heavy work in hot environments. Obesity adds strain to the respiratory system. Obese persons' decreased agility makes them more susceptible to on-the-job accidents. A. Henschel concluded that "the higher morbidity and mortality experience of obese people points to it as a major health problem."[12]

The ecology of work is the interaction of the people and the environment in which they work. Some workers are young and some are old. Some are thin and others are obese. Some people work in a safer manner than others. Certain work environments are more hazardous than others. Some people work where there is an established occupational health program; others, where there is none. What effect, if any, does having a nurse at the place of employment have on the worker's ability to work and live in a safer and more healthful manner? The null hypothesis that has not been tested to its logical and empirical consequences is:

> Workers who are taught good health practices by the occupational health nurse have no better health-related behavior than those who are not so instructed.

What is needed are studies to determine what effect the occupational health nurse has on worker health behavior and what are the interrelated variables of occupational health nursing practice.

Two editorials in the July 1975 issue of the *New England Journal of Medicine* discussed hypertension at the work place. One of those, "The Nurses' Role in Treating Hypertension," commented on a program to detect and treat hypertension at the work site. It presents an accomplished activity which serves as a prototype of how the nurse practitioner can contribute to worker safety and health.[13] The writer of the other editorial, "Detection and Treatment of Hypertension at the Work Site," says, "Backed by the union, the medical director of a large department store incorporated a screening and treatment program for the employees found to be hypertensive. At the end of the first year the blood pressures had been brought under control in 80 percent of the workers. Ninety-seven percent of those who entered into the program were still under treatment."[14] The long-term management of these workers was carried out by occupational health nurses.

In occupational health much of what happens to and for workers is carried on by nurses, but there has been too little study of this; hence there are too little objective data that can be used to describe the occupational health nursing process and to establish why nurses are effective or not effective in dealing with occupational health problems.

A research orientation—interest in and an awareness of what their colleagues in the health field are finding out—should cause occupational health nurses to gather data that are objective and measurable and to look for alternatives before drawing conclusions. Such an orientation has far-reaching implications, as it will result in records that permit an assessment of what nurses do, how they do it, and how it affects the health of workers.

The latter could be the focus of a research project to determine the nurse's contribution to worker health. Nurses who have a research orientation can design and carry on research projects in which certain things are done for one group of workers, using a similar group of workers as the control. Studies can determine if what was done for the study group did nor did not make any difference.

References

1. DHEW. *Surveys of Public Health Nursing 1968–1972*. Washington, D.C.: GPO, 1975, p. 122.
2. Hershey, N. "The Nurse Who Works Alone," *Archives of Environmental Health*, Vol. 11, No. 8, Aug. 1965, pp. 230–234.
3. Ede, L. "Legal Relations in Nursing," *Occupational Health Nursing*, Vol. 17, No. 12, Dec. 1969, pp. 9–15.
4. AMA, Council on Occupational Health. *The Legal Scope of Industrial Nursing Practice*. Chicago, 1959.
5. ANA. *Code for Nurses, with Interpretive Statements*. Kansas City, Mo.,: 1976.
6. Creek, J. L., and Johnson, M. N. "Angiosarcoma of the Liver in the Manufacture of Polyvinyl Chloride," *Journal of Occupational Medicine,* Vol. 16, No. 4 Apr. 1974, pp. 150–151.
7. Billmaire, D., Yee, H. I., Craft, B., Williams, N., Epstein, S., and Fontaine, R. "Peripheral Neuropathy in a Coated Fabric Plant," *Journal of Occupational Medicine*, Vol. 16, No. 10 Oct. 1974, pp. 665–671.
8. Sleight, R. B., Cook, K. C., and Staff Century Research Corporation, *Problems in Occupational Safety and Health: A Critical Review of Select Worker Physical and Psychological Factors*, NIOSH Pub. No. 75–124. Washington, D.C.: GPO, 1974, pp. 1–6.
9. Snook, S. H., and Cirriello, V. M. "Low Back Pain in Industry," *Journal of the ASSE*, Apr. 1972, pp. 723–725.

10. Brown, J. R. *Manual Lifting and Related Fields: An Annotated Bibliography.* Ontario: Ontario Ministry of Labor, 1972, p. 16.
11. Magora, A. "Investigation of the Relation between Low Back Pain and Occupations," *Industrial Medicine and Surgery,* Vol. 39, No. 10, p. 150–152.
12. Henschel, A. "Obesity as an Occupational Hazard," *Canadian Journal of Public Health,* Vol. 67, No. 11, Nov. 1967, pp. 491–493.
13. Finnerty, F. A., "The Nurses' Role in Treating Hypertension," Editorial, *New England Journal of Medicine,* Vol. 293, No. 2, p. 93.
14. Alderman, M. H., and Schoenbaum, E. E. "Detection and Treatment of Hypertension at the Work Site," *New England Journal of Medicine,* Vol. 293, No. 2, pp. 65–68.

Selected Readings

AAIN. *The Nurse in Industry: A History of the American Association of Industrial Nurses, Inc.* New York: AAOHN, 1976.
AAOHN. *Guide for on-the-job Orientation of Occupational Health Nurses.* New York, 1970.
AAOHN. *Guide for the Development of Functions and Responsibilities in Occupational Health Nursing.* New York, 1960.
AAOHN. *Statement on Professional Liability.* New York, 1959; revised 1977.
ABOHN. *ABOHN Bulletin.* Thousand Palms, Calif., 1977.
ANA. *Functions, Standards, and Qualifications for Occupational Health Nurses.* Kansas City, Mo., 1968.
ANA. *Standards of Nursing Practice.* Kansas City, Mo. 1973.
Bernzweig, E. P. *The Nurse's Liability for Malpractice: A Programmed Course,* 2nd Ed. New York: McGraw-Hill, 1975.
Brown, M. L. "Highlights of the Occupational Health Nursing Study," *AAIN Journal,* Vol. 13, No. 5, 1965, pp. 19–23.
Brown, M. L. "A Profile of Occupational Health Nursing," *Occupational Health Nursing,* Vol. 18, No. 2, Feb. 1970, pp. 16–18.
Charley, I. H. *The Birth of Industrial Nursing.* London: Baillière, Tindall, 1978.
Creighton, H. *Law Every Nurse Should Know.* Philadelphia: Saunders, 1975.
Flanagan, L. *One Strong Voice.* Kansas City, Mo.: ANA, 1976.
Horsley, B. "A Registered Nurse as an OSHA Compliance Officer," *Occupational Health Nursing,* Vol. 20, No. 9, Sept. 1972, pp. 7–9.
Joint Practice Committee of North Carolina Medical Society and North Carolina Nurses' Association. *Occupational Health Services,* Rep. of Task Force. Raleigh, N.C., 1976.
Lee, J. A. *The New Nurse in Industry.* Washington, D.C.: GPO, 1978.
Murchison, I., Nichols, T. S., and Hanson, R. *Legal Accountability in the Nursing Process.* St. Louis.: Mosby, 1978.
Murphy, J. F. "Role Expansion or Role Extension: Some Conceptual Differences," *Nursing Forum,* Vol. 9, No. 4, 1970, pp. 380–389.
Oda, D. "Specialized Role Development: A Three Phase Process," *Nursing Outlook,* Vol. 25, No. 6, June 1977, pp. 374–377.

Appendixes

APPENDIX A

Acronyms and Abbreviations

AA	Alcoholics Anonymous
AAIN	American Association of Industrial Nurses (now AAOHN)
AAOHN	American Association of Occupational Health Nurses
AAOO	American Academy of Ophthalmology and Otolaryngology
ABOHN	American Board for Occupational Health Nurses, Inc.
ACGIH	American Conference of Governmental Industrial Hygienists
ACOG	American College of Obstetricians and Gynecologists
ACS	American Chemical Society
ADAMHA	Alcohol, Drug Abuse, and Mental Health Administration
AFL-CIO	American Federation of Labor–Congress of Industrial Organizations
AIHA	American Industrial Hygiene Association
AJN	American Journal of Nursing
AMA	American Medical Association
ANA	American Nurses' Association
ANSI	American National Standards Institute
AOMA	American Occupational Medical Association
ARC	American Red Cross
ASA	Acoustical Society of America
ASAP	Alcohol Safety Action Program
ASSE	American Society of Safety Engineers
CDC	Center for Disease Control
CFR	Code of Federal Regulations
CIS	Center for Information Services
COHN	certified occupational health nurse
CPR	cardiopulmonary recuscitation
DHEW	Department of Health, Education, and Welfare
DHHS	Department of Health and Human Services
DOL	Department of Labor
EEOC	Equal Employment Opportunity Commission
EMS	emergency medical service
EPA	Environmental Protection Agency

ERC	Educational Resource Center (for Occupational Health Manpower)
FDA	Food and Drug Administration
FECA	Federal Employees' Compensation Act
FEPA	Fair Employment Practice Act
FEV_1	forced expiratory volume in 1 second
FVC	"forced" vital capacity
GNP	gross national product
GPO	Government Printing Office
HCM	health care management
HHE	health hazard evaluation
HMO	health maintenance organization
IAPA	Industrial Accident Prevention Association
ICDA	International Classification of Disease, Amended
IH	industrial hygienist
ILO	International Labour Organization
IUD	Industrial Union Department (of the American Federation of Labor and Congress of Industrial Organizations)
NCA	National Council on Alcoholism
NCCHR	National Commission on Confidentiality of Health Records
NCI	National Cancer Institute
NIAAA	National Institute on Alcohol Abuse and Alcoholism
NIH	National Institutes of Health
NIOSH	National Institute for Occupational Safety and Health
NJPC	National Joint Practice Commission
NLN	National League for Nursing
NSC	National Safety Council
NSPB	National Society for the Prevention of Blindness
NTIS	National Technical Information Service
OCAW	Oil, Chemical and Atomic Workers
OHI	Occupational Health Institute
OSH	occupational safety and health
OSHA	Occupational Safety and Health Act *or* Occupational Safety and Health Administration
PAT	Proficiency Analytical Testing
PL	Public Law
PHS	Public Health Service
ppm	parts per million
PSRO	Professional Standards Review Organization
rem	roentgen equivalent man
SCP	Standards Completion Program
SIC	Standard Industrial Classification
SOEH	Society for Occupational and Environmental Health

TLV^R	threshold limit value
TWA	time-weighted average
USPHS	United States Public Health Service
VA	Veterans' Administration
WC	workmen's (worker) compensation
WHO	World Health Organization

APPENDIX B

Glossary

Explanations of terms as used in occupational safety and health nursing are included here to help nurses communicate more effectively with other members of occupational safety and health teams. This list is not all inclusive; it is intended to serve as a convenient resource for nurses as they develop similar lists for inclusion in an occupational health unit's policy and procedure manual. Each industry has a special lingo, terms that are understood by those who use them but that may be incomprehensible to the outsider. As nurses increase their vocabulary, they should add the new terms to the glossary in their unit's manual.

The numbers that follow each explanation or definition refer to the following sources:

1. Occupational Safety and Health Administration (OSHA).
2. National Safety Council (NSC).
3. American Conference of Governmental Industrial Hygienists (ACGIH).
4. Environmental Protection Agency (EPA).
5. American National Standards Institute (ANSI).
6. Source immediately follows definition.
7. M. L. Brown, author of this book.

accident: that occurrence in a sequence of events which usually produces unintended injury, death, or property damage. 2

accident type: describes the occurrence in relation to injury or property damage. 2

action level: term used by OSHA and NIOSH to express that level of airborne concentration that is one-half of the TWA. When the action level is reached, the OSHA standards state what environmental monitoring and medical surveillance activities are to be carried out. 1

aerosol: an assemblage of small particles, solid or liquid, suspended in air. The diameter of the particles may vary from 100 microns down to .01 micron or less, e.g., dust, fog, smoke. 3

agency or agent: the principal object such as a tool, a machine, or equipment involved in an accident; usually the object that inflicts injury or property damage. 2

Glossary

air filter: an air cleaning device to remove light particulate loadings from normal atmospheric air before introduction into the building. Usual range: loadings up to 3 grains per thousand cubic feet (.003 grains per cubic foot). Note: Atmospheric air in heavy industrial areas and in-plant air in many industries have higher loadings than this, and dust collectors are then indicated for proper air cleaning.   3

asbestos: (1) a collective mineralogical term encompassing the asbestiform varieties of various minerals; (2) an industrial product obtained by mining and processing primarily asbestiform minerals.   3

asbestosis: a diffuse but nonuniform fibrosis of the lungs that is generally most severe in the basilar portions. As a result of the fibrosis some of the air spaces (alveoli) are not perfused with blood, and those that are perfused with blood may not be adequately ventilated because of stiff, thickened alveolar walls. The fibrosis makes the lungs less compliant, thereby increasing the energy required for breathing. Increasing impairment in diffusion of gases leads to increasing breathlessness. It is not uncommon to find thickening of the visceral pleura, sometimes very severe, by extension of the parenchymal inflammation. This causes an additional increase in the effort of breathing. The parietal pleura may show patches of severe thickening—particularly over the diaphragm and the lower portions of the chest wall—resulting in so-called pleural hyaline plaques. These may become visible in X-ray films of the chest—particularly, if they become impregnated with calcium salts. Such pleural plaques may develop from asbestos exposure in the absence of asbestosis. They cause no symptoms. Asbestosis is caused by breathing in quantities of asbestos particles of a size and type that can enter and damage the lung.   3

biological handling: how a living organism processes a substance; as the uptake, storage, metabolism, and excretion of that substance.   4

biomedical research: investigation or experimentation aimed at the discovery and interpretation of facts to be used for application in the human population.   4

biophysics: a branch of knowledge concerned with applying physical properties and methods to biological problems.   4

carbon monoxide (CO): a colorless, odorless, highly toxic gas that is a normal byproduct of incomplete combustion of carbon-containing substances such as coal, gasoline, oil, and natural gas; one of the major air pollutants; can be harmful in small amounts if breathed over a long period of time.   4

carbonyl compounds: oxidation products (products formed after combination with oxygen) of normal blood constituents; normally not present in the blood; therefore, when they are present they are easily detectable by simple chemical techniques.   4

carcinogenicity: the ability to produce or incite cancer.   4

ceiling limit: a term used by OSHA in the formulation of a TWA, a ceiling value; the level of a toxic substance in the work environment that should not be exceeded.   1

certification: the process whereby a professional association that is not a government agency determines qualifications considered to be signs of excellence. The individual practitioner must elect to undertake the required examination and to meet the other criteria before recognition of achievement, i.e., certification, can be awarded. Nurses are certified by ABOHN. The purpose is to implement and conduct the program of certification of qualified occupational health nurses. Industrial hygienists are certified by the American Board of Industrial Hygiene. Organized in 1960, this board aims to improve the practice and educational standards of the profession of industrial hygiene. Certified industrial hygienists belong to the American Academy of Industrial Hygiene. 7

chemistry: a science that deals with the composition, structure, and properties of substances and of the transformations these substances undergo. 4

chlorofluorocarbons: gases, formed of chlorine, fluorine, and carbon, whose molecules normally do not react with other substances; they are therefore useful, when compressed, as spray-can propellants because they do not alter the material being sprayed. 4

chromosome: one of a group of threadlike structures contained in the nucleus of the cell; human cells normally have 46 or 23 "pairs" of chromosomes, one of each pair contributed by the mother, the other by the father, at conception. 4

comfort zone (average): the range of effective temperatures over which the majority (50% or more) of adults feel comfortable. 4

compliance program: the plan developed by the employer utilizing engineering and work practice controls to reduce and maintain the employee's exposure to the regulated substance. The compliance program is to be a written program and shall include schedules for development and implementation of the controls. The plan shall be revised at least every 6 months to reflect the current status of the program. 1

cybernetics: the comparative study of electronic communication systems which combines the disciplines of neurophysiology, mathematics, and electrical engineering; it is concerned with the process of information flow through which the brain controls the body and through which computers control machines. It supports the hypothesis that the functioning of the human brain is similar to that of electronic control devices. 6 *Duncan's Dictionary for Nurses*, New York, Springer, 1971, p. 99.

day of disability: any day on which an employee is unable, because of injury, to perform effectively, throughout a full shift, the essential functions of a regularly established job which is open and available to him or her. The day of injury and the day on which the employee was able to return to full-time employment are not counted as days of disability; all intervening calendar days, or calendar days subsequent to the day of injury (including weekends, holidays, other days off, and other days on which the plant may be shut down) are counted as days of disability. 5

detoxication: the process whereby a toxic agent is either removed or metabolically converted to a less toxic compound. 4

dose-response relationship: the correlation of relationship between the amount of an agent (drug, chemical, etc.) to which one is exposed and the resulting effect on the body. 4

dust: small, solid particles created by the breaking up of larger particles by pro-

Glossary

cesses such as crushing, grinding, drilling, explosions, etc. Dust particles already in existence in a mixture of materials may escape into the air through such operations as shoveling, conveying, screening, sweeping, etc. 4

dust collector: an air cleaning device to remove heavy particulate loadings from exhaust systems before discharge to outdoors. Usual range: loadings 0.003 grains per cubic foot and higher. 4

electron microscopy: use of a microscope in which an electron beam, instead of light, forms an image for viewing on a fluorescent screen or for photography; capable of extremely high magnification. 4

emphysema: a condition marked by rupture of the air sacs of the lung and the consequent impairment of heart action. 4

employment: (1) all work or activity performed in carrying out an assignment or request of the employer, including incidental and related activities not specifically covered by the assignment or request; (2) any voluntary work or activity undertaken while on duty for the purpose of benefiting the employer; (3) any other activities undertaken while on duty with the consent or approval of the employer. 5

environment: the sum of all external conditions and influences affecting the life, development, and ultimately the survival of an organism. 4

environmental agents: external influences and conditions—particularly physical, biological, and synthetic and natural chemical substances found in the environment. 4

environmental health sciences: a broad range of fields of study including chemistry, toxicology, pharmacology, biometry, biophysics, biology, etc., aimed at detecting and understanding the action in humans and animals of agents in the environment which have an adverse effect on humans. 4

environment-related diseases: illnesses brought about or aggravated by environmental agents. 4

epidemiology: the study of population patterns to determine possible causes of diseases which may exhibit a prolonged latency or dormant period before they are clinically identifiable. This is the definition for chronic disease epidemiology and is applicable to occupational health. 4

first-aid cases: involve one-time treatment and subsequent observations of minor scratches, cuts, burns, splinters, etc., which do not ordinarily require medical care, even though such treatment is provided by a physician or other registered professional personnel. 1

frequency rate: the number of disabling work injuries per million man-hours of exposure. 2

fumes: small solid particles formed by the condensation of vapors of solid materials. 3

gases: formless fluids which tend to occupy an entire space uniformly at ordinary temperatures and pressures. 3

Health Hazard Evaluation (HHE) Program: Section 20 (a)(6) of the Occupational Safety and Health Act [29 USC 669(a)(6)] provides as follows: "The Secretary of Health, Education and Welfare shall . . . determine following a written request by any employer or authorized representative of employees, specifying with reasonable particularity the grounds on which the request is made, whether any substance normally found in the place of employment has potentially toxic effects in such concentrations as used or found; and shall submit such determination both to employers and affected employers as soon as possible." The conduct of each HHE usually incorporates the following five phases:(a) validation of request, (b)initial field investigation, (c) follow-up environmental-medical studies, (d) analysis and determination of toxicity, and (e) report back to requestor or employer, the union, and OSHA. A valid request for an HHE can be made by at least three workers, by the representative of the workers (i.e., the union), or by management. An HHE request form is available from NIOSH in Cincinnati, Ohio, or in Rockville, Maryland, or from any one of the 10 regional offices. An HHE should be requested when there is concern that there may be a toxic substance in the work area. 7

heavy metals: metallic elements with high molecular weights; generally toxic in low concentrations to plant and animal life; examples include mercury, chromium, cadmium, arsenic, and lead. 4

Heimlich maneuver: a technique used to dislodge food or an object from the throat of a person who is choking. Abrupt upward pressure is applied to the abdomen below the rib cage and above the navel, forcing the diaphragm upward, compressing air in the lungs, and expelling the object. 7

history: a chronological record of significant events: (1) occupational—the work experience including part-time work—(information sought includes name of employer; dates of employment; jobs held, including major responsibilities and list of possible hazards associated with each; and personal protective equipment worn, for what purpose, and frequency); (2) reproductive—number of live births, including any deformities and lost pregnancies—(information asked of both men and women); (3) smoking (questions include: At what age did the person start to smoke? Does he or she continue to smoke? What does the person smoke and how much? How often if at all has the person stopped smoking and for how long? At what age did the person increase smoking to more than one package of cigarettes a day? 7

hydrocarbons: a vast family of compounds containing carbon and hydrogen in various combinations found especially in fossil fuels such as coal, petroleum, natural gas, and bitumens; some are major air pollutants, some may be carcinogenic, and others contribute to smog. 4

incidence rate: number of injuries and illnesses, or lost workdays experienced, by 100 full-time workers. The rate is calculated as: $N/EH \times 200,000$, when N = total number of occupational injuries and illnesses, other injuries or illnesses, or lost workdays; EH = total hours worked by all employees during calendar year; and 200,000 = base for 100 full-time equivalent workers (working 40 hours per week, 50 weeks per year). The median incidence rate is the middle measure in the distribution (i.e., half of the establishments have an incidence rate more than and half less than the median rate). The middle range (interquartile) is defined by two measures: a fourth of the establishments have a rate less than the first quartile and a fourth a rate more than the third quartile rate. 5

Glossary

industrial nurse: one who gives nursing service under general medical direction to ill or injured employees or other persons who become ill or suffer an accident on the premises of a factory or other establishment. Duties involve a combination of the following: giving first aid to the ill or injured, attending to subsequent dressings of employees' injuries, keeping records of patients treated, preparing accident reports for compensation or other purposes, assisting in physical examinations and health evaluations of applicants and employees, and planning and carrying out programs involving health education, accident prevention, evaluation of plant environment, or other activities affecting the health, welfare, and safety of all personnel. 6 DOL, Bureau of Labor Statistics, Bulletin No. 1950-41.

International Classification of Diseases and Injuries (IDIC): a taxonomy designed for the classification of morbidity and mortality information for statistical purposes and for the indexing of hospital records. It is used to code diseases and operations for data storage and retrieval. This system has meaning and usefulness for the coding of occupational injuries and illnesses as well. Uniform definitions and uniform systems of classification are prerequisites of data collection on injury, illness, and death; therefore a standard classification of disease and injury for statistical purposes is essential. In the eighth revision of the IDIC the classifications are arranged in 17 main sections. The first section deals with disease caused by well-defined infective agents; this is followed by categories for neoplasms and for endocrine, metabolic, and nutritional diseases. Most of the remaining diseases are arranged according to their principal anatomic site, with special sections for mental diseases, complications of pregnancy and childbirth, certain diseases peculiar to the perinatal period, and ill-defined conditions including symptoms. The last section provides a dual classification of injuries; that is, they are classified according to the "external cause" giving rise to the injury and according to the "nature of the injury", puncture, open wound, or burn. 6 DHEW, PHS, National Center for Health Statistics. *International Classification of Diseases,* adapted for use in the United States, 8th ed. Washington, D.C., GPO, 1972.

laboratory accreditation: (1) The AIHA Laboratory Accreditation Program is designed to evaluate personnel qualifications, internal quality control procedures, equipment, facilities, and record-keeping procedures by site visitation of laboratories, in addition to evaluating proficiency testing performance. A pamphlet, "A Plan for Accreditation of Industrial Hygiene Laboratories," describing the AIHA Laboratory Accreditation Program is available by contacting: Coordinator of Laboratory Accreditation, American Industrial Hygiene Association, 475 Wolf Ledges Parkway, Akron, Ohio 44311. (2) The CDC has programs in laboratory accreditation for microbiology, immunology, immunohematology, and chemistry (includes blood lead) laboratories. Contact: Proficiency Testing Branch, Center for Disease Control, Building 6, Room 315, Atlanta, Ga. 30333. (3) The EPA provides programs in microbiology, radiochemistry, water pollution, and ambient air analysis. Contact: U.S. EPA, Environmental Monitoring and Support Laboratory, Research Triangle Park, N.C. 27711. **6 AIHA**

lost workdays: those days which the employee would have worked but could not because of occupational injury or illness. The number of lost workdays should not include the day of injury. The number of days includes all days (consecutive or not) in which, because of injury or illness the employee: (a) would have worked but could not, (b) was assigned to a temporary job, (c) worked at a permanent job less than full time, or (d) worked at a permanently assigned job but could not perform all duties normally assigned. 1

lower explosive limit: the lower limit of flammability or explosibility of a gas or vapor at ordinary ambient temperatures expressed in percentage of the gas or vapor in air by volume. This limit is assumed constant for temperatures up to 250°F. Above these temperatures, it should be decreased by a factor of 0.7 since explosibility increases with higher temperatures. 3

man-hours: The total number of hours worked by all employees in an establishment, a company, or an industry. A man-hour is the equivalent of one employee working 1 hour. 2

manometer: an instrument for measuring pressure; essentially a U-tube partially filled with a liquid, usually water, mercury, or a light oil, so constructed that the amount of displacement of the liquid indicates the pressure being exerted on the instrument. 3

medical treatment: includes treatment administered by a physician or by registered professional personnel under the standing orders of a physician. Medical treatment does not include first-aid treatment (see definition) even though provided by a physician or other registered professional personnel. 1

mesothelioma: a rare form of cancer with malignant tumors occurring on the surface of the lung or abdominal viscera. 4

metabolism: the sum of the processes by which a particular substance is handled in the living body. 4

micron: a unit of length, one-thousandth of 1 millimeter or one-millionth of a meter (approximately 1/25,000 of an inch). 3

mists: small droplets of materials that are ordinarily liquid at normal temperature and pressure. 3

mutagens: compounds causing heritable alteration in DNA that can damage egg and sperm cells prior to fertilization and damage the embryo as well. A chemical substance or physical agent may act directly on the germ cells so that fertilization does not take place, or it may cause such severe anomalies in the zygote as to result in an early, at times unrecognized, abortion. There are relatively few reports of parental exposures related to either outcome, although the risk is recognized. It is during this preconception period that both paternal and maternal exposure to mutagenic agents must be considered for both, collectively or independently, for exposure may result in the inhibition of fertilization or the production of abnormal embryos. 6 "Reproductive Toxicology and Workers," J. Messite, a paper presented at the New York Academy of Medicine, 1979.

nitrogen dioxide (NO_2): a compound produced by a chemical reaction in which oxygen combines with nitric oxide in the atmosphere; a major contributor to photochemical smog. 4

nonfatal cases without lost workdays: cases of occupational injury or illness which did not involve fatalities or lost workdays but did result in: (a) transfer to another job or termination of employment, (b) medical treatment other than first aid, (c) diagnosis of occupational illness, (d) loss of consciousness, or (e) restriction of work or motion.   1

nurse practitioner: a registered nurse who has successfully completed a formal program of study designed to prepare registered nurses to perform in an expanded role in the delivery of primary health care. Nurse practitioner functions and responsibilities are: assessing the health status of individuals, families, and communities through: (a) taking a health and medical history; performing physical examinations; and defining health and developmental problems, physical and emotional status, social and economic status, and cultural and environmental background; (b) intervention through instructing, guiding, and counseling individuals, families, and groups in the: promotion and maintenance of health; prevention of illness and disability; involvement of individuals, families, and groups in planning for their health care; institution and provision of continuity of care to clients (patients) during acute and chronic phases of illness; application of health education techniques with clients to ensure understanding of and compliance with the therapeuric regimen within established protocols; and recognition of the need for referral and referring the client to a physician, other health care providers, or community resources; (c) collaboration with other health care providers and agencies to: provide all aspects of basic health care services needed for individual and family care and to coordinate and manage all aspects of basic health care services to individuals and families.   6   HEW Guidelines for Nurse Practitioner Education Programs.

OSHA Standards: see Standards, OSHA.

occupational health nursing: the application of nursing principles in conserving the health of workers in all occupations; involves prevention, recognition, and treatment of illness and injury and requires special skills and knowledge in the fields of health education and counseling, environmental health, rehabilitation, and human relations.   6   AAOHN, "Definition of Occupational Health Nursing," 1968.

occupational medicine: medical practice concerned with the prevention of disease, the maintenance and promotion of health among employed persons in their group setting, the community's health as it is affected by industry, and the consumers' health as affected by industrial products; involves clinical medicine, toxicology, epidemiology, and administrative expertise. The Council on Medical Education and Hospitals of the AMA in June 1955 authorized certification of specialists in occupational medicine by the American Board of Preventive Medicine.   6   New York Academy of Medicine, "Statement on the Health Manpower Situation in Occupational Medicine" (1977).

ozone: (O_3): a pungent, colorless, toxic gas whose molecules are formed of three oxygen atoms; one component of photochemical smog and considered a major air pollutant.   4

ozone shield: a naturally variable layer of ozone in the earth's upper atmosphere which absorbs the most lethal wavelengths of ultraviolet radiation from the sun; it thus serves as a shield between this radiation and the inhabitants of the earth. 4

parts per million (ppm): a unit used to express concentration of a trace substance (contaminant); with vapors, ppm is expressed as a volume/volume relationship (i.e., 1 microliter SO_2 per liter air = 1 ppm SO_2); with liquids and solids, ppm usually refers to mass concentration. 4

pathology: the study of the essential nature of diseases and especially of the structural and functional changes produced by them. 4

permanent disability (synonymous with permanent impairment): includes any degree of permanent impairment of the body such as amputation, permanent impairment of vision and other permanently crippling nonfatal injuries. Permanent total disability implies permanent, complete inability to perform gainful work but also includes the amputation of both arms, both legs, both feet, or any combination of the two extremities, or the total loss of sight. Permanent partial disability implies permanent impairment of any degree less than permanent total. 2

pharmacokinetics: the study of the rate of absorption, distribution, metabolism, and excretion of substances from the body. 4

physical environmental agents: influences and conditions characterized by the forces and operations of physics—as noise, microwave radiation, vibration. 4

polycyclic aromatic hydrocarbons: organic compounds that contain carbon and hydrogen in a particular combination and that often occur in petroleum, natural gas, coal, and bitumens; some have been shown to cause cancer. 4

polymerization: the act or process of forming a compound by the combination of simpler molecules; a chemical reaction in which two or more small molecules combine to form larger molecules. 4

The Pregnancy Disability Law (PL 95–555): enacted on October 31, 1978; amends Title VII of the Civil Rights Act of 1964 by prohibiting employment discrimination against pregnant women. The law mandates that if medical benefits are provided for other disabilities then they must be provided for pregnancy-related disabilities on the same terms and conditions. Because radiation has long been recognized as a fetotoxin, problems pertaining to the transfer of pregnant employees out of positions with potential radiation exposure have surfaced in the past. In fact a 1977 report of the National Council on Radiation Protection and Measurements expressly stated that "during the entire gestation period, the maximum permissible dose equivalent to the fetus from occupational exposure of the expectant mother should not exceed 0.5 rem." 6 NIOSH No. 78-118. *Guidelines on Pregnancy and Work*, Washington, D.C. GPO, 1977, p. 23.

pressure, atmospheric: pressure due to the weight of the atmosphere; the pressure indicated by a barometer. *Standard atmospheric pressure* or *standard atmosphere* is the pressure of 29.92 inches of mercury. 3

Proficiency Analytical Testing (PAT) Program: a quality assurance service provided by NIOSH to industrial hygiene laboratories. Although one objective of PAT is to determine the analytical competence of participating laboratories that use conventional industrial hygiene analytical procedures, the primary objective of the program is to assist the participating laboratories in improving analytical performance. 7

radiation, thermal (heat): the transmission of energy by means of electromagnetic waves of very long wavelength. Radiant energy of any wavelength may, when absorbed, become thermal energy and result in an increase in the temperature of the absorbing body. 7

radiation injuries: Radiation may be absorbed by a cell and damage it genetically so that it reproduces in damaged form over a period of years or it may kill the cell. Cell damage may, over time, produce delayed health effects such as cancer, developmental abnormalities, or genetic defects. Animal studies indicate that radiation produces gene mutations which can result in genetic abnormalities in subsequent generations, but similar genetic changes in humans have not yet been demonstrated conclusively. Numerous studies have shown that radiation exposure produces—many years after exposure—some forms of cancer, most notably leukemia and thyroid, breast, and lung cancer. Our knowledge of the health effects of radiation comes primarily from human and animal studies of high-level radiation exposures (50 rem or more). The problem is how to apply this knowledge to predict the incidence of cancer from exposures at lower levels. If we assume that low dose exposures produce cancer at a rate directly proportional to the incidence at high doses, then in a population of 10,000 persons—in which one may normally expect 1,600 cases of fatal cancer to occur naturally—exposure of each of the 10,000 persons to 1 rem of radiation may be expected to produce one additional case of fatal cancer. 7

recordable case: any work-related injury case requiring more than first aid, and all occupational illnesses. Recordable cases include: (a) deaths, regardless of the time between occupational injury or illness and death; (b) all occupational illnesses; and (c) all occupational injuries resulting in any of the following: lost workdays—either days away from work or days of restricted work activity, medical treatment other than first aid, loss of consciousness, restriction of work or motion, temporary or permanent transfer, or termination of employment of ill or injured employee. 5

regularly established job: one which has not been established especially to accommodate an injured employee, either for therapeutic reasons or to avoid counting the case as a temporary total disability. 5

rem: the unit used to measure radiation dose. The rem refers to the amount of radiation required to produce a particular amount of biological damage in tissue. Because the rem is too large a unit to describe easily, the relatively low levels of many types of environmental exposure doses are often expressed in millirems: 1 rem = 1,000 millirems.

safety testing: experiments on environmental agents to determine whether they are safe or whether they could have adverse effects on human health. 4

severity rate: the total days charged for work injuries per million man-hours exposure. Days charged include actual calendar days of disability for temporary total injuries, and scheduled charges for deaths and permanent disabilities. Charges are 6,000 days for death or permanent total disability, with proportionately fewer days for permanent partial disabilities of varying degrees of seriousness. 2

smoke: an air suspension (aerosol) of particles, usually but not necessarily solid, often originating in a solid nucleus, formed from combustion or sublimation. 3

Standard Industrial Classification (SIC): a taxonomy to classify places of employment by major type of activity. Factories, businesses, and farming establishments are included. Any industrial establishment can be classified. The classification is three-tiered. A two-digit classification represents the broadest category, e.g., manufacturing. Within each two-digit classification are three- and four-digit refinements. The three-digit classifications tend to represent specific functional divisions within the greater category. The four-digit classification usually gives a more detailed breakdown of the industrial activity. "The purposes are to facilitate the collection and tabulation of data relating to establishments and to provide for uniformity and comparability in the presentation of statistical data. Each establishment is assigned an industry code on the basis of its primary activity which is determined by its principal product or group of products produced or distributed or services rendered." An establishment is an economic unit generally at a single physical location where business is conducted or where services or industrial operations are performed. An establishment is not necessarily identical with the enterprise or company, which may consist of one or more establishments. The manufacturing division includes establishments engaged in the mechanical or chemical transformation of materials or substances into new products, i.e., "food and kindred products" as a major group have a two-digit SIC of 20, "meat products" would have a three-digit SIC of 201, and "sausages and other prepared meat products" would have a four-digit SIC of 2013. In another example, "electrical and electronic machinery, equipment, and supplies"—major group 36—the three-digit SIC 362 identifies "electrical industrial apparatus," and the four-digit SIC 3635 identifies the establishment that manufactures household vacuum cleaners. 6   U.S. Bureau of the Budget, *Standard Industrial Classification Manual*, Washington, D.C., GPO, 1972, pp. 10, 59, 87.

Standards ANSI: The ANSI Z/37 Committee in its published standards uses the term *maximal acceptable concentrations*. The ANSI's time-weighted average is essentially the same as the time-weighted 8 hour average of the ACGIH's threshold limit values committee formulation procedure. The Z/37 Committee of ANSI is composed of governmental, industrial, professional society, and university-based experts in industrial toxicology, hygiene, and medicine. Assignments for standard development are given to committee members or others having experience with the material in question. The committee votes upon the standard, which is then sent forward for other institute approval and ultimate publication as a standard. Maximal acceptable concentrations are published for a number of materials as individual documents which give the basis for such judgments. In addition, analytical and sampling methods are recommended; the standard publication also describes the toxicity of the material as well as physical and chemical properties. 5   (See p. 300 for information about the availability of ANSI's publications.)

Glossary 295

Standards, OSHA: Under the Occupational Safety and Health Act, the Secretary of Labor is enpowered to promulgate standards after determining that such standards will assure safe and healthful working environments. (See Appendix D for an example of an OSHA standard.) The DOL's role in occupational safety and health standards development prior to passage of the act was limited. The Walsh-Healey Public Contracts Act of 1936, the Service Contract Act of 1965, and the Construction Safety Act of 1969 produced standards applicable only to employers and places of employment subject to the terms of federal contracts. Under the Williams-Steiger Act, as the Occupational Health and Safety Act of 1970 is sometimes called, the Secretary of Labor is empowered to issue mandatory occupational safety and health standards that he or she determines will assure safe and healthful working conditions. Basically, three procedures are provided for the development and promulgation of standards: (a) adoption of national consensus standards and established federal standards without regard to the requirements of the Administrative Procedures Act (Congress considered that these standards had already been subject to public review and comment by affected parties; the power to adopt standards by these procedures expired April 28, 1973); (b) issuance, modification, or revocation of standards under the detailed procedures of section 6(b) of the act providing for advisory committees and an opportunity for public hearings and comment; and (c) issuance of temporary emergency standards under the authority provided in section 6(c) which become effective immediately upon publication in the *Federal Register*. However, section 6(c) provides that upon the publication of an emergency temporary standard, the Secretary shall commence a rule-making proceeding in accordance with section 6(b) of the act, and that the emergency standard as published shall also serve as a proposed rule for the section 6(b) proceeding. Before an emergency standard can be adopted, it must be determined both that employees are exposed to grave danger from toxic agents or substances or new types of hazards and that the standard is necessary to protect employees from such danger. The first temporary emergency standard was for asbestos. This was issued on December 7, 1971, after a request was received from the AFL-CIO. The temporary standard reflected the maximum exposure level to asbestos dust prescribed by the American Conference of Governmental Industrial Hygienists in its notice of intended changes in 1971.   1

temperature, effective; an arbitrary index which combines into a single value the effect of temperature, humidity, and air movement on the sensation of warmth or cold felt by the human body. The numerical value is that of the temperature of still, saturated air which would induce an identical sensation.   3

temperature, wet-bulb: (1) Thermodynamic wet-bulb temperature is the temperature at which liquid or solid water, by evaporating into air, can bring the air to saturation adiabatically at the same temperature. (2) Wet-bulb temperature without qualification is the temperature indicated by a wet-bulb psychrometer constructed and used according to specifications.   3

temporary total disability: an injury which does not result in death or permanent disability but which renders the injured person unable to perform regular duties on one or more full calendar days after the day of the injury.   2

teratogenic effects: birth defects produced in the developing embryo. 4

teratogens: agents which produce structural abnormalities. They are capable of damaging the embryo by disturbing the maternal homeostatis or by direct action on embryonic tissues or organs. The first trimester, particularly the first 8-week period of embryonc organogenesis, is the time of greatest susceptibility to environmental influences, and the majority of teratological effects are induced during this period. The drug thalidomide is a documented example of a substance that produces its effects solely during this critical period. In almost every case, the embryo is more sensitive to toxins than is the maternal organism. This is attributed to more rapid cell turnover by the embryo and fetus, their relative lack of detoxification mechanisms, and their immature biological barriers. In the first 3 weeks, there is relatively little structural deformity produced but considerable lethality, while from 3 to 8 weeks as organogenesis proceeds, the embryo is highly susceptible to structural deformity. 6 Messite, op. cit.

threshold limit values (TLV®): the values for airborne toxic materials which are to be used as guides in the control of health hazards and which represent time-weighted concentrations to which nearly all workers may be exposed 8 hours per day over extended periods of time without adverse effects. Because of wide variation in individual susceptibility, however, a small percentage of workers may experience discomfort from some substances at concentrations at or below the threshold limit; a smaller percentage may be affected more seriously by aggravation of a preexisting condition or by development of an occupational illness. The TLVs of gases and vapors are expressed as ppm, meaning parts of gas or vapor per million parts of air. The TLVs of fumes and mists are expressed as milligrams per cubic meter of air and often listed as milligrams per 10 cubic meters of air to indicate total daily exposure. The TLVs of dusts are expressed in millions of particles per cubic foot of air. Three categories of TLVs are: (a) threshold limit value = time-weighted average (TLV-TWA)—the time-weighted average concentration for a normal 8-hour workday or 40-hour workweek, to which nearly all workers may be repeatedly exposed, day after day, without adverse effect; (b) threshold limit value—short-term exposure limit (TLV-STEL)—the maximal concentration to which workers can be exposed for a period up to 15 minutes continuously without suffering from (i) irritation, (ii) chronic or irreversible tissue change, or (iii) narcosis of sufficient degree to increase accident-proneness, impair self-rescue, or materially reduce work efficiency, provided that no more than four excursions per day are permitted, with at least 60 minutes between exposure periods, and provided that the daily TLV-TWA also is not exceeded; (c) threshold limit value-ceiling (TLV ^{R}-C)—the concentration that should not be exceeded even momentarily. For some substances, e.g., irritant gases, only one category, the TLV-C, may be relevant. For other substances, either two or three categories may be relevant, depending upon their physiological action. It is important to observe that, if any one of these three TLVs is exceeded, a potential hazard from that substance is presumed to exist. The TLV-TWA should be used as guides in the control of health hazards and should not be used as fine lines between safe and dangerous concentrations. The ACGIH publishes annually "TLVs Threshold Level Values for Chemical Substances and Physical Agents in the Workroom Environment." 3

time-weighted average (TWA): the term used in the OSHA Standards to express exposure limits. The TWA represents the average concentration of a hazardous substance over 8 hours. It is arrived at by taking air samples over 8 hours and dividing the amount of the substance collected in the samples by the amount of air passed through the sampling device to determine the exposure and whether the exposure falls within the limits set by the OSHA Standards. 1

toxic agents: substances that kill or injure an organism through their chemical or physical action or through altering its environment. 4

toxic substance: one which demonstrates the potential to induce cancer, to produce long-term disease or bodily injury, to affect health adversely, to produce acute discomfort, or to endanger life of human or animal. The danger to life results from exposure via the respiratory tract, skin, eye, mouth, or other routes in quantities which are reasonable for experimental animals or which have produced adverse effects in humans. 6 NIOSH, Registry of Toxic Effects.

Toxic Substance List: Section 20 (a)(6) of the Act requires that NIOSH publish annually a list of all known toxic substances and the concentrations at which such toxicity is known to occur. First published in 1971, the *Toxic Substance List* contained information on approximately 8,000 substances. This publication is now entitled *Registry of Toxic Effects of Chemical Substances*. The eighth edition contains 124,247 listings of chemical substances; of this number 33,929 are different substances and the remainder are synonyms. 7

toxicity: the degree or quality of being poisonous or harmful to plant or animal life. 4

toxicology: a science that deals with poisons, their actions, their detection, and the treatment of the conditions they produce. 4

vapor: gaseous form of substances which are normally in the solid or liquid state and which can be changed to these states either by increasing the pressure or decreasing the temperature. Vapors diffuse. 3

Wise Owl Club of America: a national program sponsored by NSPB to prevent needless loss of sight due to accidents in industry, off the job, and in school.

work injuries (including occupational illnesses): those which arise out of and in the course of gainful work. Excluded are work injuries to domestic servants and injuries occurring in connection with farm chores, both of which are classified as home injuries. 2

APPENDIX C

Occupational Safety and Health Resources

Throughout this book are references to professional associations and units of government that publish reports, books, and pamphlets; conduct studies; and provide consultation services for occupational safety and health professionals. Many reports of studies and conferences are available as well as books, pamphlets, and audiovisual materials on occupational safety and health topics that occupational health nurses can use to increase their knowledge and to help others better to understand their responsibilities and functions. In this book the word *resource* means both people and materials.

Another important concept associated with the word *resource* is expertise. Experts can and do provide consultation services and answer questions about occupational safety and health principles and practices. Among the experts available for consultation are occupational safety and health specialists; nurses employed by insurance companies, corporations, and the government; and private consultants who are available for hire. Nurses may be able to call on safety professionals or the industrial hygienists who can refer them to a particular organization (private or governmental), to a publication that is already in the unit library, or to an expert that they know they can recommend.

The following list of occupational safety and health resources, while not all inclusive, does contain the nongovernmental and governmental organizations and agencies that are most involved in occupational safety and health activities and are known to produce printed and audiovisual materials that are of special value to members of the occupational safety and health team. It is hoped that this list will be helpful to nurses as they develop resource files for their own and others' use. The examples of published materials are all presently available. They can, of course, be discontinued, and new and different ones may become available. Prices, current as of this writing can be changed without notice.

Nongovernmental Agencies

Acoustical Society of America (ASA)
  335 East 45th Street
  New York, N.Y. 10017

Founded in 1929 to increase and diffuse the knowledge of acoustics and promote its practical application. *Catalogue of Acoustical Standards* published annually. Example:

ANSI S3.21 - 1978
American National Standard Method for Manual Pure-Tone Threshold
Audiometry $8.75

ANSI S1.1 1960 (R 1976)
American Standard Acoustical Terminology $7.00

American Association of Occupational Health Nurses (AAOHN)
575 Lexington Avenue
New York, N.Y. 10022

Membership organization for occupational health nurses. The official journal is *Occupational Health Nursing*. A list of publications is available. Examples:

1. *Guide for Setting up a Record System*, $1.50.
2. *A Guide for the Preparation of a Manual of Policies and Procedures for the Occupational Health Services*, $8.00.
3. AAOHN Committee Reports, available for purchase.

American Chemical Society (ACS)
1155 16th Street, N.W.
Washington, D.C. 20026

This professional organization for chemists has a section for occupational health and safety professionals. It publishes a wide variety of technical materials and tape recordings of symposia. A list of printed matter and audiovisual presentations is available. One example is a tape recording on chemical carcinogens, an in-depth look at the problem of hazardous substances by experts from NIOSH, EPA, and the NCI.

American Conference of Governmental Industrial Hygienists (ACGIH)
2205 South Road
Cincinnati, Ohio 45238

Membership organization founded in 1942 for OSH professionals who work in either governmental or nonprofit organizations. Has for many years had a Threshold Limit Value Committee which establishes the TLV®s that are used in codes and laws around the world as a reference for airborne levels of toxic substances. Publishes reports on organized conferences. An annual list of publications is available. It also has a paid subscription service for those who are not ACGIH members. Examples of publications:

1. *Industrial Ventilation, a Manual of Recommended Practice*, 16th ed., 1978. Available from the Committee on Industrial Ventilation, P.O. Box 16153, Lansing, Mich. 48901, $10.00.
2. Current-year edition of the TLV® booklet, $2.00.
3. *Guide for Control of Laser Hazards*, 1976, $3.25.
4. *History of the Development of Industrial Hygiene Sampling, Instruments and Techniques*, $5.00.*

*Examples 2, 3, and 4 are available from the Cincinnati office at the address given above.

American Industrial Hygiene Association (AIHA)
475 Wolf Lodge Parkway
Akron, Ohio 44313

Membership organization for industrial hygienists. The official journal is the *American Industrial Hygiene Association Journal*. Publishes a wide selection of guides and other aids for industrial hygienists. A list of publications is available. Examples of resource materials available:

1. Analytical Guides, sold as a set at $60.00; selected ones individually at $1.50.
2. Ergonomic Guides: *Guide to Manual Lifting*, $1.50; *Guide to Assessment of Physical Work Capacity*, $1.50.
3. The AIHA conducts the accreditation program for industrial hygiene laboratories, using the PAT Program, and publishes a list of those accredited. Request information from the Coordinator of Laboratory Accreditation.
4. The AIHA also conducts training courses. Contact the Akron office for information.

American Medical Association (AMA)
Department of Environmental Public and Occupational Health
535 North Dearborn Street
Chicago, Ill. 60610

Membership organization for physicians. The association publishes *Journal of the American Medical Association, Archives of Environmental Health*, and reports of committees. Single copies of the latter are available free; others are for sale at a nominal price. A list of publications and a price list are available. Examples:

1. *Guide to Small Plant Occupational Health Programs*, 1973 rev. ed.
2. *The Legal Scope of Industrial Nursing Practice*, 1959.
3. *Scope, Objectives, and Functions of Occupational Health Programs*, 1971 rev. ed.

American National Standards Institute (ANSI)
1430 Broadway
New York, N.Y. 10018

A federation of leading trade, technical, and professional organizations, government agencies, and consumer groups; founded in 1918. Its principal function is to act as a clearinghouse for coordinating the work of standards development in the private sector currently carried on by nearly 400 different organizations. Through its procedures, competent, efficient, and timely development of standards is made possible, and a neutral forum is provided to consider and identify needed changes in standards. A list of publications including a price list is available. Examples of published standards:

1. *Z4.1—Requirements for Sanitation in Places of Employment*, 1968, $3.25.
2. *Z87.1—Occupational and Educational Eye and Face Protection*, 1968, $5.75.

American Nurses' Association (ANA)
2420 Pershing Road
Kansas City, Mo. 64108

The professional organization for registered nurses. The official journal is the *American Journal of Nursing*, published by the American Journal of Nursing Company. The AJN Company conducts continuing education programs utilizing self-study. For information address the American Journal of Nursing Company, 555 West 57th Street, New York, N.Y. 10019. Examples of publications:

1. *Perspective on the Code for Nurses*, $2.00.
2. *Roles, Responsibilties and Qualifications for Nurse Administrators*, $1.50.
3. *Functions, Standards, and Qualifications for an Occupational Health Nurse in a One-Nurse Service*, $1.50.

American Occupational Medical Association (AOMA)
150 North Wacker Drive
Chicago, Ill. 60606

The membership organization of occupational health physicians. The official journal is the *Journal of Occupational Medicine*.

American Society for Safety Engineers (ASSE)
850 Busse Highway
Park Ridge, Ill. 60608

A membership organization primarily for safety professionals; founded in 1911. The official journal of the association is *Professional Safety*. A list of publications is available.

Chamber of Commerce of the United States
1615 H Street, N.W.
Washington, D.C. 20062

Example of publications: *An Analysis of Workers' Compensation Laws*, published annually, single copy, $5.00.

Channing L. Bete Company
South Deerfield, Mass. 01373

Publishes scriptographic booklets that deal with occupational and environmental topics. Useful adjuncts to a health education training program in that the presentation is nontechnical, uses simple illustrations, and is in comic book format. A list of publications is available. Examples:

1. *Asbestos*
2. *What Everyone Should Know about Stress*
3. *What Everyone Should Know about OSHA Programs for Federal Employees*

Comprehensive Health Planning Council of Southeastern Michigan
1200 Book Building
Detroit, Mich. 48226

In 1977 the council published a revised edition of the *First Aid Guide for Small Business or Industry*, first published by the Detroit First Aid Advisory Committee. Based on the American Red Cross and the American Heart Association's first-aid procedures, it was prepared by experienced physicians and nurses who know the needs of industry and how first aid can and should be provided for the worker who is injured or ill; priced at $1.00.

Hazelden Foundation, Inc.
P.O. Box 176
Center City, Minn. 55012

Active in the field of alcoholism prevention. Conducts workshops and publishes a wide variety of books and pamphlets on the subject. List of publications and prices available from the Hazelden Literature Department.

Health Communications, Inc.
2119-A Hollywood Boulevard
Hollywood, Fla. 33020

Affiliated with the *U.S. Journal of Drug and Alcohol Dependence*. This company distributes a wide variety of publications on drugs and alcohol. Examples:

1. *Alcohol in the Workplace*, $3.50.
2. *The Supervisor's Handbook on Substance Abuse*, $.75.
3. *Employee Assistance Education and Training Programs*, $20.00.

Health Education, Inc.
79 East 55th Street
New York, N.Y. 10022

Publishes materials on health education. Contact the Company for information as to availability and cost. Examples:

1. A series of six video cassette presentations, written by an occupational health nurse and entitled "Occupational Health Nursing Practice" was developed with advice from practicing occupational health nurses. Available as a series or singly from the McGraw-Hill Publishing Company, 1221 Avenue of the Americas, New York, N.Y. 10020.
2. A series of video cassette presentations entitled "The First Thirty Minutes" was developed primarily for physicians working in hospital emergency rooms. Available for purchase.

Illuminating Engineering Society and Illuminating Engineering Research Society
345 East 47th Street
New York, N.Y. 10017

List of publications is available. Example: *RP-7 Industrial Lighting*, $6.50.

Industrial Accident Prevention Association
2 Vloor Street, E., 9th floor
Toronto, Ontario, M4W IA8 Canada
Phone (416) 965-8888

Membership organization of Ontario industries. Provides industrial accident prevention services for member companies. Publishes wide variety of safety and accident prevention materials.

International Labour Office (ILO) and *International Occupational Safety and Health Information Center (CIS)*
1211 Geneva 22 Switzerland

An intergovernmental agency, the ILO was established in 1919 and entered into relationship with the United Nations as a specialized agency in 1946. Works to improve the safety and health of workers all over the world. Established the CIS in 1959 with the support of various national and international bodies active in the field of occupational safety and health. The aim is to ensure systematic collection and utilization of all valuable information relating to occupational safety and health. National centers all around the world transmit abstracts and documents to the Geneva office. A guide for users of the CIS classifications is available upon request.

Lead Industries Association, Inc.
292 Madison Avenue
New York, N.Y. 10017

A nonprofit organization of lead-mining, smelting, refining, and fabricating companies throughout the free world. Published in 1979 *Occupational Lead Poisoning—It Needn't Be: A Manager's Manual.*

Medical Society of Wisconsin
330 East Lakeside Street Box 1109
Madison, Wisc. 53713

Publishes *Occupational Health Guide for Medical and Nursing Personnel*, which was prepared jointly with the State Nurses' Association, the State Board of Health, and the Medical Society, priced at $10.00

National Council on Alcoholism (NCA)
1917 I Street, N.W., Suite 201
Washington, D.C. 20006

A national voluntary health organization that works against the disease of alcoholism; founded 1945. Comprises a network of 195 local alcoholism councils throughout the United States. Services include public information, identfication, intervention, referral, advocacy, prevention, and education. Publishes materials particularly useful in professional and worker health education. Examples:

1. Harrison Trice, *Alcoholism in Industry, Modern Procedures.*
2. "Advances in Secondary Prevention of Alcoholism through the Cooperative Efforts of Labor and Management in Employer Organizations."
3. "Company/Union Programs for Alcoholics."

National Commission on Confidentiality of Health Records, Inc. (NCCHR)
1211 Connecticut Avenue, N.W., Suite 504
Washington, D.C. 20036

The only national group devoted exclusively to confronting problems regarding confidentiality of health information; it represents all to whom health records are an issue: health professionals, hospitals, clinics, third-party payers, and consumers. Founded in 1976. Assembles and disseminates information through a newsletter and in meetings, conferences, and policy papers. Their publications are for sale from the Washington office.

National Joint Practice Commission (NJPC)
35 East Wacker Drive, Suite 1990
Chicago, Ill. 60601

An interprofessional organization established by the AMA and the ANA to improve health care; funded by these organizations and the W. K. Kellogg Foundation. Has defined joint primary care practice and recommended guidelines for primary care joint practice by nurses and physicians. State joint practice committees have been set up. The Joint Practice Committee of North Carolina Task Force report, *Occupational Health Services*, is available from the North Carolina Nurses' Association or from the Medical Society office in Raleigh, N.C.

National League for Nursing (NLN)
10 Columbus Circle
New York, N.Y. 10019

Membership organization for nurses and nonnurses; all who are concerned about patient care are eligible. Is concerned primarily with nursing education, nursing services, and community planning for nursing care. An annual catalog of publications is available. Examples:

1. Pub. No. 15-1555, "Who is the Nurse Practitioner?" $.50.
2. Pub. No. 14-1644, *The Role of the Nurse as Employee: A Case of Mutual Responsibility*, $1.95.

National Safety Council (NSC)
444 North Michigan Avenue
Chicago, Ill. 60611

A nonprofit, nongovernmental, privately supported public service organization dedicated to reducing both the number and severity of accidents. Founded in 1913 and chartered by the United States in 1953. The council gathers, analyzes, and distributes safety information nationally and internationally through a variety of publications and programs. It is the most authoritative source of information about safety. Members receive a balanced program of safety materials each year, including books, magazines, newsletters, training aids such as booklets and posters, technical reports, and announcements of new items. The annual congress, held in Chicago, is highlighted by an exposition consisting of scientific and educational exhibits; hundreds of commercial exhibits of products and devices for safety, fire prevention, first aid, and training are displayed. A special session for occupational health nurses is held during the congress. The council publishes a wide variety of professional and worker oriented books, pamphlets, films, and posters. Examples:

1. *National Safety News*.
2. *Journal of Safety Research*.
3. *General Materials Catalogue;* lists the resources of the organization including films, books, pamphlets, and training courses.
4. Films: "Toxic Hazards in Industry," 23 minutes, color, for sale or rent; "Human Factors in Safety," a series dealing with the human element in accident prevention; "Big Lift," showing proper techniques for lifting.
5. Industrial Data Sheet Library. Over 300 data sheets, each of which examines a single industrial accident topic.
6. Newsletter for occupational health nurses; available to nu   es whose company is a member of the NSC.
7. Books: *Accident Prevention Manual for Industrial Operations; Industrial Nurse and Hearing Conservation; Fundamentals of Industrial Hygiene; Supervisors' Safety Manual*.

The National Society for the Prevention of Blindness (NSPB)
79 Madison Avenue
New York, N.Y. 10016

A voluntary health agency committed to the reduction of needless blindness; founded in 1908. A list of publications is available. Examples:

1. *The Occupational Health Nurse and Eye Care*, 2nd ed., 1972, $.50.
2. *Eyes in Industry—a guide to Better Industrial Testing*, $.25.
3. "The Wise Owl Club of America," single copy free.
4. *Glaucoma Alert Program Guide*, $5.00.

Occupational Health Institute (OHI)
150 North Wacker Drive
Chicago, Ill. 60606

An organization founded many years ago by the Industrial Medical Association for the purposes of studying problems pertaining to the practice of medicine as applied to the needs of industry and to encourage the development of safety and health services and educational programs. Example of publications: *Organization and Operation of an Occupationa Health Program*, $.50.

Wellness Resource Center
42 Miller Avenue
Mill Valley, Calif. 94941

Publishes:
1. John W. Travis, M.D., *The Wellness Workbook*, 1977.
2. *The Wellness Inventory*.

Work in America Institute, Inc.
700 White Plains Road
Scarsdale, N.Y. 10583

A nonprofit, nonpartisan organization founded in 1975 to advance productivity and improve the quality of working life. Aims to accomplish these purposes through the publication of such items as the monthly *World of Work Report* as well as books and topical studies.

World Health Organization (WHO)

A specialized agency of the United Nations with primary responsibility for international health matters and public health. Publications, including a catalog, are available from WHO Publications Center, U.S.A., 49 Sheridan Avenue, Albany, N.Y. 12210. Examples:

1. No. 89, *Expert Committee on Health Education of the Public*, SW fr. 6.*
2. No. 568, *Smoking and Its Effects on Health*, SW fr. 9.
3. No. 571, *Early Detection of Health Impairment in Occupational Exposure to Health Hazards* Vol. 1, *Manual on Radiation*, SW fr. 8.
4. *Protection in Hospitals and General Practice: Basic Protection Requirements*, SW fr. 8.

Governmental Departments and Agencies

Of the eleven major federal departments each headed by a Secretary appointed by the President and approved by the Senate, the two that are primarily concerned with the health and safety of workers and of the industrial environment are the Department of Health and Human Services (DHHS) and the Department of Labor (DOL).

Department of Health and Human Services (DHHS)

This department has 10 regional offices. On the staff of each office is an occupational safety and health consultant who represents the National Institute of Occupational Safety and Health (NIOSH) in that region. This is the person to contact for help with an occupational health or safety problem. The industrial hygienist assigned to the region takes part in the HHE Program of NIOSH. Representatives of both NIOSH and OSHA are available to answer questions about the agencies' programs and have their publications available for free distribution. When the free supply is exhausted the regional consultant can furnish information as to availability

---

*Swiss franc, but WHO publications can be paid for in equivalent U.S. dollars.

and cost. The consultant can also supply the form on which to request NIOSH to do an HHE. The industrial hygienist provides consultation on environmental sampling and monitoring questions. Locations of the regional offices of DHHS follow. The states served by each office can be identified on the map in Figure 1.

Region I
JFK Building
Boston, Mass. 02203
(617) 223-6668/9

Region II
26 Federal Plaza
New York, N.Y. 10007
(212) 264-2485/8

Region III
3525 Market Street
P.O. Box 13716
Philadelphia, Pa. 19019
(404) 881-4474

Region IV
101 Marietta Tower, Suite 502
Atlanta, Ga. 30303
(404) 221-2396

Region V
300 South Wacker Drive
Chicago, Ill. 60607
(312) 886-3881

Region VI
1200 Main Tower Building, Room 1700-A
Dallas, Tex. 75245
(214) 665-3081

Region VII
601 East 12th Street
Kansas City, Mo. 64107
(816) 374-5332

Region VIII
19th and Stout Streets
9017 Federal Building
Denver, Colo. 80202
(303) 837-3979

Region IX
50 Fulton Street (223 FOB)
San Francisco, Calif. 94102
(415) 556-3781

Region X
1321 Second Avenue (Arcade Building)
Seattle, Wash. 98101
(206) 442-0530

Figure 1 Ten Standard Federal Regions

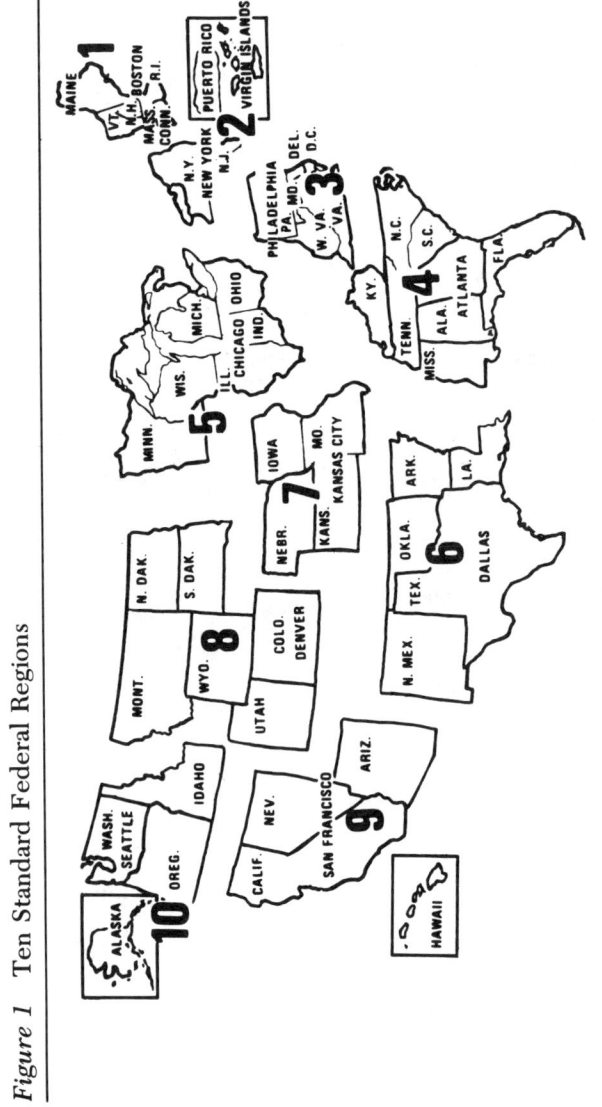

Region	States	Region	States
1	Conn, Maine, Mass, NH, RI, Vt	6	Ark, La, NM, Okla, Tex
2	NJ, NY, Puerto Rico, Virgin Islands	7	Iowa, Kan, Mo, Neb
3	Del, DC, Md, Pa, Va, W Va	8	Colo, Mont, ND, SD, Utah, Wyo
4	Ala, Fla, Ga, Ky, Miss, NC, SC, Tenn	9	Ariz, Calif, Guam, Hawaii, Nev, Trust Territory of the Pacific Islands*
5	Ill, Ind, Mich, Minn, Ohio, Wis	10	Alaska, Idaho, Ore, Wash

*Caroline Islands, Mariana Islands, Marshall Islands

Occupational Safety and Health Resources

The Public Health Service (USPHS) is the name given to the health part of the DHHS which was formerly called the Department of Health, Education and Welfare (DHEW). The USPHS was established in 1798 to provide health and medical care for seamen, and it still administers the network of public health hospitals. The Center for Disease Control (CDC) is a part of the USPHS, as are NIOSH and the Food and Drug Administration (FDA).

Food and Drug Administration
5600 Fishers Lane
Rockville, Md. 20857

Protects the public health of the nation as it may be impaired by foods, drugs, biological products, cosmetics, medical devices, ionizing and nonionizing radiation-emitting products, and substances, poisons, pesticides, and food additives. The Bureau of Radiological Health is part of the FDA. It is responsible for protecting the public health by reducing unnecessary exposure to ionizing and nonionizing radiation. The EPA, created in 1970, has the responsibility for environmental radiation problems and programs as it does for water and air pollution control programs. The FDA publishes a wide variety of reports and memos; for example, "Mercury Vapor and Metal Halide Lamps," a consumer memo.

National Cancer Institute (NCI)
Building 31, 900 Bethesda
Rockville Park, Md. 20014

One of 10 institutes that make up the National Institutes of Health (NIH), which was created by Congress as the major health research arm of the government. The NCI maintains some 20 Comprehensive Cancer Centers (CCC) which serve as sources of information on cancer problems. Examples of publications:

1. *Breast Cancer Digest*, a list of resources for use by program planners, employees, patients, and their families. This is an activity in an NCI program on breast cancer that also includes a slide presentation available in black- or white-family version and is for sale by the National Audiovisual Center at $23.40.
2. *National Cancer Program Review for Communicators*, designed for those who provide cancer information to the public, the press, and the health practitioner at every level.
3. Booklets for health professionals and the general public: "Asbestos Exposure: What It Means, What to Do," "Asbestos Exposure: A Desk Reference for Communicators," "Clearing the Air—A Guide to Quitting Smoking." Free copies of these booklets and of "Smoking and Health" and "Asbestos and Health" are available from The Cancer Information Clearinghouse, National Cancer Institute, 7910 Woodmont Avenue, Bethesda, Md. 20014.

National Institute for Occupational Safety and Health (NIOSH)
5600 Fishers Lane
Rockville, Md. 20857

ALSO: Cincinnati Laboratory
4676 Columbia Parkway
Cincinnati, Ohio 45226
AND: Morgantown Laboratory
944 Chestnut Ridge Road
Morgantown, W.Va. 26505

The principal federal agency engaged in research to eliminate on-the-job hazards to the health and safety of workers. Identifies hazards and recommends changes in regulations limiting them; trains occupational health personnel; conducts the health program set forth in the Federal Coal Mine Health and Safety Act of 1969 (PL 91-173). Under the Occupational Safety and Health Act it conducts research on new occupational safety and health standards and transmits its recommendations to the DOL, which has the responsibity for developing, promulgating, and enforcing the standards. Publishes a wide variety of material, which is printed by the GPO. Examples:

1. *List of Publications of the National Institute for Occupational Safety and Health,* a most useful reference. To obtain a free copy, send request to the Information Office, Technical Information, National Institute for Occupational Health and Safety, Public Health Service, U.S. Department of Health and Human Resources, Cincinnati, Ohio 45226. To facilitate response include a self-addressed label.
2. NIOSH Pub. No. 78-132, *Comprehensive Bibliography on Pregnancy and Work,* GPO:017-33-00288-6, $3.00.
3. NIOSH Pub. No. 77-152, *Criteria for a Recommended Standard: Occupational Exposure to Fibrous Glass,* GPO: 017-033-00214-2, $3.50.
4. NIOSH Pub. No. 77-201, *Good Work Practices for Electroplaters,* GPO: 017-033-00240-1, $1.40.
5. *The Pocket Guide to Chemical Hazards,* published in 1978, is no longer available for free distribution. Can be obtained from the GPO as a GPO publication, No. 017-33-00542, $5.00.

Department of Labor (DOL)

Occupational Safety and Health Administration (OSHA)
200 Constitution Avenue, N.W.
Washington, D.C. 20210

Created by the Occupational Safety and Health Act of 1970, the function of this agency is to promulgate standards that will accomplish the purpose of PL 91-596. These standards are first published in the *Federal Register*. It also prepares statements that spell out the intent of the standards or the administrative directives that are to be used to enforce the standards. Copies of these statements are available from the GPO and from OSHA's Regional Office. Examples of available publications:

1. Program and Policy Series: OSHA 2098, *OSHA Inspections,* 1975; OSHA 2265, "Material Safety Data Sheet," 1977.

2. Job Health Hazard Series: OSHA 2224, *Carbon Monoxide*, 1975; OSHA 2230, *Lead*, 1975; OSHA 2277, *Hot Environments*, 1976.
3. Safe Work Practice Series: OSHA 2237, *Handling Hazardous Materials*, 1975; OSHA 2236, *Essentials of Material Handling*, 1978; OSHA 2227, *Essentials of Machine Guarding*, 1977.
4. Safety Management Series: OSHA 2231, *Organizing a Safety Committee*, 1975; OSHA 2254, *Training Requirements of OSHA Standards*, 1976; OSHA 2209, *OSHA Handbook for Small Businesses*, 1979; *Compliance Manual; The OSHA Industrial Hygiene Field Operations Manual*, GPO: 029-000-00371-8, $8.50.

OSHA 2206, General Industry, Safety and Health Regulations: Part 1910 GPO 029-015-0054-6, $8.50.

OSHA Regional Offices and Their Staffs

For an office close to you, check your telephone directory under U.S. Government or dial (800) 555-1212 and ask for the toll-free number of the OSHA office nearest you.

Region I
JFK Building, Room 1804
Boston, Mass. 02203
(617) 223-6712/3

Region II
1515 Broadway (1 Astor Plaza), Room 3445
New York, N.Y. 10036
(212) 944-3430/1

Region III
15220 Gateway Center, 3535 Market Street
Philadelphia, Pa. 19104
(215) 596-1201

Region IV
1375 Peachtree Street, N.E., Suite 587
Atlanta, Ga. 30309
(404) 526-3573/4 or 2281/2

Region V
230 S. Dearborn (32nd Floor)
Chicago, Ill. 60604
(312) 353-4716/7

Region VI
555 Griffin Square Building, Room 602
Dallas, Tex. 75202
(214) 749-2477/8 or 4716/7

Region VII
Federal Building, Room 3000
811 Walnut Street
Kansas City, Mo. 64106
(816) 374-5861

Region VIII
Federal Building, Room 15010
1961 Stout Street
Denver, Colo. 80202
(303) 837-3883

Region IX
9470 Federal Building
450 Golden Gate Avenue
P.O. Box 36017
San Francisco, Calif. 94102
(415) 566-0584

Region X
6048 Federal Office Building
909 First Avenue
Seattle, Wash. 94174
(206) 442-5930

Department of Commerce

National Technical Information Service (NTIS)
Springfield, Va. 22161

A unit of the U.S. Department of Commerce that provides as a service the duplication of a wide variety of reports, prepared by various federal agencies, many of which are not available from any other source. A list of available publications and how to use NTIS is available for free distribution. Examples of NTIS materials are: *Seminar on Marketing* and *The Occupational Alcholism Programs: New Ideas and Approaches*. P.B. 248-809/AS, $5.00.

General Services Administration

National Audiovisual Center
Reference Section RL
Washington, D.C. 20409

Created under the aegis of the National Archives and Records Service of the General Services Administration to serve as the central clearinghouse for all federal audiovisual materials and to make them available for public use through information and distribution services. Example of publications: *Reference List of Audiovisual Materials*, published by the U.S. Government, 1978. Lists over 6,000 materials selected from over 10,000 programs produced by 175 federal agencies covering a wide variety of subjects of interest to occupational safety and health professionals. Order from the GPO, priced at $15.00.

Government Printing Office (GPO)

The GPO publishes and sells a wide variety of pamphlets, books, and reports, some of which are very technical, others very simple. When an agency of the federal government wishes to publish a report or other material, it prepares the manuscript for the GPO, pays the GPO for the cost of production, and then buys from the GPO a predetermined number of copies, which it distributes at no cost. When the supply of free copies is exhausted the items may be purchased from the NTIS of the U.S. Department of Commerce (see p. 317). The GPO also has the right to sell the publication. Both the GPO and the NTIS publish a list of the publications they have for sale. Examples:

1. The GPO publishes a monthly catalog of publications which describes and gives the catalog number and cost of each item; it also previews major publications not yet off the press. Annual subscription fee, $27.00.
2. The *Federal Register*, published by the GPO Monday through Friday, except on legal holidays. This is the official source of all OSHA Standards (for an example see Appendix D). Subscription price, $50.00; single copies also available from the GPO. The *Federal Register* is also the official source of executive orders and announcements of rules and regulations of the government.
3. The GPO maintains the Occupational Safety and Health Subscription Service of Standards, Interpretations, Regulations and Procedures. This service supplements the *Federal Register* by providing the standards, interpretations, regulations, and procedures in a loose-leaf form punched for a three-ring binder. Notices of changes and additions are sent to subscribers to keep the information current.
4. The GPO publishes summaries of publications that are currently available. It is possible to have one's name placed on the mailing list to receive these items at no cost.

Other Sources of Information about OSH and OSHA Topics

Consultants

Most professional organizations and governmental organizations listed employ professionals who can and will respond to substantive questions concerning prevention or treatment activities, the availability of research and field studies results, and how to do certain procedures. Membership organizations have local and state chapters whose members frequently are experts in their field of practice and hence are a source of expert help for nurses who, for example, need direction as to where to find an industrial hygiene consultant or to find out who can do an industrial hygiene survey. One rule of thumb is to start with the closest unit of the organization. If there is a local office, ask the executive or one of the members of the board for information. When working with the federal government turn to the staff of the regional office. If the assistance you need is not available, someone there will refer you to the pertinent department at the federal level.

Another rule of thumb is to check with the state health and labor department to identify what services are available from them that can be used to increase staff effectiveness. A state which has a state OSHA plan will have OSHA staff members who have been certified by federal OSHA as being competent to carry out the intent of PL 91-596. The industry must meet the state standards. The DOL provides funds to support, in part, state consultation programs. A request to the staff of the state consultant program can result in an OSHA-type inspection that does not include first-time sanction. This resource is provided for the management of small establishments.

The use of professional consultants to provide such service is increasing. Contracts are signed and the member of a counseling service provides the industry with a report after having done the required work. The contract should be specific and should not be signed until both sides understand what is wanted, what can be provided, and in what time frame. The professional experience and education of the consultant should of course be considered when selecting a consultant.

Health Agencies

The following list includes, in addition to governmental agencies, private nonprofit organizations and professional associations which produce a wide variety of materials that nurses can use as they develop health and safety education programs for workers. Many also produce reports of a technical nature that nurses can use as they assist their employers and answer workers' questions about health and safety.

The clearinghouses listed are in-house units of the several agencies and are set up primarily as information centers and retrieval sources for the agencies' staffs. The clearinghouse will respond to requests for a literature search; they must be in writing and specific. For example, if one wants information about what is available concerning the effects of impact noise on the health of workers, a specific request will result in a computerized printout of all references in the system coded under *impact noise* along with an annotation of each article, report, or book. A similar service is available on alcoholism and drug abuse from the federal agencies that deal with these two areas.

Alcoholics Anonymous
   General Services Office (6th Floor)
   468 Park Avenue South
   New York, N.Y. 10016
   (212) 686-1100
   ATTN: Public Information Department

American Dental Association
   Bureau of Health Education and Audiovisual Services
   American Dental Association
   211 East Chicago Avenue
   Chicago, Ill. 60611
   (312) 440-2593

American Cancer Society
   Public Information Department
   777 Third Avenue
   New York, N.Y. 10017
   (212) 371-2900, ext. 254
   (or local chapter)

American College of Obstetricians and Gynecologists
Resource Center
1 East Wacker Drive, Suite 2700
Chicago, Ill. 60601
(312) 222-1600
American College of Sports Medicine
1440 Monroe Street
Madison, Wis. 53706
(608) 262-3632
American Heart Association
7320 Greenville Avenue
Dallas, Tex. 75231
(214) 750-5300
(or local chapters)
American Lung Association
1740 Broadway
New York, N.Y. 10019
(212) 245-8000
(or local chapter)
American Red Cross
National Headquarters
18th and E Streets, N.W.
Washington, D.C. 20006
(202) 857-3555
American Social Health Association
260 Sheridan Avenue
Palo Alto, Calif. 94306
(415) 321-5134
Blue Cross and Blue Shield Associations
Public Relations Office
840 North Lake Shore Drive
Chicago, Ill. 60611
(312) 440-5955
Center for Disease Control
Chronic Diseases Division
Bureau of Epidemiology
Building 1, Room 5127
Center for Disease Control
Atlanta, Ga. 30333
(404) 329-3165
Bureau of Health Education
Building 14
Center for Disease Control
Atlanta, Ga. 30333
(404) 329-3111

Center for Disease Control
Dental Disease Prevention Activity (E107)
Center for Disease Control
Atlanta, Ga. 30333
(404) 262-6631

Clearinghouse for Occupational Safety and Health
National Institute for Occupational Safety and Health
Center for Disease Control
Robert A. Taft Laboratory
4676 Columbia Parkway
Cincinnati, Ohio 45226
(513) 684-8326

Consumer Information Center
Consumer Information Center
Pueblo, Colo. 81009
(303) 544-5277, ext. 370

Consumer Product Safety Commission
Consumer Education and Awareness Division
5401 Westbard Avenue
Washington, D.C. 20207
(202) 492-6576
(or local Poison Control Centers)

Department of Transportation
General Services Division (NAD-42)
National Highway Traffic Safety Administration
Department of Transportation
400 Seventh Street, S.W., Room 4423
Washington, D.C. 20590
(202) 426-0874

Environmental Protection Agency
Office of Public Awareness
Environmental Protection Agency
401 M Street, S.W.
Mail Code: A-107
Washington, D.C. 20460
(202) 755-0700

Food and Drug Administration
Office of Consumer Communications (HFG-10)
Food and Drug Administration
Room 15B32, Parklawn Building
5600 Fishers Lane
Rockville, Md. 20857
(301) 443-3170

Mental Health Association
 1800 North Kent Street
 Arlington, Virginia 22209
 (or local chapters)
 (703) 528-6405
National Center for Health Education
 211 Sutter Street (4th Floor)
 San Francisco, Calif. 94108
 (415) 781-6144
National Clearinghouse on Alcohol Information
 P.O. Box 2345
 Rockville, Md. 20852
 (301) 468-2600
National Clearinghouse on Drug Abuse Information
 Room 10A53, Parklawn Building
 5600 Fishers Lane
 Rockville, Md. 20857
 (301) 443-6500
National Clearinghouse for Family Planning Information
 6110 Executive Boulevard, Suite 250
 Rockville, Md. 20852
 (301) 881-9400
National Clearinghouse for Mental Health Information
 National Institute of Mental Health
 Room 11A33, Parklawn Building
 5600 Fishers Lane
 Rockville, Md. 20857
 (301) 443-4517
National Council on Alcoholism
 733 Third Avenue
 New York, N.Y. 10017
 (212) 986-4433
National Family Planning and Reproductive Health Association, Inc.
 425 Thirteenth Street, N.W., Suite 350
 Washington, D.C. 20004
 (202) 783-1560
National Foundation—March of Dimes
 Public Health Education Department
 1275 Mamaroneck Avenue
 White Plains, N.Y. 10605
 (914) 428-7100
National Heart, Lung, and Blood Institute
 Public Inquiries Office
 Room 4A21, Building 31

National Institutes of Health
Bethesda, Md. 20205
(301) 496-4236

National High Blood Pressure Information Center
7910 Woodmont Avenue, Suite 1300
Bethesda, Md. 20014
(301) 652-7700

National Institute of Allergy and Infectious Diseases
Office of Research Reporting and Public Response
Room 7A32, Building 31
National Institutes of Health
Bethesda, Md. 20205
(301) 496-5717

National Institute of Child Health and Human Development
Office of Research Reporting
Room 2A34, Building 31
National Institutes of Health
Bethesda, Md. 20205
(301) 496-5133

National Institute of Dental Research
Public Inquiries Office
Room 2C34, Building 31
National Institutes of Health
Bethesda, Md. 20205
(301) 496-4261

National Institute of Environmental Health Sciences
National Institutes of Health
Post Office Box 12233
Research Triangle Park, N.C. 27709
(919) 541-3345

National Nutrition Education Clearinghouse
2140 Shattuck Avenue, Suite 1110
Berkeley, Calif. 94704
(415) 548-1363

Office of Cancer Communications
National Cancer Institute
Room 10A18, Building 31
National Institutes of Health
Bethesda, Md. 20205
(301) 496-5583

Office of Health Information and Health Promotion
Office of the Surgeon General
U.S. Department of Health and Human Resources (Room 721B HHH)
200 Independence Avenue, S.W.
Washington, D.C. 20201
(202) 472-5370

Office of Maternal and Child Health
  Program Services Branch
  Bureau of Community Health Services
  Health Services Administration
  Room 7A20, Parklawn Building
  5600 Fishers Lane
  Rockville, Md. 20857
  (301) 443-4273
Planned Parenthood Federation of America, Inc.
  810 Seventh Avenue
  New York, N.Y. 10019
  (212) 541-7800
President's Council on Physical Fitness and Sports
  U.S. Department of Health and Human Resources
  Room 3030 Donohoe Building
  400 Sixth Street, S.W.
  Washington, D.C. 20201
  (202) 755-7947
Public Affairs Committee, Inc.
  Room 1101
  381 Park Avenue South
  New York, N.Y. 10016
  (212) 683-4331
Technical Information Center for Smoking and Health
  Office on Smoking and Health
  U.S. Department of Health and Human Resourcese
  Room 1-16, Park Building
  5600 Fishers Lane
  Rockville, Md. 20857
  (301) 443-1690
U.S. Department of Agriculture
  Human Nutrition Center SEA
  Room 421A
  U.S. Department of Agriculture
  Washington, D.C. 20250
  (202) 447-7854
VD National Hot Line
  260 Sheridan Avenue
  Palo Alto, Calif. 94306
  (800) 227-8922

Newsletters

Several newsletters are published regularly and are available on an annual subscription basis:

1. *The Occupational Safety and Health Reporter*. Covers the occupational safety

and health scene with in-depth, timely reports on legislation, enforcement, regulations, research, standards, and decisions. Published by the Bureau of National Affairs, Inc., 1231 25th Street, Washington D.C. 20037.

2. *Occupational Safety and Health Letter.* A semimonthly, 8- to 10-page letter that summarizes and comments upon pertinent events of interest to occupational safety and health professionals. Published by Gershon W. Fishbein, 1097 National Press Building, Washington, D.C. 20045.

APPENDIX D

Sample OSHA Standard

This is a copy of Standard 1910.1007—Vinyl Chloride—as it appears in the General Industry Standards and Interpretations as published by the GPO. The only official source of a standard is the *Federal Register* reference (39 F.R. 41848, December 3, 1974).

1910.1017—Vinyl Chloride

(a) Scope and application.

(1) This section includes requirements for the control of employee exposure to vinyl chloride (chloroethene), Chemical Abstracts Service Registry No. 75014. [39 F.R. 41848, December 3, 1974].

(2) This section applies to the manufacture, reaction, packaging, repackaging, storage, handling or use of vinyl chloride or polyvinyl chloride, but does not apply to the handling or use of fabricated products made of polyvinyl chloride.

(3) This section applies to the transportation of vinyl chloride or polyvinyl chloride except to the extent that the Department of Transportation may regulate the hazards covered by this section.

(b) Definitions.

(1) "Action level" means a concentration of vinyl chloride of 0.5 ppm averaged over an 8-hour work day.

(2) "Assistant Secretary" means the Assistant Secretary of Labor for Occupational Safety and Health, U.S. Department of Labor, or his designee.

(3) "Authorized person" means any person specifically authorized by the employer whose duties require him to enter a regulated area or any person entering such an area as a designated representative of employees for the purpose of exercising an opportunity to observe monitoring and measuring procedures.

(4) "Director" means the Director, National Institute for Occupational Safety and Health, U.S. Department of Health, Education, and Welfare (now the Department of Health and Human Services), or his designee.

(5) "Emergency" means any occurrence such as, but not limited to, equipment failure, or operation of a relief device which is likely to, or does, result in massive release of vinyl chloride.

(6) "Fabricated product" means a product made wholly or partly from polyvinyl chloride, and which does not require further processing at temperatures, and for times, sufficient to cause mass melting of the polyvinyl chloride resulting in the release of vinyl chloride.

(7) "Hazardous operation" means any operation, procedure, or activity where a release of either vinyl chloride liquid or gas might be expected as a consequence of the operation or because of an accident in the operation, which would result in an employee exposure in excess of the permissible exposure limit.

[39 F.R. 41848, December 3, 1974.]

(8) "OSHA Area Director" means the Director for the Occupational Safety and Health Administration area office having jurisdiction over the geographic area in which the employer's establishment is located.

(9) "Polyvinyl chloride" means polyvinyl chloride homopolymer or copolymer before such is converted to a fabricated product.

(10) "Vinyl chloride" means vinyl chloride monomer.

(c) Permissible exposure limit.

(1) No employee may be exposed to vinyl chloride at concentrations greater than 1 ppm averaged over any 8-hour period, and

(2) No employee may be exposed to vinyl chloride at concentrations greater than 5 ppm. averaged over any period not exceeding 15 minutes.

(3) No employee may be exposed to vinyl chloride by direct contact with liquid vinyl chloride.

(d) Monitoring.

(1) A program of initial monitoring and measurement shall be undertaken in each establishment to determine if there is any employee exposed, without regard to the use of respirators, in excess of the action level.

(2) Where a determination conducted under paragraph (d)(1) of this section shows any employee exposures, without regard to the use of respirators, in excess of the action level, a program for determining exposures for each such employee shall be established. Such a program:

(i) Shall be repeated at least monthly where any employee is exposed, without regard to the use of respirators, in excess of the permissible exposure limit.

(ii) Shall be repeated not less than quarterly where any employee is exposed, without regard to the use of respirators, in excess of the action level.

(iii) May be discontinued for any employee only when at least two consecutive monitoring determinations, made not less than 5 working days apart, show exposures for that employee at or below the action level.

(3) Whenever there has been a production, process or control change which may result in an increase in the release of vinyl chloride, or the employer has any

Sample OSHA Standard 323

other reason to suspect that any employee may be exposed in excess of the action level, a determination of employee exposure under paragraph (d)(1) of this section shall be performed.

(4) The method of monitoring and measurement shall have an accuracy (with a confidence level of 95 percent) of not less than plus or minus 50 percent from 0.25 through 0.5 ppm, plus or minus 35 percent from over 0.5 ppm through 1.0 ppm and plus or minus 25 percent over 1.0 ppm. [Methods meeting these accuracy requirements are available in the "NIOSH Manual of Analytical Methods"].

(5) Employees or their designated representatives shall be afforded reasonable opportunity to observe the monitoring and measuring required by this paragraph.

(e) Regulated area.

(1) A regulated area shall be established where:

(i) Vinyl chloride or polyvinyl chloride is manufactured, reacted, repackaged, stored, handled or used; and

(ii) Vinyl chloride concentrations are in excess of the permissible exposure limit.

(2) Access to regulated areas shall be limited to authorized persons. A daily roster shall be made of authorized persons who enter.

(f) Methods of compliance.

Employee exposures to vinyl chloride shall be controlled to at or below the permissible exposure limit provided in paragraph (c) of this section by engineering, work practice, and personal protective controls as follows:

(1) Feasible engineering and work practice controls shall immediately be used to reduce exposures to at or below the permissible exposure limit.

(2) Wherever feasible engineering and work practice controls which can be instituted immediately are not sufficient to reduce exposures to at or below the permissible exposure limit, they shall nonetheless be used to reduce exposures to the lowest practicable level, and shall be supplemented by respiratory protection in accordance with paragraph (g) of this section. A program shall be established and implemented to reduce exposures to at or below the permissible exposure limit, or to the greatest extent feasible, solely by means of engineering and work practice controls, as soon as feasible.

(3) Written plans for such a program shall be developed and furnished upon request for examination and copying to authorized representatives of the Assistant Secretary and the Director. Such plans shall be updated at least every six months.

(g) Respiratory protection.

Where respiratory protection is required under this section:

(1) The employer shall provide a respirator which meets the requirements of this paragraph and shall assure that the employee uses such respirator, except

that until April 1, 1976, wearing of respirators shall be at the discretion of each employee for exposures not in excess of 25 ppm, measured over any 15-minute period. Until April 1, 1976, each employee who chooses not to wear an appropriate respirator shall be informed at least quarterly of the hazards of vinyl chloride and the purpose, proper use, and limitations of respiratory devices.

[40 F.R. 13211, March 25, 1975.]

(2) Respirators shall be selected from among those jointly approved by the Mining Enforcement and Safety Administration, Department of the Interior, and the National Institute for Occupational Safety and Health under the provisions of 30 CFR Part 11.

(3) A respiratory protection program meeting the requirements of 1910.134 shall be established and maintained.

(4) Selection of respirators for vinyl chloride shall be as follows:

STANDARDS AND INTERPRETATIONS

Atmospheric concentration of vinyl chloride	Required apparatus
(i) Unknown, or above 3000 ppm	Open-circuit, self-contained breathing apparatus, pressure demand type, with full facepiece.
(ii) Not over 3,600 ppm	(a) Combination type C supplied air respirator, pressure demand type, with full or half facepiece, and auxiliary self-contained air supply; or (b) Combination type C, supplied air respirator continuous flow type, with full or half facepiece and auxiliary self-contained air supply.
(iii) Not over 1,000 ppm	Type C, supplied air respirator continuous flow type, with full or half facepiece, helmet or hood.
(iv) Not over 100 ppm	(a) Combination type C supplied air respirator demand type, with full facepiece, and auxiliary self-contained air supply; or (b) Open-circuit self-contained breathing apparatus with full facepiece, in demand mode; or (c) Type C supplied air respirator, demand type, with full facepiece.

Sample OSHA Standard 325

(v) Not over 25 ppm	(a) A powered air-purifying respirator with hood, helmet, full or half facepiece, and a canister which provides a service life of at least 4 hours for concentrations of vinyl chloride up to 25 ppm, or (b) Gas mask, front or back-mounted canister which provides a service life of at least 4 hours for concentrations of vinyl chloride up to 25 ppm.
(vi) Not over 10 ppm	(a) Combination type C supplied air respirator, demand type, with half facepiece, and auxiliary self-contained air supply; or (b) Type C supplied air respirator, demand type, with half facepiece; or (c) Any chemical cartridge respirator with an organic vapor cartridge which provides a service life of at least 1 hour for concentrations of vinyl chloride up to 10 ppm.

[39 F.R. 4148, December 3, 1974.]

(5)

(i) Entry into unknown concentrations or concentrations greater than 10,000 ppm (lower explosive limit) may be made only for purposes of life rescue; and

(ii) Entry into concentrations of less than 36,000 ppm, but greater than 3,600 ppm may be made only for purpose of life rescue, firefighting, or securing equipment so as to prevent a greater hazard from release of vinyl chloride.

(6) Where air-purifying respirators are used:

(i) Air-purifying cannisters or cartridges shall be replaced prior to the expiration of their service life or the end of the shift in which they are first used, whichever occurs first, and

(ii) A continuous monitoring and alarm system shall be provided where concentrations of vinyl chloride could reasonably exceed the allowable concentrations for the devices in use. Such system shall be used to alert employees when vinyl chloride concentrations exceed the allowable concentrations for the devices in use.

(7) Apparatus prescribed for higher concentrations may be used for any lower concentration.

(h) Hazardous operations.

(1) Employees engaged in hazardous operations, including entry of vessels to clean polyvinyl chloride residue from vessel walls, shall be provided and required to wear and use;

(i) Respiratory protection in accordance with paragraphs (c) and (g) of this section; and

(ii) Protective garments to prevent skin contact with liquid vinyl chloride or with polyvinyl chloride residue from vessel walls. The protective garments shall be selected for the operation and its possible exposure conditions.

(2) Protective garments shall be provided clean and dry for each use.

(i) Emergency situations.

A written operational plan for emergency situations shall be developed for each facility storing, handling, or otherwise using vinyl chloride as a liquid or compressed gas. Appropriate portions of the plan shall be implemented in the event of an emergency. The plan shall specifically provide that:

(1) Employees engaged in hazardous operations or correcting situations of existing hazardous releases shall be equipped as required in paragraph (h) of this section;

(2) Other employees not so equipped shall evacuate the area and not return until conditions are controlled by the methods required in paragraph (f) of this section and the emergency is abated.

(j) Training.

Each employee engaged in vinyl chloride or polyvinyl chloride operations shall be provided training in a program relating to the hazards of vinyl chloride and precautions for its safe use.

(1) The program shall include:

(i) The nature of the health hazard from chronic exposure to vinyl chloride including specifically the carcinogenic hazard.

(ii) The specific nature of operations which could result in exposure to vinyl chloride in excess of the permissible limit and necessary protective steps;

(iii) The purpose for, proper use, and limitations of respiratory protective devices;

[39 F.R. 41848, December 3, 1974].

(iv) The fire hazard and acute toxicity of vinyl chloride, and the necessary protective steps;

(v) The purpose for and a description of the monitoring program;

(vi) The purpose for, and a description of, the medical surveillance program;

(vii) Emergency procedures;

Sample OSHA Standard

(viii) Specific information to aid the employee in recognition of conditions which may result in the release of vinyl chloride; and

(ix) A review of this standard at the employee's first training and indoctrination program, and annually thereafter.

(2) All materials relating to the program shall be provided upon request to the Assistant Secretary and the Director.

(k) Medical surveillance.

A program of medical surveillance shall be instituted for each employee exposed, without regard to the use of respirators, to vinyl chloride in excess of the action level. The program shall provide each such employee with an opportunity for examinations and tests in accordance with this paragraph. All medical examinations and procedures shall be performed by or under the supervision of a licensed physician, and shall be provided without cost to the employee.

(1) At the time of initial assignment, or upon institution of medical surveillance;

(i) A general physical examination shall be performed, with specific attention to detecting enlargement of liver, spleen or kidneys, or dysfunction in these organs, and for abnormalities in skin, connective tissues and the pulmonary system (See Appendix A)

(ii) A medical history shall be taken, including the following topics:

(a) Alcohol intake;

(b) Past history of hepatitis;

(c) Work history and past exposure to potential hepatotoxic agents, including drugs and chemicals;

(d) Past history of blood transfusions and

(e) Past history of hospitalizations.

(iii) A serum specimen shall be obtained and determinations made of:

(a) Total bilirubin;

(b) Alkaline phosphatase;

(c) Serum glutamic oxalacetic transaminase (SGPT); and

(d) Serum glutamic pyruvic transaminase (SGPT); and

(e) Gamma glustamyl transpeptidase.

(2) Examinations provided in accordance with this paragraph shall be performed at least;

(i) Every 6 months for each employee who has been employed in vinyl chloride or polyvinyl chloride manufacturing for 10 years or longer; and

(ii) Annually for all other employees.

(3) Each employee exposed to an emergency shall be afforded appropriate medical surveillance.

(4) A statement of each employee's suitability for continued exposure to vinyl chloride including use of protective equipment and respirators, shall be obtained from the examining physician promptly after any examination. A copy of the physician's statement shall be provided each employee.

(5) If any employee's health would be materially impaired by continued exposure, such employee shall be withdrawn from possible contact with vinyl chloride.

(6) Laboratory analyses for all biological specimens included in medical examinations shall be performed in laboratories licensed under 42 CFR Part 74.

(7) If the examining physican determines that alternative medical examinations to those required by paragraph (k)(1) of this section will provide at least equal assurance of detecting medical conditions pertinent to the exposure to vinyl chloride, the employer may accept such alternative examinations as meeting the requirements of paragraph (k)(1) of this section, if the employer obtains a statement from the examining physician setting forth the alternative examinations and the rationale for substitution. This statement shall be available upon request for examination and copying to authorized representatives of the Assistant Secretary and the Director.

(l) Signs and labels.

(1) Entrances to regulated areas shall be posted with legible signs bearing the legend:

CANCER–SUSPECT AGENT AREA
AUTHORIZED PERSONNEL ONLY

[39 F.R. 41848, December 3, 1974]

(2) Areas containing hazardous operations or where an emergency currently exists shall be posted with legible signs bearing the legend:

CANCER–SUSPECT AGENT IN THIS AREA
PROTECTIVE EQUIPMENT REQUIRED
AUTHORIZED PERSONNEL ONLY

[39 F.R. 41848, December 3, 1974]

(3) Containers of polyvinyl chloride resin waste from reactors or other waste contaminated with vinyl chloride shall be legibly labeled:

CONTAMINATED WITH
VINYL CHLORIDE
CANCER–SUSPECT AGENT

Sample OSHA Standard

[39 F.R. 4148, December 3, 1974.]

(4) Containers of polyvinyl chloride shall be legibly labeled:

POLYVINYL CHLORIDE (OR TRADE NAME)
CONTAINS
VINYL CHLORIDE
VINYL CHLORIDE IS A CANCER-SUSPECT AGENT

(5) Containers of vinyl chloride shall be legibly labeled either:

(i)

VINYL CHLORIDE
EXTREMELY FLAMMABLE GAS
UNDER PRESSURE
CANCER-SUSPECT AGENT

or

(ii) In accordance with 49 CFR Parts 170–189, with the additional legend:

CANCER-SUSPECT AGENT

applied near the label or placard.

[39 F.R. 41848, December 3, 1974.]

(6) No statement shall appear on or near any required sign, label or instruction which contradicts or detracts from the effect of, any required warning, information or instruction.

(m) Records.

(1) All records maintained in accordance with this section shall include the name and social security number of each employee where relevant.

(2) Records of required monitoring and measuring, medical records, and authorized personnel rosters, shall be made and shall be available upon request for examination and copying to authorized representatives of the Assistant Secretary and the Director.

(i) Monitoring and measuring records shall:

(a) State the date of such monitoring and measuring and the concentrations determined and identify the instruments and methods used;

(b) Include any additional information necessary to determine individual employee exposures where such exposures are determined by means other than individual monitoring of employees; and

(c) Be maintained for not less than 30 years.

(ii) Authorized personnel rosters shall be maintained for not less than 30 years.

(iii) Medical records shall be maintained for the duration of the employment of each employee plus 20 years, or 30 years, whichever is longer.

(3) In the event that the employer ceases to do business and there is no successor to receive and retain his records for the prescribed period, these records shall be transmitted by registered mail to the Director, and each employee individually notified in writing of this transfer.

(4) Employees or their designated representatives shall be provided access to examine and copy records of required monitoring and measuring.

(5) Former employees shall be provided access to examine and copy required monitoring and measuring records reflecting their own exposures.

(6) Upon written request of any employee, a copy of the medical record of that employee shall be furnished to any physician designated by the employee.

(n) Reports.

(1) Not later than 1 month after the establishment of a regulated area, the following information shall be reported to the OSHA Area Director. Any changes to such information shall be reported within 15 days.

(i) The address and location of each establishment which has one or more regulated areas; and

(ii) The number of employees in each regulated area during normal operations, including maintenance.

(2) Emergencies, and the facts obtainable at that time, shall be reported within 24 hours to the OSHA Area Director. Upon request of the Area Director, the employer shall submit additional information in writing relevant to the nature and extent of employee exposures and measures taken to prevent future emergencies of similar nature.

(3) Within 10 working days following any monitoring and measuring which discloses that any employee has been exposed, without regard to the use of respirators, in excess of the permissible exposure limit, each such employee shall be notified in writing of the results of the exposure measurement and the steps being taken to reduce the exposure to within the permissible exposure limit.

[39 F.R. 41848, December 3, 1974.]

(o) Effective dates.

(1) Until April 1, 1975, the provisions currently set forth in 1910.93q of this Part shall apply.

(2) Effective April 1, 1975, the provisions set forth in 1910.93q of this Part shall apply.

[40 F.R. 13211, March 25, 1975.]

APPENDIX A—SUPPLEMENTARY MEDICAL INFORMATION

When required tests under paragraph (k)(1) of this section show abnormalities, the tests should be repeated as soon as practicable, preferably within 3 to 4 weeks. If tests remain abnormal, consideration should be given to withdrawal of the employee from contact with vinyl chloride, while a more comprehensive examination is made.

ADDITIONAL TESTS WHICH MAY BE USEFUL:

A. For kidney dysfunction: urine examination for albumin, red blood cells, and exfoliative abnormal cells.

B. Pulmonary system: Forced vital capacity. Forced expiratory volume at 1 second, and chest roentgenogram (posterior-anterior, 14 × 17 inches).

C. Additional serum tests: Lactic acid dehydrogenase, lactic acid dehydrogenase isoenzyme, protein determination, and protein electrophoresis.

D. For a more comprehensive examination on repeated abnormal serum tests: Hepatitis B antigen, and liver scanning.

[39 F.R. 35889, October 4, 1974.]

APPENDIX E

Excerpts from Public Law 91-596

AN ACT

"Be it enacted by the Senate and House of Representatives of the United States of America in Congress assembled, That this Act may be cited as the "Occupational Safety and Health Act of 1970."

CONGRESSIONAL FINDINGS AND PURPOSE

"Sec. (2) The Congress finds that personal injuries and illnesses arising out of work situations impose a substantial burden upon, and are a hindrance to, interstate commerce in terms of lost production, wage loss, medical expenses, and disability compensation payments.

(b) The Congress declares it to be its purpose and policy, through the exercise of its powers to regulate commerce among the several States and with foreign nations and to provide for the general welfare, to assure so far as possible every working man and woman in the Nation safe and healthful working conditions and to preserve our human resources—

(1) by encouraging employers and employees in their efforts to reduce the number of occupational safety and health hazards at their places of employment, and to stimulate employers and employees to institute new and to perfect existing programs for providing safe and healthful working conditions;

(2) by providing that employers and employees have separate but dependent responsibilities and rights with respect to achieving safe and healthful working conditions;

(3) by authorizing the Secretary of Labor to set mandatory occupational safety and health standards applicable to businesses affecting interstate commerce, and by creating an Occupational Safety and Health Review Commission for carrying out adjudicatory functions under the Act;

(4) by building upon advances already made through employer and employee initiative for providing safe and healthful working conditions;

(5) by providing for research in the field of occupational safety and health, including the psychological factors involved, and by developing innovative methods, techniques, and approaches for dealing with occupational safety and health problems;

(6) by exploring ways to discover latent diseases, establishing conditions, and conducting other research relating to health problems, in recognition of the

fact that occupational health standards present problems often different from those involved in occupational safety;

(7) by providing medical criteria which will assure insofar as practicable that no employee will suffer diminished health, functional capacity, or life expectancy as a result of his work experience;

(8) by providing for training programs to increase the number and competence of personnel engaged in the field of occupational safety and health;

(9) by providing for the development and promulgation of occupational safety and health standards;

(10) by providing an effective enforcement program which shall include a prohibition against giving advance notice of any inspection and sanctions for any individual violating this prohibition;

(11) by encouraging the States to assume the fullest responsibility for the administration and enforcement of their occupational safety and health laws by providing grants to the States to assist in identifying their needs and responsibilities in the area of occupational safety and health, to develop plans in accordance with the provisions of this Act, to improve the administration and enforcement of State occupational safety and health laws, and to conduct experimental and demonstration projects in connection therewith;

(12) by providing for appropriate reporting procedures with respect to occupational safety and health which procedures will help achieve the objectives of this Act and accurately describe the nature of the occupational safety and health problem;

(13) by encouraging joint labor-management efforts to reduce injuries and disease arising out of employment."

INSPECTIONS, INVESTIGATIONS, AND RECORDKEEPING

"Sec. 8(a) In order to carry out the purposes of this Act, the Secretary, upon presenting appropriate credentials to the owner, operator, or agent in charge, is authorized—

(1) to enter without delay and at reasonable time any factory, plant, establishment, construction site, or other area, workplace or environment where work is performed by an employee of an employer; and

(2) to inspect and investigate during regular working hours and at other reasonable times, and within reasonable limits and in a reasonable manner, any such place of employment and all pertinent conditions, structures, machines, apparatus, devices, equipment, and materials therein, and to question privately any such employer, owner, operator, agent, or employee."

Index

Accident, industrial, 46–55
  causes of, 50–51
  prevention, 18, 33, 51–54
  proneness, 54
Administration, occupational health unit. *See* Occupational health unit, management of
AFL-CIO, 22, 23
  industrial union department, 23
  occupational safety and health concerns, 23
Alcohol, 129
  abuse of, 178, 179, 180
  related disability, 180–181
Alcoholic, 178, 179, 180
Alcoholics Anonymous, 185–186
  affiliated groups, 187
Alcoholism and the worker, 178–190
  causal factors, 178
  federal legislation regarding, 181–182
  Law Enforcement Assistance Act, 181
  programs for prevention, treatment, rehabilitation, 181–182, 187
  recognition of, 178, 184
  statistics on, 178
Amalgamated Association of Iron and Steel Workers, 22
American Academy of Ophthalmology and Otolaryngology, 104
American Association of Industrial Nurses, 104
American Association of Occupational Health Nurses, 104, 271, 299
American Board of Occupational Health Nurses, Inc., 270
American College of Obstetricians and Gynecologists, 63, 90
American Federation of Labor, 21
American Industrial Hygiene Association, 16, 34, 300
American Medical Association, 116, 300
  Council on Occupational Health, 102
  Department of Environmental, Public, and Occupational Health, 15
  guide for industrial nurses, 108
  guidelines for medical examinations, 71
American National Standards Institute, 39, 150, 300
  aims and functions of, 150
  code for compiling records, 150
  Standards, 294
American Nurses' Association, 271, 301
American Occupational Medical Association, 271, 301
American Red Cross, 122, 123
  first-aid courses, 122, 123
Angiosarcoma, 125, 131
Asbestos, 65, 91, 131, 285
  Asbestos Standard Code of Federal Regulation, 91, 92
  medical surveillance required, 91
Asbestosis, 130, 285
Assessment, health, 71–85
  for executives, 75–76
  final, 76
  fitness-for-work, 75
  legal aspects, 72–73
  periodic, 72, 74–75
  preplacement, 71, 72, 73–74
  records, 82–84
  reporting findings, 82
  screening programs, 78–81
  special, 71

Benzene, poisoning, 130
Biomechanics, 33
Blue Cross, Blue Shield, 24, 191
Bronchitis, 130
Bureau of Industrial Hygiene, 126
Bureau of Mines, 46, 122
Byssinosis, 114

Cancer, 126, 127, 129, 134
  death rate in, 126
  lung, 125, 131

335

Capacity, ventilatory, 80–82
  screening for, 80–82
Carbon monoxide, 129, 285
  protocol for care in poisoning, 240–241
Carbon tetrachloride, 130
Carcinogenesis, occupational, 126, 127
Carcinogens, 41, 83, 110, 131
Cardiovascular disease, 158, 199
Ceiling limit, 285
Center for Disease Control, 36, 108
Certification, 270, 285
Chemist, industrial, 33, 36
Cigarette smoking, 65, 73
  and lung cancer, 131
Civil Rights Act, 72
Clinical laboratories Improvement Act, 36
Code for Nurses, 272
Commission on Chronic Illness, 78
Committee on Conservation of Hearing, 104
Communication, intrastaff, 205
Community health nursing, 6, 9–10
  resources for, 6
Compliance
  program, 286
  with OSHA Standards, 98, 109–110
Confidentiality, 83, 184
  of health assessment records, 83, 84
  in programs for alcoholism, 184
Congress of Industrial Organizations, 22
Conservation, of occupational health, programs for, 98, 107–110
  dermatitis control, 98, 106–107
  hearing conservation, 98, 103–104
  immunization programs, 98, 108–109
  respiratory disease control, 98, 104–106
  substances harmful to workers' progeny, control of, 98, 107–108
Consultant, occupational health, 18, 63, 64, 170, 227
  part-time, 7
Corrective actions, 37–41
  isolation, 38
  occupational toxicology, 40–41
  personal protective equipment required, 39–40
  substitution, 38
  ventilation, 38–40
Cotton dust, 114
Crisis intervention, by nurse, 3, 5, 172
Criteria Documents (NIOSH), 90, 92
Cybernetics, 286

Defenders, ear. See Hearing
Department of Health, Education, and Welfare, 14
Department of Health and Human Services, 13, 306–310

Department of Interior, 122
Department of Labor, 6, 13, 47, 50, 144, 145, 310–312
Department of Transportation, Office of Alcohol Countermeasures, 181
Dermatitis, occupational, 106–107
  causative agents, 106
  control programs for, 106–107
  nursing care in, 105–107
  protocol for care, 236–237
  workers at risk, 105–106
Disability
  alcohol related, 179, 180–181
  permanent, 292
  temporary total, 295
Disaster plan, 123–124
Disease, occupational, defined, 125
Division of Nursing Resources Administration, 16
Doctor-nurse relationship, 113, 114
Dose-response curve, 40–41, 286
Drug abuse, 168–169

Ecology, occupational, 56–67
  activities associated with, 56, 57
  clues to health hazards, 58
  environmental monitoring, 28, 56–58
  environmental sanitation, 58–61, 127
  nurse's involvement in, 66–67
  preventive practice, 57
Education for health and safety, 199–217
  aids for, 212, 213
  factors influencing learning, 201, 202
  health education committee, role of, 204
  plan for, sample, 206–208
  programs for, industrial, 204–211
  resources for, 203
  workers and, 3, 60–61, 99, 103, 106, 127
Emergency Medical Service, 123
Employers' right to know, 253
Environment, occupational,
  control of, 41–42
  evaluation of, 35–36
  health physics in, 41–43
  monitoring of, 28, 31–37
  nurses' involvement in, 43–44
  sampling, 36
  surveys of, 37–41
Epidemiologist, 65
Epidemiology, 64–66, 287
  studies in, 65–66
Equal Employment Opportunity
  the Act, 72
  Commission on, 72
  for women, 90

Index

Ergonomics, 42–43
  application in industry, 42–43
Ergonomist, 33
Exercise programs, for executives, 75–76

Fair Employment Practice Act, 72
Fair Labor Standards Act, 22
Federal Radiation Council, 135
Federal Register, 90
First aid, 47, 115, 121, 287. See also Primary care
First-aider, in occupational settings, 121–124
  in disaster situations, 123–124
  functions and role, 122
  textbook for, 123
Food and Drug Administration, 309
Fumes, 165, 287

Gompers, Samuel, 21
Good Samaritan laws, 121
Government Printing Office, 312

Handicap, defined, 72
Hazards, to safety and health, 7, 13, 35, 36, 37, 56, 90, 287
  anesthetics, 129
  asphyxiants, 129
  carcinogens, 131
  chemical, 127–128, 129, 130
  dermatitis-producing agents, 130
  irritants, 129, 130
  narcotics, 129
  nonchemical, 132–133
  pneumoconiotic agents, 130
  radiation, occupational, 41–42, 134
  stress, environmental, 134
  systemic toxins, 130
Headache, protocol for care, 239–240
Health Maintenance Organizations, 6, 192, 193
  group-practice type, 193
  individual-practice type, 193
  principles of, 192
Health, occupational
  expenditures for, 157
  third party payments, 157
Health Physics Society, 41
Hearing
  audiometric testing for, 103–104
  conservation programs for, 103–104
  ear defenders, 103
Heimlich maneuver, 288
History, 9, 80, 288
Human factors engineering, 73, 100
Hydrocarbon, 130, 131, 288

Hygiene
  occupational, 33–45
  personal, 127
Hygienist, industrial, 16, 18, 25, 33–37, 40, 57, 92, 94
Hypertension, 156

Illness, occupational, 125–135
  hazardous agents and, 127–135
  nursing diagnosis, 137–138
  OSHA reporting system for, 150
  rehabilitation, 139–141
Immunization, programs
  for influenza, 108–109
  for tetanus, 109
  for travelers, 109
Incidence rate, 288
Injury, occupational, 135–143
  nursing care in, 136–141
  OSHA reporting system for, 150
  protocols for care, 136
  recording requirements, 135
  rehabilitation, 140–141
  statistics on, 136
Insurance, health, 191–196
  basic hospital, 193
  basic medical-surgical, 193
  Blue Cross/Blue Shield, 191
  comprehensive major medical, 194
  for dental care, 191
  disability income, 194
  major medical, 194
  Medicaid, 157, 191, 192
  Medicare, 157, 191, 192, 195
  national health, 191
  prepaid group-practice, 194
  for uniformed services, 191
  Veterans Administration, 191
International Classification of Diseases and Injuries, 5, 289
International Ladies Garment Workers Union, 23
International Union of Electrical Workers, 25
International Union of Machinists, 25
Isolation, as a corrective action, 38

Job-fitness ratings, classification of, 82

Labor Management Relations Act, 22
Labor Safety and Health Institute, 24
Laboratory, occupational health, 225
  accreditation of, 289
Laceration, protocol for care, 238–239
Laser beam, 134
Lead, 125, 303
  poisoning, 120, 130, 303
Lighting, for work areas, 101

Maintenance, of occupational health, 98–110
Management, of occupational health units and programs, 219–265
  administrator, functions of, 221
  budgeting for, 222, 225, 232
  communications, intrastaff, 229
  consultants, functions of, 224, 225
  laboratory services, 225
  medical director, 222, 224
  nurse's functions, 222, 228
  nursing service personnel, 226
  organization of unit, 223
  physicians role in, 222, 223, 224
  protocol development, 236–243
  safety and hygiene specialists, 224
  staffing for unit, 222
  supervisors, functions of, 228, 229
  technicians, role in unit, 225
Medical practice acts, 113
Medicine, occupational, 291
Mental health, occupational, 163–177
  in industrial settings, 163–166
  nurse's role in, 163–175
  psychiatric illness, 166–170
  psychogenic illness episodes, 164–166
Mercury, 125, 126, 139
Mesothelioma, 131, 290
Methadone clinic, 169
Monitoring
  hygiene, occupational, 33–45
  lifetime, health, 77
  safety, occupational, 46–55
  of work areas, 57, 58. *See also* Assessment, health; Ecology

National Advisory Committee on Occupational Safety and Health, 14
National Advisory Council on Alcohol Abuse and Alcoholism, 182
National Cancer Institute, 309
National Commission on State Workmens Compensation laws, 14
National Council for Industrial Safety, 46
National Council on Alcoholism, 187, 303
National Council on Compensation Insurance, 147
National Institute on Alcohol and Alcoholism, 181
National Institute for Occupational Safety and Health (NIOSH), 13, 39, 63, 81, 83, 98, 148, 213, 272, 309–310
National Labor Relations Act, 22
National Occupational Safety and Health Review Commission, 14
National Safety Council, 46, 304
National Society for Prevention of Blindness, 79, 102, 305

NIOSH. *See* National Institute for Occupational Safety and Health
Noise, 103, 133, 165
Nonoccupational health problems 154–162
  factors influencing care, 156–157
  special programs for, 155–156
  workers' families and, 158–159
Nurse, occupational health
  accountability of, 271
  as a person and a professional, 269–277
  as ombudsman, 198
  as workers' advocate, 158–159
  certification, 270
  code of conduct, 271–272
  in occupational mental health programs, 163–166, 170–175
  job description for, 227–228
  legal issues and, 270
  nursing role in occupational illness and injuries, 138
  role in accident prevention, 53–54
  role in alcoholism programs, 186–187
  role as consultant, 62, 64, 227
  role as counselor, 170–175
  role on the health team, 17, 18
  role in immunization programs, 98, 108–109
  role in medical surveillance programs, 93–96
  role in monitoring programs, 31–32, 56, 57
  role in nursing research, 273–276
  role as occupational health educator, 216
  role in special-emphasis programs, 98, 99, 102, 103–4, 107
Nurse practice acts, 113
Nurse practitioner, 117, 291
Nursing diagnosis, 117–119, 137, 160
Nursing, occupational health, and community health nursing, 4, 6, 9–10, 11

Occupational health, as a field of practice, 12–30
  basic principles of, 12–29
  care team, 3–4, 14–16
  clinics, 6
  Institute, 305
  laboratories, 16
  nurse. *See* Nurse, occupational health
Occupational Health Unit, 3, 12, 135
  administrator, 221, 225, 227, 230
  budgeting for, 222, 232
  equipment for, 233
  maintenance of, 231–233
  management of, 221–244
  medical director, 222, 224
  physical facilities, 233

Index

policy and procedure manual, 233–235
protocols for care in, 3, 101, 114, 236–243
reports required, 4
staffing for, 219, 222–227, 231, 232
supervision of, 228–229
Occupational Safety and Health Act, 6, 12, 13, 15, 21, 27, 33, 62, 90, 128
  excerpts from, 332, 333
Occupational Safety and Health Administration (OSHA), 6, 7, 13, 14, 36, 39, 46, 71, 76, 81, 83, 98, 119, 135
  General Industry Standards, 39–40
  inspection rights of, 14
  responsibilities of, 13
  standards (OSHA), 39–40, 71, 98, 110, 127, 128, 138, 295, 321–329
Office of Workers Compensation, 144
Oil, Chemical, and Atomic Workers, 25
Ophthalmologist, 100, 101
OSHA. *See* Occupational Safety and Health Administration

Personal protective equipment, 39–40, 53, 57, 105–106, 127, 200, 202
Physician, occupational health, 18, 92, 113, 126, 165
PL 91-596. *See* Occupational Safety and Health Act
Pregnancy Disability Law, 292
Primary care, 3, 9, 28, 237
  in alcoholism, 178–190
  in first-aid cases, 121–124
  for nonoccupational health problems, 154–161
  occupational, 113–120
  in occupational illness, 125–135
  in occupational injury, 135–141
  in workmens compensation cases, 144–153
Professional Standards Review Organization Act, 271
Proficiency Analytical Testing Program, 292
Protocols, 115, 116, 117, 122, 136, 139, 156, 235
  examples of, 236–243
Public health nursing survey, 16, 17

Radiation, 41–42, 134, 293
  safety standard for, 134–135
Record keeping, 257–264
  essentials of, 258–260
  record storage, 262–264
Records, occupational health, 251–265
  completeness, importance of, 82, 251
  confidentiality of, 83, 259–262
  correctness, importance of, 82, 251
  facts to be recorded, 251
  forms and how to use them, 253–257

log of occupational illnesses and injuries, 257–258
  protection of, 259–262
  Workmens Compensation, 258
Reference library, 96
Referrals, 155, 179, 184
Rehabilitation, for industrial workers, 140–141
Reports, occupational health unit
  administrative, 245–246
  annual, 246–247
  health assessment, 82
  memoranda, 249–250
  monthly, 246, 247
Research, in industrial safety, 54
Resources, for occupational safety and health information, 298–313
Respirator, 105, 106, 127
Respiratory disease, 104–106, 125
  protective equipment, 105, 106
  spirometry in, 104–105

Safety
  department, functions of, 47–48
  director of, 48, 49
  occupational, 46–55
  professionals, 18, 20, 33, 48, 49, 56, 57, 103
Sampling, 36
Screening, 78–82
  for glaucoma, 78, 208, 209
  for hearing, 80
  for hypertension, 78
  mass, 78
  multiphasic, 78
  selective, 78
  for ventilatory capacity, 80–82
  for visual defects, 78
Secretary of Labor, 13, 14, 150
Solvents, 129, 165
Spirometry, 81–82, 104–105
Spotlight on Health and Safety, 23
Standard Industrial Classification, of places of employment, 294
Standards Completion Program, 90, 96
Standing orders, 155
Substances, hazardous, 125, 127–128
  OSHA regulated, 98
  toxic, 96, 114, 124, 167–168, 297
Substitution, as a corrective measure, 38
Supervisor, 20, 51, 103, 179, 184, 211, 228–229
Surveillance programs
  guidelines for, 96
  occupational health, 28, 69–110
  protocols for, 93, 96
  for well adults, 77

Surveillance programs *(continued)*
  for women at work, 90–91
  of work area, 57–58
Surveys
  compliance, 37
  industrial hygiene, 165
  preventive, 37
  trouble-shooting, 37

Taft-Hartley Act. *See* Labor Management Relations Act
Teratogens, 107, 131–132, 296
Tetanus, 109, 241–243
Threshold limit values, 35, 296
  Time weighted averages, 35, 297
Toxic substances reference file, 235
Toxicology, occupational, 40–41, 297

Ulcer, chrome, 125
Unions, labor, 21, 23, 24, 25, 126
United Auto Workers, 25
U.S. Bureau of Labor Statistics, 46–47, 135, 150
U.S. Public Health Service, 56

Ventilation, 38–39
Vinyl chloride, 110, 125, 131
  Standard for, 83, 92, 214, 321–329
Vision, 98, 100–102

Wagner Act. *See* National Labor Relations Act
Walk-through inspections, 35, 36
Wise Owl Club of America, 101, 102, 297
Women in industry, 42, 63–64, 90–91, 292
Workers Bill of Rights, 21
Workers' right to know, 61, 62, 197, 201, 203
Workmens Compensation, 9, 46–47, 119, 144–152, 258
  administration of, 148–149
  Federal Employees Compensation Act, 144
  legal implications of, 252–253
  National Commission on State Compensation Laws, 151
  nurse's responsibility in, 152
  premium rates, 147–148
  second injury compensation, 149–150
  state compensation laws, 146–148
  U.S. laws, current, 146–147
World Health Organization, 127, 306, Expert Committee on Environmental Sanitation, 58

X-rays, 134